PROSTHESES FOR THE BRAIN

PROSTHESES FOR THE BRAIN

Introduction to Neuroprosthetics

ANDREJ KRAL
Cluster of Excellence Hearing4All, Hannover, Germany
Hannover Medical School, Hannover, Germany
Macquarie University, Sydney, NSW, Australia

FELIX APLIN
Cluster of Excellence Hearing4All, Hannover, Germany
Hannover Medical School, Hannover, Germany

HANNES MAIER
Cluster of Excellence Hearing4All, Hannover, Germany
Hannover Medical School, Hannover, Germany

ELSEVIER

ACADEMIC PRESS
An imprint of Elsevier

Academic Press is an imprint of Elsevier
125 London Wall, London EC2Y 5AS, United Kingdom
525 B Street, Suite 1650, San Diego, CA 92101, United States
50 Hampshire Street, 5th Floor, Cambridge, MA 02139, United States
The Boulevard, Langford Lane, Kidlington, Oxford OX5 1GB, United Kingdom

Library of Congress Cataloging-in-Publication Data
A catalog record for this book is available from the Library of Congress

British Library Cataloguing-in-Publication Data
A catalogue record for this book is available from the British Library

ISBN: 978-0-12-818892-7

For information on all Academic Press publications
visit our website at https://www.elsevier.com/books-and-journals

Publisher: Mara Conner
Acquisitions Editor: Fiona Geraghty
Editorial Project Manager: Isabella Silva
Production Project Manager: Poulouse Joseph
Cover Designer: Miles Hitchen

Typeset by SPi Global, India

Contents

Preface *xi*

PART 1 Introduction

1. The historic preconditions of neural prostheses **3**

Historic roots of biomedical technology 4

History of computer technology 5

Development of electrophysiology 12

The concept of a neural prosthesis 15

Brief summary 17

Key literature and further reading 17

2. History of neuroprostheses **19**

Historical attempts at electrical stimulation 19

Mapping the brain 20

Deep brain stimulation 21

Invention of the implantable pacemaker 22

Early brain prostheses 25

Development of the cochlear implant 26

Contemporary neuroprostheses 28

Brief summary 30

Key literature and further reading 30

3. Ethics and technology development **33**

Ethical perspectives 34

Ethical aspects of technology development 35

Medical technology 37

Ethical aspects for general design considerations 43

Brain implants as human "extension"? 47

Brief summary 50

Key literature and further reading 50

PART 2 Principles

4. Neuronal excitation **55**

Neuronal excitation 62
Propagation of excitation 65
Dynamic properties of the neuronal membranes: Time and length constants 70
Thresholds in excitation 73
Macroanatomy of the nervous system 73
Brief summary 74
Key literature and further reading 75

5. Electrode-tissue interface **77**

The water hose analogy 80
Electrode configurations 82
Electric models of the double layer 89
Brief summary 92
Key literature and further reading 93

6. Artificial electrical stimulation: Principles, efficacy, and safety **95**

Charge, current, and thresholds 95
Materials for electrostimulation 97
Faradaic charge transfer 100
AC/DC stimulation 102
Safety limits 103
Microelectrodes 109
Electrode surface and electrode impedance 110
Other surface materials 111
Brief summary 111
Key literature and further reading 112

7. Stimulation rules **115**

Geometry of the electric field and the neurons 115
Previous activation history: Temporal adaptation phenomena 126
Signal forms 127
Energy requirements 132
Brief summary 133
Key literature and further reading 133

8. Tissue reaction to neuroprostheses **135**

Surrounding tissue adaptations: The implant as a foreign body 135
Electrode impedance and its clinical value 137
Infection of the implants 145

Summary 147
Brief summary 148
Key literature and further reading 148

9. Brain adaptations to neuroprostheses 149
Neuronal plasticity and neuroprosthetic devices 149
Forms of neuronal plasticity 150
Plasticity and brain structures 154
Brain plasticity affects outcomes of prosthetic therapy 157
Plasticity in adult age 162
Adaptation in senior age 163
Detecting adaptations and maladaptations to the implant 163
Brief summary 164
Key literature and further reading 164

10. Advanced concepts physical chemistry: Electrodes and electrolytes 167
Introduction 167
Faraday constant 168
Specific conductivity 169
Conductivity of strong electrolytes 170
Strong and weak electrolytes 171
Ion mobilities and solvation of ions 173
Conductivity and mobility of ions 175
Hittorf transport numbers 176
Conductometric titration 176
The tissue-electrode interface: Electrochemical processes 178
Chemical surface charges 182
Mathematical treatment of the interface impedance 184
Non-polarizing electrodes 188
Brief summary 207
Key literature and further reading 208

PART 3 Applications

11. Auditory neuroprostheses 211
Hearing loss 219
The cochlear implant 222
Auditory brainstem implants 241
Auditory midbrain implants 246
Brief summary 248
Key literature and further reading 248

12. Visual neuroprostheses **251**
The retina 251
Information processing in the visual system 255
The post-retinal visual pathway 258
Vision loss 260
Retinal remodeling 265
Animal models of blindness 267
Retinal implants: Basic principles 268
Optic nerve implants 277
Cortical and lateral geniculate nucleus visual implants 278
Data processing and stimulation strategies 282
Clinical outcomes 286
Brief summary 288
Key literature and further reading 289

13. Pacemaker for the brain: Deep brain stimulation **291**
Parkinson's disease 294
Mechanism of deep brain stimulation 296
Design of the stimulator 298
The electrode 299
Stimulation configuration 299
Clinical approaches 300
Concluding remarks 301
Brief summary 302
Key literature and further reading 302

14. Peripheral nerve and spinal stimulation **305**
Physiology of the nociceptive and somatosensory periphery 305
Neurophysiology of the spinal cord and dorsal horn 308
Information processing principles in peripheral/spinal nociception 311
Chronic neuropathic pain 314
Pain neuromodulation 317
Measuring clinical outcomes 325
Brief summary 327
Key literature and further reading 327

15. Sensing implants **329**
Non-invasive BCI 335
Invasive BCI 338
Electrocorticographic and endovascular recording 338
Single-unit recording arrays 340

Decoders 346
Brief summary 351
Key literature and further reading 351

16. Future directions **353**
Emerging neural interface therapies 353
Upcoming technological innovations 370
Brief summary 384
Key literature and further reading 385

Index *387*

Preface

Science is systematized knowledge.

Throughout history, knowledge has expanded exponentially. While centuries ago it was possible for a single gifted person to embrace all scientific fields, now science encompasses so much knowledge that is impossible to be mastered by any one scientist alone. Concurrently, the tools used in research have also become more demanding; some complex devices require the technical expertise of a dedicated person. The combination of artistic gift and scientific knowledge, important in the time of Alexander von Humboldt to document biological observations by their accurate drawings, has been replaced by the ability to use technology, particularly computers and their software. Without knowledge of computer programming, most state-of-the-art systems neuroscience is no longer possible to do. Using such powerful tools has allowed us to reach a more profound understanding of the world. Additional to the complex equipment that requires skilled handling, we also need to know and process more facts. Thus, science and its tools have substantially transformed, most prominently in the last 50 years.

Most areas of modern science require experts from several disciplines to team together. Neuroprosthetics is such a field. In the domain of neuroprostheses, medical doctors, engineers, computer experts, material researchers, physicists, as well as nonmedical clinicians (audiologists, speech therapists, physiotherapists, etc.) must interact. Since the start of the lead author's own research career at the Institute of Sensory Neuroscience at J.W. Goethe University, Frankfurt am Main, Germany, where he worked on cochlear implants, the lack of an introductory textbook on neuroprosthetics providing the knowledge base from these different disciplines was glaringly obvious. For example, he found older introductory texts on physical chemistry and electrophysiology surprisingly more helpful than more recent literature, which leaves behind most readers (particularly students) and instead targets experts from the same field.

This is a particular issue when there is wide clinical use of neural prostheses, for example, with cochlear implants that have penetrated otolaryngology and audiology, or deep brain stimulation approaches that are widespread in neurology. Our Institute of AudioNeuroTechnology in Hannover, Germany, is focused on technology in the auditory domain, including cochlear and brain implants. We have scientists from many scientific domains among us. We have a correspondingly multidisciplinary team of PhD students with diverse backgrounds. This multidisciplinary environment, particularly the education of a great diversity of PhD students, required a common knowledge base and underscored the lack of an introductory textbook.

Furthermore, education in such an environment faces the problem of how to introduce scientific subjects to students with such different backgrounds. This not only requires acquisition of knowledge from different disciplines but also different ways of education. Some disciplines have a different approach to problem solving. The challenge is to make an introductory text readable for students with diverse backgrounds, providing new insights for each of them to generate a common knowledge base required for communication between the specialized fields. We decided to tackle this challenge and write a textbook dedicated to this goal. Our volume conveys respect to and enhances understanding of the strengths and problems of the disciplines involved, creating a common base for scientific exchange.

Our main aim was to synthesize and systematize the information available in many papers and different neuronal systems into common principles that explain neuroprosthetic applications and their successful designs. As such, we want to contribute to the introduction of the science of neuroprosthetics as systematized knowledge on implantable prostheses for the brain.

Our attempts date back to 2011, when Andrej Kral and Hannes Maier started to teach an elective course on neuroprosthetics. This gave us the framework for putting together the information and material for this book. Felix Aplin joined us later and, in addition to his own research project, worked with us on this textbook. It was a creative time with many discussions that shaped the concepts contained herein. We discussed every chapter in detail with Felix, and the text profited substantially from these discussions. Andrej drafted **Chapters 1–9, 11, and 13**. Felix wrote the chapters on visual prostheses (**Chapter 12**), prostheses for pain treatment (**Chapter 14**), and future technologies (**Chapter 16**) and helped us to improve our English grammar. Hannes took care of the advanced concepts in physical chemistry (**Chapter 10**) and sensing implants (**Chapter 15**). Together, we discussed, commented, edited, and approved all chapters. Thus, the book is the intellectual child of all of us.

We want to apologize to the readers for any potential inaccuracies in the text that may have gone unnoticed. Although we put effort into covering all key topics and taking care of all details, errors are an inevitable side effect of any human striving; this includes writing a textbook. Please do not hesitate to inform us if you encounter any so that we can correct them in the future. Any suggestions of topics not covered are also very much welcome.

The authors want to thank Prof. Thomas Lenarz, MD, the chairman of the Clinics of Otolaryngology, Hannover School of Medicine, Germany (Fig. 1), for founding our infrastructure in Hannover. He has remarkable persistence in following his vision, especially in times when the climate does not favor our discipline. The positions for all authors are in some ways related to Thomas' efforts, and later to the Cluster of Excellence Hearing4All of the Deutsche Forschungsgemeinschaft, which he co-chairs. The broad scope of expertise collected at the Institute of AudioNeuroTechnology, and its technological

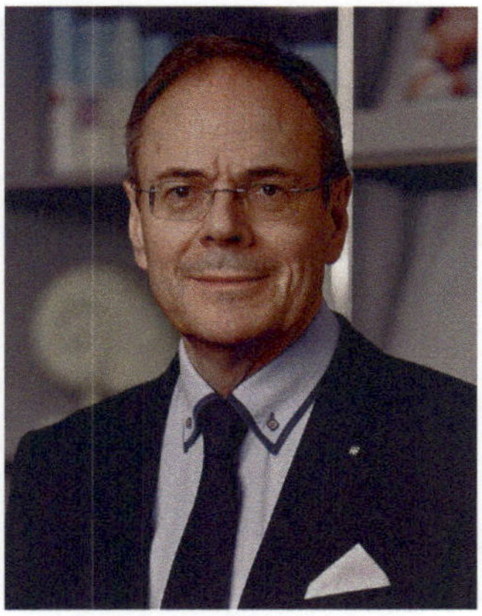

Fig. 1 Thomas Lenarz, MD.

and laboratory infrastructure, allowed us to undertake research that helped us to better understand hearing, hearing loss, and prosthetic devices. Thomas provided us full-time researchers with clinical perspectives. Without his generous support in many ways, our work would have been much more difficult, if not partly impossible. This book would have not been written without him.

We are grateful to the auditory community for its friendly and supportive atmosphere. The biannual Conference on Implantable Auditory Prostheses (CIAP) organized by changing chairs under the administrative and ideal leadership of Prof. Robert V. Shannon, PhD (Fig. 2), helped to shape many of our views. Bob Shannon is a pioneer of cochlear implants with numerous seminal contributions to the understanding of normal hearing, particularly the development of cochlear implants and their application in humans. Bob has never been competitive. His "child" CIAP explicitly encourages

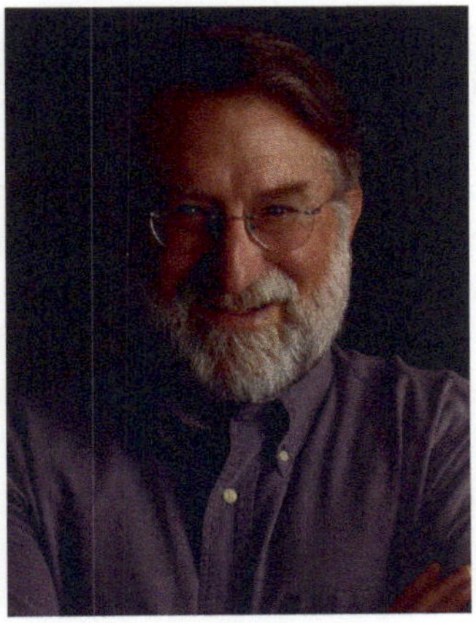

Fig. 2 Robert V. Shannon, PhD.

interaction and provides the platform for meeting colleagues in an informal atmosphere. CIAP allowed us to have intensive interaction with the leaders in auditory prosthetics like Bob himself, Ingeborg and Erwin Hochmair, Michael F. Dorman, Gerald M. O'Donoghue, Bryan Pfingst, David B. Pisoni, Robert K. Shepherd, Blake S. Wilson, and many more that we unfortunately cannot all name here. We have had the joy of co-authoring publications with several of these individuals and have spent a lot of time in intense discussions. Bob Shannon, Peter Roland, Edwin Rubel, and Helge Rask-Andersen were always very generous in sharing knowledge and data. Bob, with support of his wife Elaine Minehart, has frequently been the "center of gravity" of our scientific community. Many of his students became professors at universities around the globe. From him we learned that good science is cooperative. For all of this, we want to say thank you.

Andrej is further grateful to his teachers, particularly Dr. Rainer Hartmann, an engineer by training, who introduced him to neuroengineering. Andrej especially profited from the mathematics and computer science skills he acquired at his secondary school (Gymnasium Jura Hronca, Bratislava), and the follow-up university courses of higher mathematics that he visited with Prof. V. Majernik, PhD, DSc, from the Institute of Mathematics, Slovak Academy of Sciences, Bratislava. This, together with his work in the lab of Rainer Hartmann, Frankfurt am Main, provided the tools and technical background he needed for this book. It also spurred his interest in the different disciplines shared with the readers of this textbook. Additionally, Andrej wants to thank Jochen Tillein, Anu Sharma, Steve Lomber, Jos Eggermont, Rob Shepherd, Blake Wilson, Gerry O'Donoghue, and Karen Gordon for many years of friendship and collaboration. He also profited from his secondary appointment at Macquarie University, its generosity in support of his travels, and numerous discussions at the Australian Hearing Hub.

Hannes thanks Dr. Fritz A. Sauer from the Max Planck Institute of Biophysics, Frankfurt, whom he owes for his understanding of theoretical physics and the necessity of experimental validation. He also wishes to thank Claus-Peter Richter, MD, PhD, and Anthony W. Gummer, PhD, who triggered his interest in auditory research and enabled him to transition into this completely new field.

The authors wish to thank the team at the Department of Experimental Otology, Hannover Medical School, for their support. They participated in scientific discussions on many occasions and shaped the views presented in this textbook. Several figures used in this book were developed following these discussions or were part of the research performed at our department. In particular, the authors wish to thank Dr. Peter Baumhoff, Daniela Beyer and Janet Cheung for generously providing some of the illustrations. Daniela and Eddy Kühne, our technicians, and our secretary, Manuela Chambers, helped us keep our "backs free" of many administration and technical issues while working on this textbook.

Finally, the authors want to thank Dr. Jens Grosche from Effigos AG, Leipzig, Germany (https://effigos.com), for generously providing several excellent illustrations in the book, including the cover figure.

We are grateful to our spouses Julia, Janet, and Chris for the time that we invested in this project. This included many weekends of work that otherwise would be dedicated to our families.

We hope that this book will ignite interest from our readers in the quickly advancing area of biomedical technology. May they share our fascination for it and help the field to grow further; may they expand and deepen what we know. Finally, may they find solutions to unsolved problems that we failed to find, to the benefit of those that require medical support.

Andrej Kral, MD, PhD[a,b]
Felix Aplin, PhD[a]
Hannes Maier, PhD[a]
[a]Cluster of Excellence Hearing4All, Hannover Medical School, Hannover, Germany
[b]Macquarie University, Sydney, NSW, Australia

PART 1

Introduction

CHAPTER 1

The historic preconditions of neural prostheses

We are often not aware of changes that take place within our society. While changes that overturn everyday life may in retrospect appear as revolutions, on a day-by-day basis they may be small and incremental. Such incremental changes eventually fundamentally impact society. Sociologists call small changes leading to large leaps in societal structure baseline shifts.

Today we experience such a change. The digitization of our lives progresses constantly and influences daily life in form of the Internet, smart phones, and tablets. We use them to buy tickets for the bus, plane, or train, to watch movies, stream TV programs and listen to our favorite music, and to navigate through unknown places. We are digitizing our culture. This revolution, with its positive and negative consequences, affects medicine in a fundamental way. It has provided us with one of the mightiest tools that science has developed: the computer and information technology.

This revolution is affecting the treatment of nervous system diseases in particular. Many new treatments rest on the success of the field of **bionics** (biologically inspired engineering). By mimicking nature, bionics leads to the design of supportive devices that can subsequently enhance or replace the function of the original biology (**prosthetics**). Since the brain is an information-processing device, progress in computer technology and prosthetic devices will lead to the treatment of many neural diseases, and potentially to the extension of brain capabilities. However, development of neural prostheses is complex. It requires (1) an understanding of nervous system function, (2) an understanding of how to interface with the nervous system using technology, and (3) a level of technical development that allows for the fabrication of devices that imitate, compensate, or replace nervous system function.

In clinical neuroscience there has been a baseline shift in the application of bionics to the treatment of disease, since we are now able to intervene in conditions that were at the border of science fiction only a few years ago. We can treat deaf subjects with cochlear implants, can alleviate symptoms of Parkinson's disease using deep brain stimulation, can help to reduce chronic pain, and regain control of lost bladder function. Many new applications are in clinical use or rapidly approaching it. How did this field come so far in such a short time, and where were the fundamental roots of these approaches?

Prostheses for the Brain
https://doi.org/10.1016/B978-0-12-818892-7.00005-5

Historic roots of biomedical technology

Knowledge about the brain has accumulated over decades of neuroscientific research, primarily driven by experimentation on animal (model) systems. This allowed us to understand the fundamental principles of nervous function. In the past, the brain was regarded as a syncytium: a tissue where individual cells fused into a huge mesh without clear delineation of their original border and with extensive communication of the intracellular space (this is indeed partly true in the heart or for the placenta of an unborn child). Histologists Camillo Golgi (1843–1926) and Santiago Ramon y Cajal (1852–1934) studied the brains of animals and deceased humans. Golgi developed a method that stains individual nerve cells (**neurons**, Fig. 1.1). Using this method he overturned the theory that brain is a syncytium

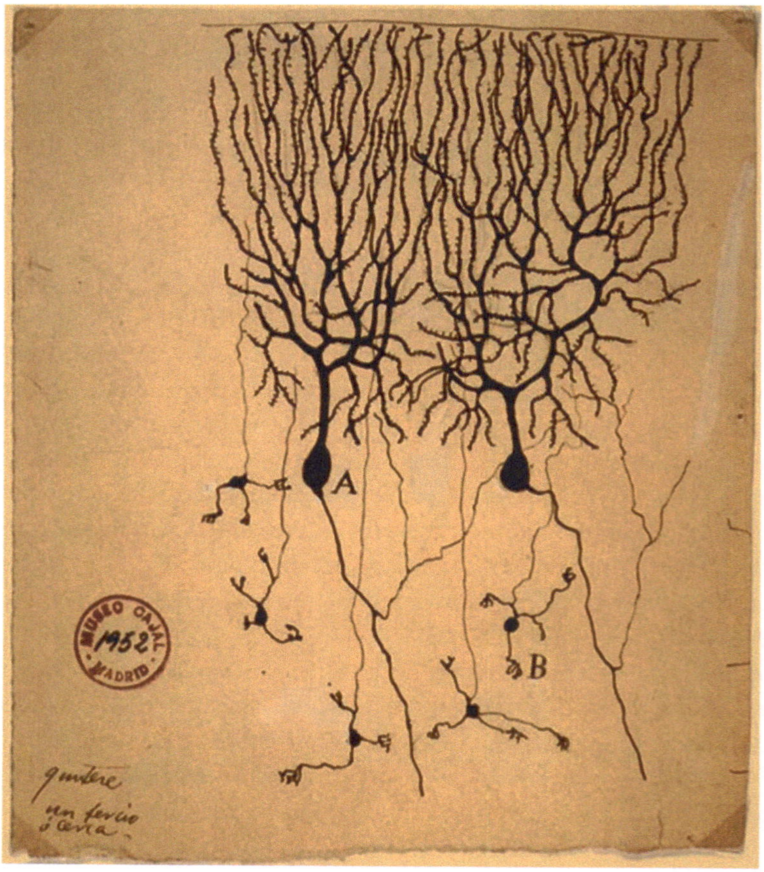

Fig. 1.1 Drawn traces of neurons stained using the Golgi method from the cerebellum, drawings by S. Ramon y Cajal. The Golgi method showed conclusively that the brain contained nerve cells, or neurons, that are part of an interconnected web. From Museo Cajal in Madrid, Spain, public domain.

and demonstrated that cells in the brain are separated and distinct (**Chapter 4**). From this we learned that the brain is an intricate structure of an immense number of such neurons (estimations for human brain go to 10^{11}), each of them being connected with thousands of other neurons (in some cases up to 100,000 or more). It was Ramon y Cajal who then explicitly formulated the **neuron doctrine**: that individual neurons are the elementary processing elements of the brain. Neurons are cells specialized to process information, coded in an electrical signal on their neuronal membrane, and processed in the chemical contacts between neurons (the synapses). We have subsequently understood that a network of such cells can process information in a complex way; not only can it perform logical operations, as Warren McCulloch and Walter Pitts showed in the 1940s, but it can also store information in a distributed way via the pattern of network connections, rather than in individual cells. A neuronal network can process information, generate sequences of events (like as required for motor action), and a multi-layered neuronal network can learn in a desired (supervised) way; deep learning artificial intelligence is inspired by this and has become a part of our daily cell phone usage when, for example, transcribing spoken language into a text or talking to Siri. Over the centuries we have also learned that the brain is the seat of our mind, our feelings, and our perceptions. Now the principles of action of the brain have allowed computers and electronics to extend back into the body and communicate with organic tissue.

To reach this point, two streams of science had to come together: the concept of virtual representations and virtual instructions (information theory and computers) and the knowledge of electric fields and bioelectricity. Both of these were equally important and, interestingly, also started in parallel. They involved two different branches of knowledge: technology and natural science.

History of computer technology

The separation of information from its signal, and the storage of this information, started millennia ago with the invention of written words. Clay tablets from Mesopotamia (around 2000 BCE) allowed for the first time the storage of information and usage of this information to artificially combine signs and develop new meanings. This information could be conserved by transforming its form, that is, separating information from the signals transmitting it. Over centuries this principle developed into the alphabet that we use today, including centuries of development of writing instruments and the evolution of clay tablets to papyrus or metal rolls, and leather to paper. At the same time, mathematicians realized that devices used to store mathematical information, such as the abacus, could also be used to simplify the calculation (i.e., processing) of said information. These concepts form the groundwork for what would become information technology: the study of systems and devices that store, convert, and process information.

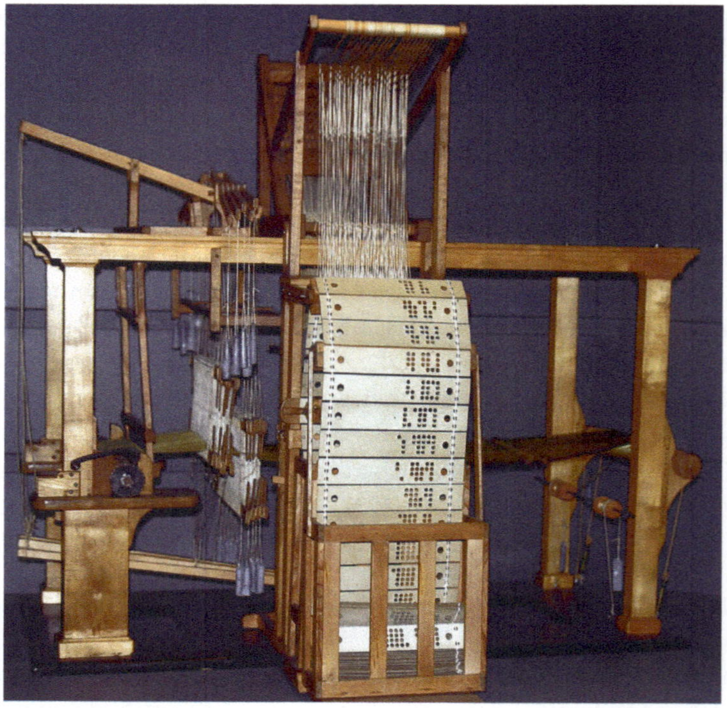

Fig. 1.2 Loom of Jean Baptiste Falcon, a predecessor of the famous Jacquard loom, with the wooden punch cards in front. Thread could be fed down through a system of punch cards to convert stored information into patterned weaving. This eliminated the need for error-prone humans to follow complex weaving patterns and is the first modern example of a computing machine. *(Photograph by Rama, Wikimedia Commons, Cc-by-sa-2.0-fr.)*

The roots of modern computing technology arose in France and in England in the eighteenth century. The device that initiated the development of a computing machine was the loom controlled by punch cards (Fig. 1.2), the most famous built in 1804 by Joseph Marie Jacquard (1752–1834) in Lyon, France, to allow efficient manufacturing textiles with complex patterns like brocade or damask that otherwise required extensive manual work and were prone to error. Introduction of the Jacquard loom sped up weaving of complex fabric substantially. Using punch cards, a production pattern was predefined (and could be modified nearly at will) for the machine to "read out" and execute. It was the first time that a machine followed an algorithmic instruction that could be varied to produce different outcomes. By this, the Jacquard loom and its less famous predecessors were the first devices that physically separated instructions (programs) from the machine hardware. The loom revealed that information could be extracted, abstracted, stored, and then fed back into a system to reproduce the original output. This invention proved that computing technology was not only academically interesting but also a useful technique for practical economic applications.

The Jacquard loom is the predecessor to machines produced, for example, by IBM that were initially used to simplify population counting and store large amounts of information. These devices were used to replace human "computers" (a term signifying employees who manually performed mathematical calculations; usually women[a]). The oldest human computers were probably Hipparchus of Nicaea (180–125 BCE) and Claudius Ptolemy (90–165 CE), generating tables for the tracing of celestial objects. Human computers were popular in the sixteenth through nineteenth centuries; they were used to calculate tables to track celestial objects over time, to determine the movement of comets, for the navigation of ships, for military purposes, in banks for performing financial calculations, and so on. Human computers developed mathematical tables for computing goniometric functions or logarithms, an essential tool for all students until ~30 years ago. Further innovation towards a computing machine capable of following sequences of instructions at a rate faster and less error-prone than a human was necessary to enable greater insight into neuroscience.

One essential step of development of computers was the development of the machine code. The initial contribution came from the German polymath Gottfried Wilhelm Leibniz (1646–1716, Fig. 1.3) by developing binary calculus. Inspired by old Chinese writings and some contemporary works, he formalized computation in binary numbers, anticipating information theory as well as the development of computing machines. Using his work, Leibniz laid the concepts of computer science and cybernetics (in addition to other monumental contributions in the fields of mathematics, physics, and other sciences).

The genuine ideas of real computing machines, however, date to Charles Babbage (1791–1871, Fig. 1.4), who imagined and designed a plan for mechanical machines that were to follow a "program" and perform mathematical computations (an "Analytical Engine" and a "Difference Engine"). While he designed the principles of such machines, including a punch card system inspired by the Jacquard loom, he never built a functional prototype. His successors much later built a machine similar to Babbage, and eventually proved the applicability of the design.

Babbage was very skilled in selling his ideas and receiving funding for his work. Even though his machines were never built, they inspired the theory of computation and led to many subsequent inventions. For example, Ada Lovelace (1815–1852, Fig. 1.5), a mathematician interested in Babbage's work, conceptually designed the first computer program for Babbage's Engines that already included subroutines and conditional terms. By that, she can be considered the first software developer. Since Babbage's machine was never built,

[a] Buzz Aldrin, the second man on the moon, when mistrusting outcomes of computer programs insisted that the human computers check whether the calculations performed by technical devices are correct. Only recently did it became publicly clear how essential the contribution was that women played in the success of the landing on the moon by designing software and computing trajectories, etc. (compare, e.g., www.space.com/women-of-apollo.html).

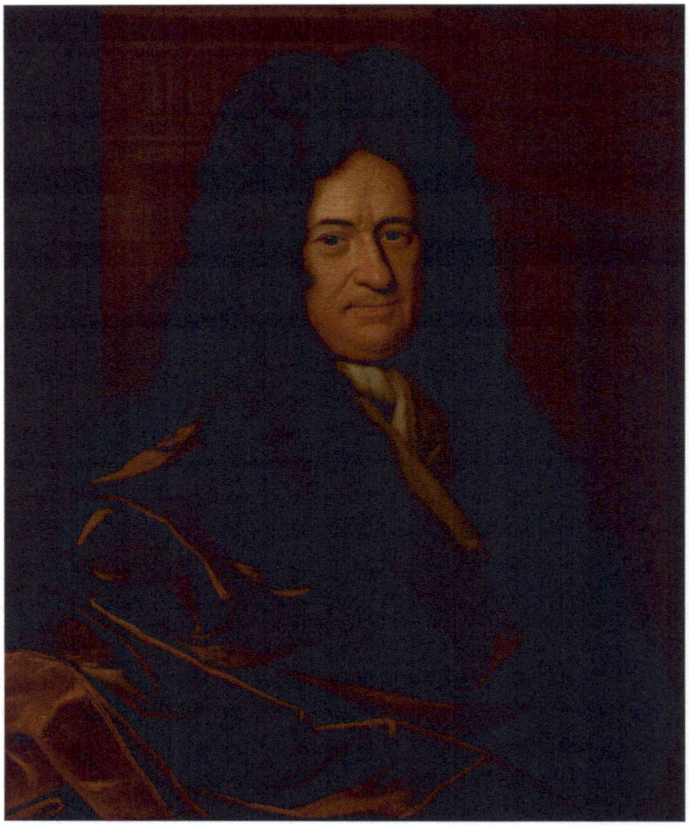

Fig. 1.3 Gottfried Wilhelm Leibniz (1646–1716). German polymath and inventor of binary calculus. By his formalization of calculation with binary numbers he formed the mathematical basis of machine code used in present-day computers. *(Painting by Christoph Bernard Francke.)*

these programs were never practically tested and used during Lovelace's life, although subsequently they were proven functional. To honor the contribution of Lovelace to computer technology, her name was selected for a programming language, "Ada," developed for the company Honeywell Bull; it shared some similarity with the more popular language Pascal widely used for nearly two decades on many computer systems.

It further took further nearly 200 years until Alan Turing (1912–1954, Fig. 1.6) wondered what happens in the mind of human computers; is human nature and consciousness really necessary to perform complex mathematical computations? In his influential 1936 paper "On computable numbers, with an application to the Entscheidungs problem,"[b] he provided parts of the answer. He realized that the human computers simply follow a

[b] This paper is in fact on the question of undecidability in computation (whether an algorithm will finish the computational process or continue infinitely; the so-called Halting problem).

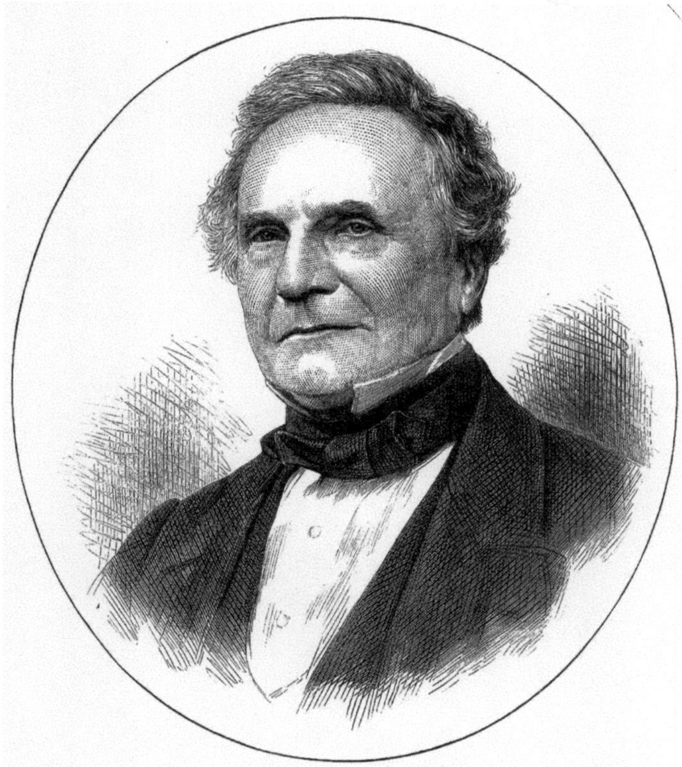

Fig. 1.4 Charles Babbage (1791–1871). Inventor of the first mechanical computer.

set of rules (instructions) and operate them on provided data. Thus a virtual machine (the **universal Turing machine**) could perform the same tasks provided it had enough memory and a processor following a sequence of instructions. In this sense Alan Turing followed the ideas of Lovelace, Jacquard, and others and constructed a formal mathematical background for computer science.

In parallel with the development of information theory, technological innovation fostered the quantification and miniaturization of information flow.[c] Punch cards were bulky physical objects that had to be mechanically transported from place to place. This is too slow a technique for most practical applications of information interchange. Samuel Thomas Sommering (1755–1830) was an influential anatomist (he discovered the corpus luteum in the retina) and a famous inventor. Building on the inventions in the field of electricity, he suggested the use of electrical signals to transmit written information. The received information was made visible by electrochemical reactions leading to bubble formation in a fluid that also caused acoustic signals. The codes used were complex

[c] Parts of these historical views are discussed in the BBC documentary "Order and Disorder."

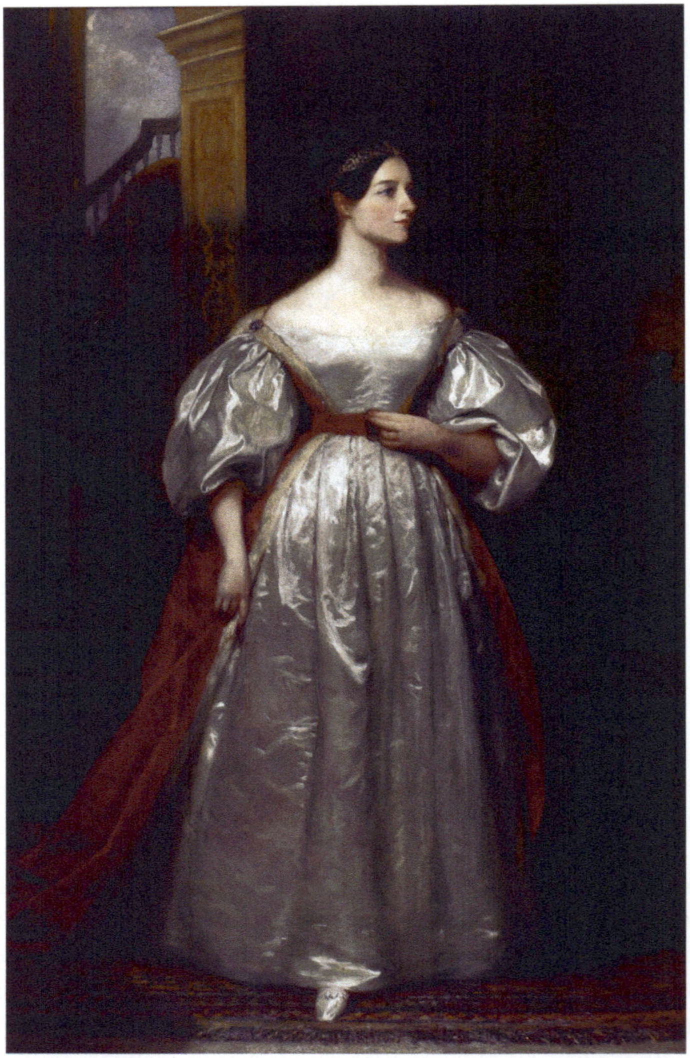

Fig. 1.5 Ada Lovelace (1815–1852). Founder of software. Ada Lovelace formulated the basic ideas related to computer programs. Subroutines and conditional terms are also her invention.

and not practical, but Samuel F. B. Morse (1791–1872) improved the transmission speed substantially by transforming the alphabet to binary signals based on duration (short and long signals), using the frequency of occurrence to further boost transmission speed (e.g., the most frequent letter "E" was coded by the shortest signal). The invention of Morse code allowed a fast transmission of information and finally to the practical use of the telegraph. The invention of the telephone by Alexander Graham Bell (1847–1922) and many follow-up inventions in his Bell Laboratories, together with the wireless telegraphy developed by Guilermo Marconi (1874–1937) and Karl F. Braun (1850–1918; Braun also

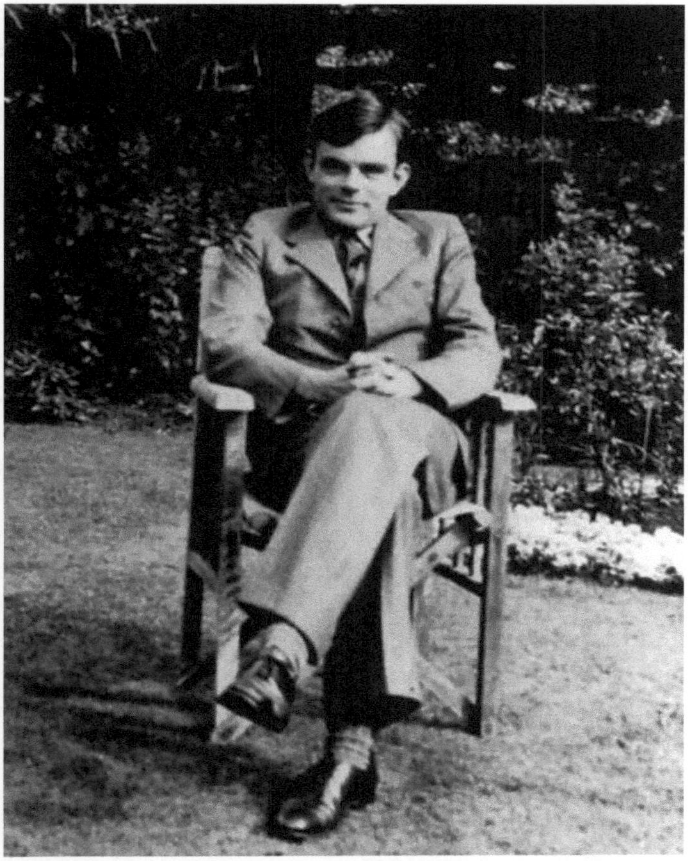

Fig. 1.6 Alan Turing (1912–1954). Pioneer of computer science.

built the first cathode-ray tubes that were the basis for television sets), revolutionized and sped up information interchange over large distances.

The final essential step in information theory took place in the famous Bell Laboratories. These laboratories provided scientists with extensive academic freedoms, similar to the traditional academic freedoms of university professors in some countries, with a very solid financial funding of Bell Telephone Company (later renamed to American Telephone & Telegraph Company, AT&T). The scientists in Bell Laboratories were allowed to follow any idea they considered important, and were only obliged to respond to the requests of other scientists and members of Bell's company. One of these scientists was Claude E. Shannon (1916–2001); he made excellent use of these freedoms and decided to focus on measuring information. Bell's invention, by that time already in world-wide use, was transmitting information, but nobody could measure (quantify) it. Claude Shannon realized that a measure of information is not related to the interpretation (meaning), but to the amount of how surprising (unexpected) the information is. To measure information it is sufficient to measure the *change* or *variance* in a signal, that is, the part of the signal that is "surprising" or unexpected.[d] Only the unexpected is true (new) information. In his 1948 paper "A mathematical theory of computation," based on the binary calculus developed by Leibniz, he measured information using entropy (the measure of the "disorder" used in thermodynamics[e]). Here the elementary amount of information, the informational atom, was one "binary digit," abbreviated "bit." Using his formalisms he eventually transformed information into an exact science. From this, the technological development of computing machines was purely a matter of the physical development and miniaturization of components that allow "computational" processing of electrical information, such as the transistor and later the integrated circuit.

These developments established the concept that information processing can be separated from a substrate on which it is running, and that complex electrical or mechanical machines can then interpret and transform this information based on a set of pre-programmed rules. While our brains do not work identically to computers, they are also responsible for the transmission and transformation of information, and neuroscience required an understanding of information theory to progress as a field. This background was essential for development of active prostheses that process some kind of input information and convert this into output signals that finally stimulate neurons. Thus, these prostheses are controlled by dedicated "computers" and stimulate neurons of our brain. For this, computers had to become small, cheap, and easy to implement. Therefore, development of computers initiated the development of prosthetics that control, based on some kind of input, neuronal activity. They need to process the input and transform it to a signal that can be meaningfully processed by the brain.

Development of electrophysiology

The second root of neuroprosthetics, bioelectricity, originated in Italy. The electrical revolution was initiated by Alessandro Volta (1745–1827, Fig. 1.7) who described static electricity and subsequently he and others observed similar phenomena in nervous tissue: the discovery of bioelectricity. Luigi Galvani (1737–1798, Fig. 1.8) used static electricity to stimulate the muscle of a frog and his bimetal experiments paved the way for the invention of the battery. More importantly, his frog experiments proved that animals use electricity in their bodies. This was the period of great electrical inventions, and electricity was a controversial and popular topic of the time similar to today's smartphones. A product of this time was also the novel from Mary Goodwin (later Shelley)

[d] A general and well-written introduction to information theory is W. Ross Ashby's monograph *An Introduction to Cybernetics*, Chapman & Hall Ltd., 1957.

[e] James Clerk Maxwell (1831–1879) speculated about the relation of temperature and information; he suggested that information can create order, and thus linked thermodynamics, energy, and information. While at this time he could not finally resolve the issues he discovered, he outlined these directions already.

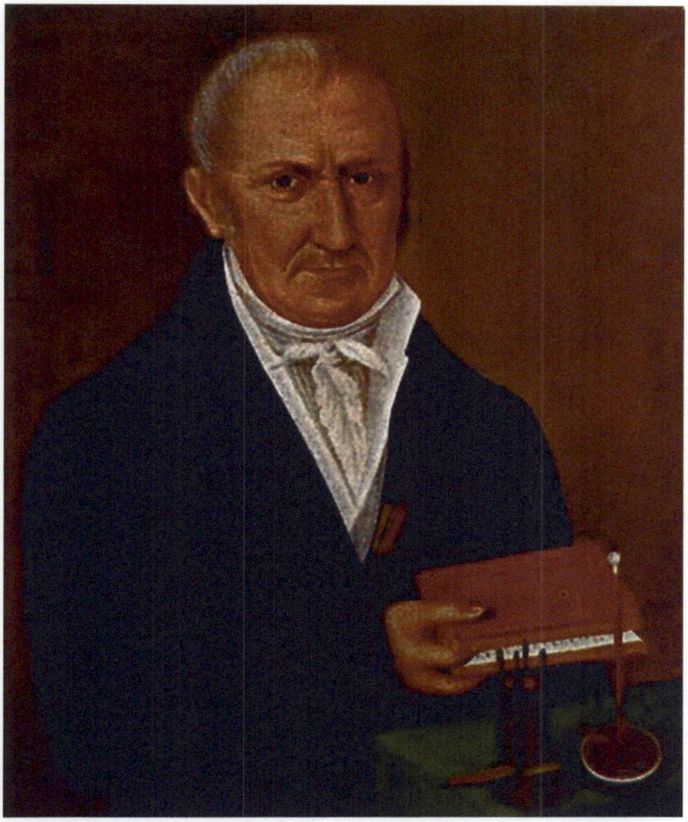

Fig. 1.7 Alessandro Volta (1745–1827). Described static electricity and bioelectricity.

(1797–1851) called *Frankenstein* or *The Modern Prometheus*. Here electricity played a key role; the body constructed from parts of dead men was brought to life by an igniting electric shock. Thus, electricity was considered the source of the "spark" of life. These early ideas proved false, but such fascination for electricity allowed for further innovation.[f]

[f] Interestingly, the roots of electrical phenomena in the brain and of information theory converged by coincidence in 1816. When Mary Goodwin wrote the *Frankenstein* novel, she and her partner Percy Bysshe Shelley were visiting a friend, Lord George Gordon Byron, in Villa Diodati at the Geneva Lake (Switzerland). The above company were trapped inside the house by cold and rain. To entertain themselves, they invented horror stories. It was a productive vacation. In addition to the famous novel of Mary Goodwin Shelley, Byron's physician John Polidori wrote another novel, *The Vampyre*, which inspired Bram Stoker's *Dracula*. In 1815, a year before these events happened, Lord Byron fathered a girl, but left his pregnant wife in England; it is said that he never met his daughter. This gifted girl later, as a young woman, made very a key contribution to information science and technology; her name was Ada Lovelace.

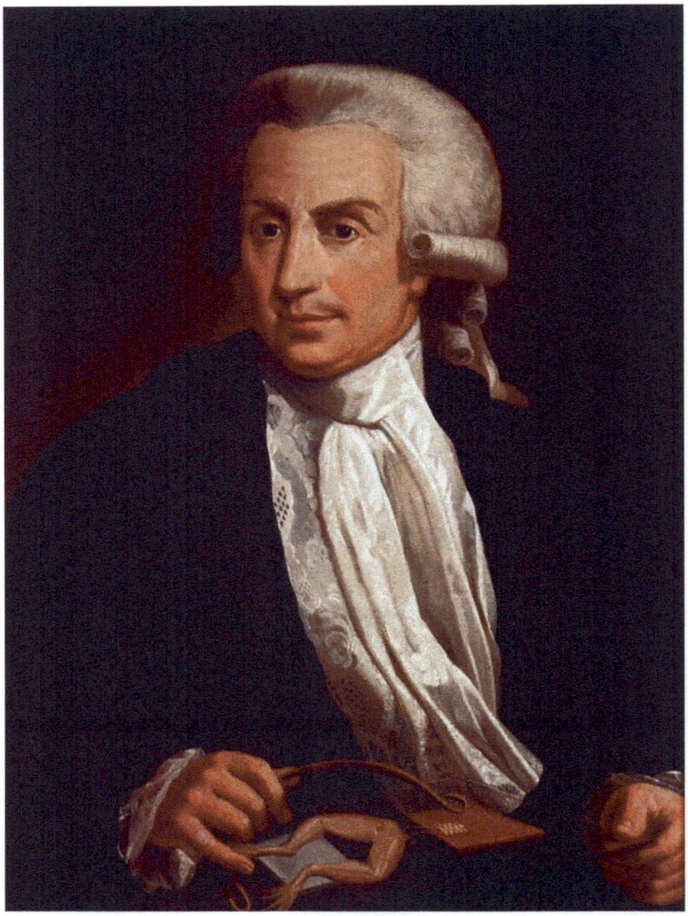

Fig. 1.8 Luigi Galvani (1737–1798). Performed the first muscle stimulation experiments with electricity.

While a link between electricity and the body was proven from the onset of electrical science, at that time technology was insufficient to explore the electrical processes in the brain in more detail. Nearly 100 years of further technological development finally enabled the recording of electrical phenomena in individual neurons. The first recording of electrical signals from the human brain, the electro-encephalogram (and also electrocardiogram) was measured by Emil Heinrich du Bois-Reymond (1818–1896), followed in 1868 by recording of nerve potentials by Julius Bernstein (1839–1917) and much later Edgar Douglas Adrian (1898–1977) together with Keith Lucas (1879–1916). The latter developed the "capillary electrometer," a technical device that recorded action potentials extracellularly from the sciatic nerve of a frog. This technological development initiated the series of studies by Adrian. Subsequently, Joseph Erlanger (1874–1965) and Herbert Spencer Gasser (1888–1963) followed this approach in the first decades of 1900. Recording of electrical phenomena allowed for the calculation of nerve fiber conduction velocity, which revealed that anatomically similar neurons were further differentiated according to their functional properties. Many features used in clinical neurology today still refer to these observations.

The nervous system, as these researches could demonstrate, and today‘s computers share aspects of information processing and use electrical signals to convey this information. In the brain, pulse-like depolarizations of the cell‘s outer membrane, lasting ~1–2 ms and having an amplitude of ~90 mV, called action potentials, serve this function (see **Chapter 4**). In modern technical equipment, e.g., transistor-transistor logic (TTL) pulses is one way to perform a similar function. Alan L. Hodgkin (1914–1998) and Andrew F. Huxley (1917–2012) finally mathematically described the physiological process behind action potentials and their work allowed us to understand the molecular mechanisms of action potentials.

In parallel, neuroscience begun to understand that the function of the brain was separated into different processing streams, which were sometimes physically discreet. Pierre Paul Broca (1824–1880) documented a specific loss of language function following damage in a distinct brain region (the area is now called "Broca's area"). This was followed by the work of Gustav Theodor Fritsch (1838–1927) and Julius Eduard Hitzig (1838–1907) who in 1870 documented that electrical stimulation of a certain brain region (now called motor cortex) caused limb movements on the opposite side of the body in a dog. A similar technique has been repeatedly used to delineate the function of human brain regions, most widely exploited by the neurosurgeon Wilder Penfield (1891–1976) to identify language areas. This was of key importance in prevention of damage to these areas during brain operations, to prevent the loss of a key cognitive function: language. Penfield realized another cardinal aspect of this technique: it allowed him to better localize different neuronal functions to distinct brain regions. This had huge impact on both neuroscience and neurology.

Using these developments, it was established that **the brain uses electrical phenomena for processing of information**, both for generating perceptions and for controlling muscle activity. This knowledge, combined with the general principles of coding within sensory organs, allows us to transfer information between technology and neural tissue.

The concept of a neural prosthesis

Since we now know how to manipulate and transform information across different signals, and we understand that the brain also processes and stores information, we can in theory use technology to convey information from a constructed device to the brain, and vice versa. That is the basic concept of a neural prosthesis.

Diseases of the nervous system remained unrecognized for a long time in human history. This was partly due to the limited ability of humans to localize the seat of the human mind, and the director of our body, to the brain. Traditionally, the heart had been considered the organ where feelings are generated, and many famous philosophers, including Aristotle, failed to recognize the brain as the center of our thinking. For this reason, treatments involving the brain are relatively new in medical practice. After scientists discovered the principles of electricity, it became possible to reveal electric phenomena in the brain, and understand that neurons control muscles that exert physical force. Particularly during World War I, brain damage became a subject of medical research and diagnosis. While the principles of brain stimulation, as used by Fritsch and Hitzig, were already known, the technology was very underdeveloped and precluded any practical use of such techniques beyond diagnostic features. Here electrophysiology increasingly involved direct electrical stimulation, as currently performed to test peripheral nerves (the H-reflex).

The brain, as any other organ of the body, is subject to degeneration and disease. Inborn metabolic disease can affect the function of neurons, as can inflammation and infection, injury, intoxication, vascular disease, and tumors. The brain can be affected locally or globally and damage to its structures means that functions cannot be executed effectively. This may involve our sensory systems, our motor system, or also the integrative function of the brain that combines several individual functions into one. Perception and cognition are examples of such functions. The brain is a differentiated tissue with discreet neuronal and regional functions that in contrast to some species (like lizards) does not regenerate after injury in humans. While the growth of new neurons has been discovered in some parts of the brain, the numbers are far too low to provide the brain with the substrate for regeneration. Individual nerve cells can change their function and connective structure to some extent (this is the substrate for learning), but they cannot replace lost neurons due to injury. Controlling the process of regeneration has been an elusive goal of molecular biology and we cannot yet encourage parts of the brain to regrow. However, an understanding of brain function provides us with the possibility to interfere using artificial systems, that is, to replace the lost function by a technical device (a prosthesis). Prosthetic devices can alleviate the consequences of some brain diseases or injuries. Prostheses do not directly treat the disease, but can partially (or ideally fully) replace some of the lost function.

It has required the substantial progress in science and technology outlined in this chapter to allow for the manipulation of the human nervous system in a way that is pragmatically useful for replacing some lost function in patients. Today we know that this is possible, and the potential of this technology is still growing. This field has remained focused on replacing degenerated or underdeveloped sensory functions, motor disease, and modulating pathologic behaviors. As shown in this introductory book, this typically requires "active implants" that are implanted into the body and can sense neuronal activity or stimulate neurons. These devices are highly complex and must be biologically inert (do not undergo chemical reactions when placed in the body, and do not disassemble); some such implants have to be hermetically packed to prevent any interaction between the technology and the bodily fluids. Active implants interact with neurons using electrical fields, and this can influence the health of the surrounding tissue. Electric current may dissolve the implant material and cause further chemical reactions in the tissue. Eventually, such reactions may lead to tissue damage. Therefore, neural prostheses are complex and potentially dangerous devices that must be carefully developed, evaluated, and implemented in order to provide useful benefit to patients. The combination of such a diverse set of scientific concepts necessary to produce these implants means that scientists, engineers, and clinicians working on these devices must have a broad base of knowledge. This book thus provides an overview of the biology, engineering, and clinical applications that are necessary to properly understand neural prosthesis development.

Brief summary

- Neural prostheses are devices that replace or enhance the function of the nervous system.
- The modern understanding of neural prostheses relies on the complementary development of medical and information technologies.
- Information and signal can be separated and information can be stored independently of the original signal.
- The brain transforms, processes, and stores information using a combination of electrical and chemical signals.
- In conjunction with computer technology, it is possible to accurately record and decode bioelectrical signals.
- Artificial electrical signals can be used to generate bioelectrical signals.

Key literature and further reading

Ashby, W.R., 1957. An Introduction to Cybernetics. Chapman & Hall, Ltd.

Cooper, S., van Leeuwen, J., 2013. Alan Turing: His Work and Impact, 1st ed. Elsevier Science.

Davis, M., Sigal, R., Weyuker, E.J., 1994. Computability, Complexity, and Languages: Fundamentals of Theoretical Computer Science, 2nd ed. Academic Press.

Essinger, J., 2004. Jacquard's Web: How a Hand-Loom Led to the Birth of the Information Age. Oxford University Press, Oxford.

Finger, S., 2001. Origins of Neuroscience: A History of Explorations into Brain Function. Oxford University Press, US.

Finger, S., 2004. Paul Broca (1824–1880). J. Neurol. 251, 769–770.

Hyman, A. (Ed.), 1989. Science and Reform: Selected Works of Charles Babbage. Cambridge University Press, Cambridge, England.

Hammerman, R., Russell, A.L., 2015. Ada's Legacy: Cultures of Computing from the Victorian to the Digital Age. Morgan & Claypool.
Johnston, J.B., 1906. The Nervous System of Vertebrates. P. Blakiston's Son & Co., Philadelphia.
Pancaldi, G., 2003. Volta, Science and Culture in the Age of Enlightenment. Princeton University Press.
Posselt, E.A., 1887. The Jacquard Machine, Analyzed and Explained: With an Appendix on the Preparation of Jacquard Cards, and Practical Hints to Learners of Jacquard Designing. Dando Printing and Publishing Co., Philadelphia.
Shannon, C.E., 1948. A mathematical theory of communication. Bell Syst. Technol. J. 27, 379–423, 623–656.
Turing, A.M., 1936. On computable numbers, with an application to the Entscheidungs problem. J. Math. 58, 230–265.
Verkhratsky, A., Krishtal, O.A., Petersen, O.H., 2006. From Galvani to patch clamp: the development of electrophysiology. Pflugers Arch. 453 (3), 233–247.

CHAPTER 2

History of neuroprostheses

Historical attempts at electrical stimulation

Probably the first historic mention of the medical use of electrical current is from 76 CE, when Pedianos Dioscurides (exact life dates unknown)[a] described attempts to use electric rays (that generate electric fields to anesthetize fish) in therapy of epileptic seizures in his *De materia medica*. Subsequently, Avicenna (979–1037) in his *Canon of Medicine*, most likely following the suggestions of Galenos of Pergamon (~128–199 CE), suggested use of the same rays in the therapy of chronic headache. While they were not aware of the nature of electricity, they intuitively coupled anesthetic effects and neurological disorders. It required millennia for science and technology (**Chapter 1**) to progress enough for more mechanistic approaches.

Galvani's observation of neuronal excitability, as discussed in detail in **Chapter 1**, did not have any contemporary practical uses. Volta's attempts to self-stimulate the auditory and visual organs were in principle the beginning of modern concepts of neurostimulation. However, the application of the current was uncontrolled and clearly dangerous. Even Volta himself did not dare to start systematically investigating it. Despite these early discoveries, many scientists still did not believe that the brain was excitable by electric current. It took the combined effort of multiple scientists to demonstrate the relationship between electricity and human perception. Charles Le Roy (1726–1779) first documented the application of current to the forehead of a blind subject to stimulate the eye electrically. While his intervention did not cure the blindness of the subject, the subject clearly described visual perceptions from the apparatus that most probably stimulated the optic nerves or the remaining tissue of the retinae.

Concurrently, the work of Galvani's nephew Giovanni Aldini (1762–1834) focused on experiments on heads of executed criminals and demonstrated that facial muscles could contract following electrical stimulation of the exposed cerebral cortex if performed in close succession of the execution; some believed that Aldani could bring life back to dead. Aldini instead suggested that electrical stimulation of the head might be a method for treatment of melancholy. This could be seen as a predecessor of the electroconvulsive therapy ("electroshock therapy") used in psychiatry, for example, in intractable depression and psychotic diseases. Throughout the nineteenth century, electric stimulation became very popular as a "cure-all" for many medical conditions, the vast

[a] Little is known about his life; only that he resided in Tarsos and is considered the father of pharmacology.

Prostheses for the Brain
https://doi.org/10.1016/B978-0-12-818892-7.00009-2

majority of which were likely fraudulent or ineffective. The development of more sophisticated, evidenced-based approaches required the maturation of modern medicine and a better understanding of nervous system anatomy and function.

Mapping the brain

More focused stimulation approaches required a map of the functions of individual regions of the brain. Luigi Ronaldo (1773–1831) was probably the first to use galvanic currents to stimulate the cortex (brain surface) of animals in attempts to understand their function. This was followed up by the work of Gustav Th. Fritsch (1838–1927) and Eduard Hitzig (1838–1907). Fritsch and Hitzig stimulated the motor cortex of dogs and established that specific locations in the cerebral cortex are responsible for particular body parts (then called muscle regions). These were the first findings supporting a representation of the body surface in cortical maps, further extended by David Ferrier (1843–1928), who mapped out the motor cortex of monkeys. Studies on humans were rare at that time, but already Fritsch and Hitzig reported in one subject that cortical stimulation in the posterior parts of the cortex leads to eye movements. Some of the early studies were on subjects following injuries with freely accessible brain, or in children with encephalocele (brain or cerebrospinal fluid prolapse through the skull due to developmental deficits in skull bone formation). With such subjects Robert Bartholow (1831–1904), Ezio Sciamanna (1850–1905), and Alberto Alberti (1856–1913) performed the motor cortex mapping experiments. It was Hermann Munk (1839–1912) who proposed that there is also a point-to-point mapping of the retina ("retinotopy") to the occipital cortex, which was later confirmed by studies on injured soldiers during World War I by Gordon M. Holmes (1876–1965). Most interesting were studies on subjects who suffered from epilepsy following gunshots to the head, with skull fragments disposed towards the brain. The surgeons, after removing the fragments and foreign bodies, stimulated the occipital cortex electrically. The subjects reported flickering lights, expanding rings of light, and stars, even in subjects that were otherwise partly or fully blinded. This showed it was possible to cause visual sensations even in the part of the brain that mapped to the blind portion of the retina.

Otfrid Foerster (1873–1941) continued with more detailed stimulation studies, confirmed the Holmes' retinotopy, and extended this to the periphery of the occipital pole. These attempts finally led to the comprehensive mapping of the human cortex performed by Förster's student Wilder G. Penfield (1891–1976) on more than 300 subjects. Wilder Penfield (Fig. 2.1) used electrical current to identify and ablate epileptic foci in the 1930s (the "Montreal Procedure"). He additionally used electrical stimulation at the cortical surface to map out the brain functions. Since the brain has no nociception (pain receptors), brain surgery can be performed when subjects are conscious. It is essential that neurosurgery on the dominant hemisphere avoids damage to language regions; however,

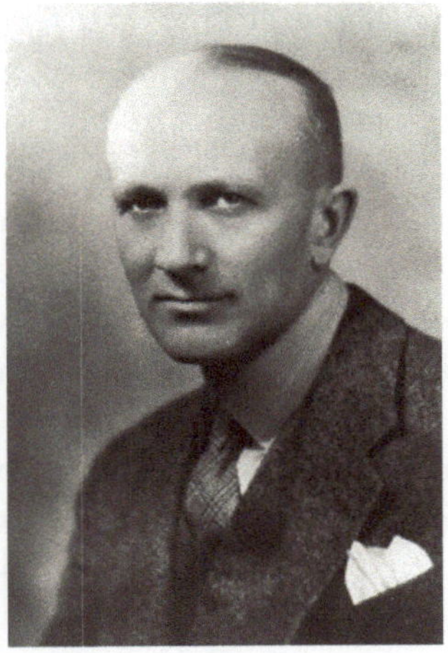

Fig. 2.1 Wilder Penfield (1891–1976). The pioneer of electrostimulation of the cortex and neurosurgical cortical interventions. His work has led to a modern understanding of functional organization in the human cerebral cortex.

their exact location varies between patients. Functional mapping is therefore still used to determine where they are represented in the cortex in the individual subject. The patient is subjected to a linguistic task (like reading a text aloud) while an electrical pulse train is applied at different places at the cerebral cortex. When the electrical stimulation interferes with the linguistic task, the area stimulated is likely involved in the task. During the surgery, these areas are then marked by placing a tag at the surface of the cortex before, for example, brain tumors are removed. Penfield also used this method to map linguistic regions of the brain. Over time, the idea of mapping sensory features and motor functions to distinct regions of the brain has been substantially extended by electrophysiological methods in animals and functional magnetic resonance imaging in humans in the last two decades. This was not only an essential step in preventing complications of neurosurgical interventions, but it also provided essential data on functional anatomy of the cerebral cortex.

Deep brain stimulation

An early attempt to use lesioning therapeutically was the development of surgical frontal lobotomy by Antonio Egnas Moniz (1874–1955). The procedure surgically disconnected the frontal lobe from the rest of the brain and by that reduced positive (active) symptoms of some psychiatric diseases. In the time before modern pharmacological antipsychotic therapy, this addressed a great financial burden of healthcare in the United States, and in 1949, Moniz was awarded with the Nobel Prize for physiology and medicine.

However, as recognized later, lobotomy also introduced a massive impact on the cognitive capabilities of the subject. The procedure substantially and irreversibly affected the lives of many patients, who were sometimes simply restless housewives or hyperactive children. This intervention has thus been abandoned. However, there remained interest in the use of focal brain lesions as a means to treat intractable neurologic disorders if this could be achieved without widespread damage and subsequent personality changes.

Early neural stimulation attempted to use focused electric current for therapeutic deep brain stimulation in neurologic disorders, including pain management and movement disorders. This concept grew from studies showing that lesioning specific parts of the brain could alleviate some symptoms of disease. Ernst Spiegel (1895–1985) and Henry Wycis (1911–1971) introduced the first human stereotactic frame (modified from the original Clarke and Horsley apparatus for animals) in 1947. Stereotactic frames allowed the determination of Cartesian coordinates for deep brain structures, and so enabled reliable access to these structures. Targeted ablations were the initial application. They required the exact identification of deep structures responsible for the neurologic condition. The paradigm in all these experiments was similar: electric stimulation was used to assess the potential symptom reduction of anatomical ablation. When a suitable location was found, anatomical ablation followed. A period of extensive experimentation on human subjects using the stereotactic approach increased medical understanding of neuronal structures. However, as discussed in **Chapter 3**, this kind of experimentation continued to raise ethical issues, especially as many of these interventions were irreversible and performed on psychiatric patients that could not give free consent.

One outcome from this work was an interesting observation in patients with Parkinson's disease. During the pre-lesion experimentation with electric current (used as means to determine which brain structure needs to be removed to relieve the symptoms) it was noted that stimulation of parts of the basal ganglia with frequencies greater than 120 pulses per second suppressed or improved tremor in Parkinson patients. This created a potential therapeutic niche for the electrical stimulation component of surgery without the need for anatomical ablation. The discovery of levodopa, a drug that is effective at treating Parkinsonian tremor, stopped further electrical current experiments by the end of the 1960s. In conjunction, the ethical issues associated with anatomical lesions reduced the political palatability of the approach. Only a few centers in the United States and Europe continued to use electrical stimulation in cases of intractable pain and in non-responsiveness to levodopa. It was not until after the success of other implantable devices such as the pacemaker and cochlear implant did deep brain stimulation see a resurgence in popularity.

Invention of the implantable pacemaker

The next major step in the development of neural prostheses was the commercial introduction of a portable cardiac pacemaker (Fig. 2.2). Subjects suffering from severe heart

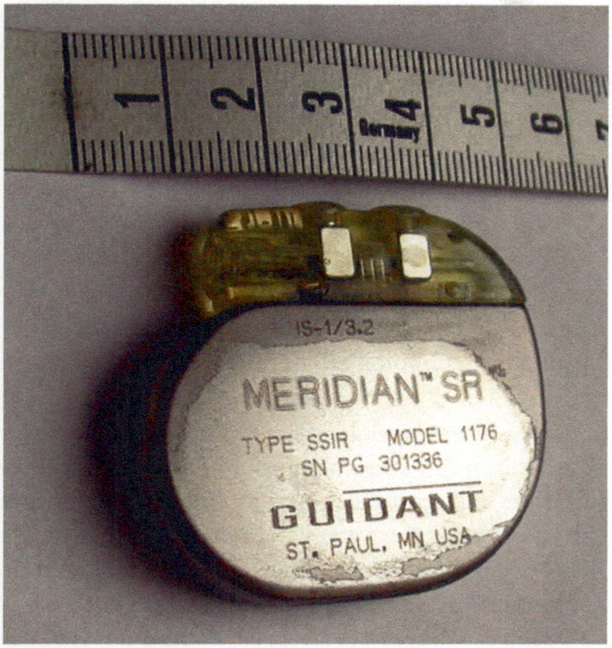

Fig. 2.2 An implantable cardiac pacemaker. Pacemakers are implantable devices, placed in the chest or abdomen, that stimulate the heart with electrical pulses. Their primary usage is for the treatment of heart arrhythmias (abnormal heart rhythms). Their widespread adoption popularized the concept of implantable stimulators and accelerated the development of neural prostheses. *(Image by J. Heuser (2005).)*

arrhythmias were treated with devices that were the size of a television set and connected to the power mains. After a power outage in 1957, a child died because of the blackout. Medtronic Comp., Minnesota, USA, run by Earl Bakken (1924–2018), originally a medical equipment repair shop, started its interest in portable pacemakers. Together with the surgeon Clarence Walton Lillehei (1918–1999), they developed the first wearable pacemaker with a percutaneous connection to the subcutaneous electrodes, and with an external battery pack.

The first fully implantable pacemaker was developed by Rune Elmquist (1906–1996) and implanted by Ake Senning (1915–2000) in 1958 in Sweden. It was fully implanted in the abdomen. The first device functioned only a few hours in a human subject and had to be replaced the next morning. In February 1960, a redesigned architecture lasted for a few months, and the first Swedish subject consequently received many replacements of pacemakers throughout his life (he lived to be 86 years old). In parallel, Wilson Greatbatch (1919–2011) in the United States pursued the same idea. Greatbatch was developing a device for recording heartbeat sounds when he noticed that the circuit he had been testing had erroneously generated a series of electric pulses. He realized that this could be used as a stimulating device and began developing a pacemaker with the surgeon William M. Chardack (1915–2006). Their final implant consisted of a simple two-transistor oscillator circuit run by a mercury battery, encapsulated in epoxy resin. Chardack implanted such a device in the first human subject in April 1960, and it worked for many months. This Chardack–Greatbatch pacemaker was commercialized by Medtronic Comp., and its small size, simplicity, and durability made it an instant clinical success. Greatbatch realized that the key remaining issue was battery lifespan of the implant, and in 1970 he founded a company, Greatbatch Ltd., that produced batteries for pacemakers. The pacemaker became a great success of biomedical technology (with more than 200 million devices implanted since 1960) and the first real step towards modern implantable neuroprostheses by establishing the technology of hermetic sealing and chronic, pulsed electric stimulation of excitable tissue.

While the pacemaker was not stimulating neural tissue per se, the applications of the concept for neurological disorders were obvious. A pacemaker autonomously generates electric pulses at high rates and, particularly in cases where such stimulation suppressed neuronal activity, provided a good reversible alternative to irreversible lesions. This in turn substantially simplified the previously discussed experimental approaches in neurology. Numerous experiments by Natalia P. Bekthereva (1924–2008), C. Norman Shealy (1932–present), and Irving S. Cooper (1922–1985) during the 1970s showed the potential therapeutic benefit of a neural pacemaker in epilepsy, motor disorders, and chronic pain. Finally, Medtronic (and other pacemaker companies) developed a dedicated neural stimulator. Medtronic trademarked the abbreviation DBS ("deep brain stimulation"). The medical device market had finally come under the supervision of the Food and Drug Administration (FDA) in the United States in 1976. DBS technology had been widely used, but the criteria for successful intervention were not yet clearly defined and mostly based on the individual opinion of the surgeon. Overall, these devices were still prone to failure and were not yet proven safe or efficacious. Thus, this technology remained underutilized for many years until a team in Grenoble, France, led by Alim-Louis Benabid, showed that DBS in the thalamus could reliably relieve the symptoms of Parkinson's disease, as had been suspected in the 1960's. Benaid and Medtronic together designed multi-center clinical trials for this condition. After solving safety issues, the FDA approved DBS targeting the subthalamic nucleus in Parkinson's disease in 2002. Up to date, around 100,000 subjects benefit from DBS.

In parallel, Walter Rudolf Hess (1881–1973) used electrical stimulation in cats to control emotions. His discovery of the diencephalic role in autonomic regulation was awarded with the Nobel Prize in 1949 together with Moniz. Jose M. R. Delgado (1915–2011) continued his work. He implanted electrode arrays into the brains of animals and used a radio frequency transmission to activate them or used patterns of activity recorded through the electrodes in the brain to stimulate the brain (he called this device "stimoceiver"). Using this approach he could determine behavioral consequences of electrostimulation in deep brain structures. He could also evoke emotional reactions using this device when stimulating the amygdala or hippocampus, such as preventing a bull from attacking him or reducing the aggression of a monkey. This was one of the first uses of a closed-loop system (**Chapter 16**). Furthermore, he invented an implantable device that released a controlled amount of substance to the brain ("chemitrode"). Clinically, he also used his electrostimulation on subjects suffering from epilepsy or schizophrenia. In the 1970s he made suggestions for emotional control devices as a means to cure psychiatric illness and proposed the use of this technology in healthy subjects. His philosophical ideas were extreme and met with a hostile response from a US society that had recently been confronted with CIA attempts to medically control subjects. Ultimately he faced scandal and rejection. Consequently, Delgado had to resign from his professorship in the United States. He was subsequently appointed professor in Spain, but his work was obviously affected by the circumstances. This forgotten pioneer of electrostimulation has written many hundreds of papers on this topic. It may be that the extreme nature Delgado's philosophy led to the censorship of his scientific ideas, and this may have delayed the beneficial development of neuroprostheses. Only more recently has there been renewed interest in the use of, for example, DBS for conditions other than motor diseases.

Early brain prostheses

The perception of light elicited from occipital lobe stimulation prompted the idea that one could use cortical stimulation as a prosthetic device for the blind. In 1955, a patent was issued to Joseph D. Shaw, Joseph C. Button, and Tracey Putnam for the implantation of a simple device and two stainless-steel stimulation electrodes into the visual cortex of a patient to evoke visual sensations (phosphenes of red and white color). They intended to perform implantation of several hundred electrodes, but this was never realized. These first attempts at restoration of vision were subsequently extensively debated in the United States, but it took a further 10 years before the first multi-electrode stimulation was attempted in a human subject by Giles Brindley.

Giles S. Brindley has been an exceptionally inventive scientist. Brindley's goal was to provide the capacity to read a written text to a blind patient, and calculated he would need to stimulate ~50 to 600 electrodes. He also recognized that with only few electrodes their location would be critical, which was confirmed in later studies. Brindley proceeded systematically by first developing a device that could communicate through the skin using electromagnetic transmission; this method, based on a transmission and receiver coil, is still used in modern-day prosthetic devices. Brindley and Lewin further realized that the device would have to be chronically implanted and therefore performed extensive (yearslong) experiments on baboons to test the integrity of the system over time. After proving the stability of the system in animals, they transferred the approach to blind humans in 1967. The system consisted of eighty square platinum surface electrodes with area of 0.64 mm^2 implanted in the occipital cortex. While in these subjects nearly half of the electrodes generated useful perceptions of light (phosphenes), their location in the visual field was highly variable, did not allow for reading, and were of limited everyday use for the subjects. As such, the project was eventually abandoned.

William H. Dobelle (1941–2004) continued this line of research with a different design of the device and with less rigorous animal testing; this stimulation system had a percutaneous connection. The decision against the technology invented by Brindley led to serious problems; the percutaneous connection caused many medical issues, including leaks of cerebrospinal fluid and risk of serious infections. Ultimately, this and other technical issues meant that the system did not last a year in chronic testing. Importantly, cortical stimulation intermittently produced severe seizures in some patients, probably because of overstimulation. These and other recurrent problems lead the National Institute of Health to abandon this direction of research on human subjects entirely as the risks were considered too high for the potential benefits. This refocused neuroprosthetic development away from the visual system and towards more straightforward medical approaches in the peripheral nervous system.

Development of the cochlear implant

The modern era of interest and proliferation of neural prostheses began in earnest with the commercialization of the most successful neuroprosthetic device: the cochlear implant. The idea of electrical stimulation of the ear has existed since Alessandro Volta, who stimulated his ear with current shocks in 1790. While he perceived sounds during stimulation (he described it as the sound of a boiling thick paste), he also realized that such stimulation might be dangerous for the brain and refrained from further tests. In the 1930s, A.M. Andreev and his team used electrical stimulation to provide hearing to a profoundly deaf patient for the first time. Follow-up experiments were performed by Andre Djorno and Charles Eyries in 1957, validating this approach. Djorno worked on stimulation coils for a device that stimulated the diaphragm in paralyzed patients who could not breathe without support. During a facial nerve surgery, Djorno observed that a long-deaf patient could hear sounds while he operated the electric thermal knife close to the auditory nerve. The patient, an engineer, later called Eyries and asked whether it was possible to exploit this phenomenon to regain hearing. Given the early work of Ernest G. Weaver and Charles Bray on electric signals from the auditory nerve in cats ("cochlear microphonics") this was a physiologically plausible request. Therefore Eyries contacted Djourno and together they developed an electrode connected to a coil, and used this to stimulate the remaining auditory nerve. Indeed, the subject could hear with this device, and even differentiate a few words. In their report, Djourno and Eyries predicted the development of a cochlear implant. This research was picked up by William House and the brothers John and Jim Doyle. They developed the first electrode for implantation into the cochlea. House inserted a test electrode array into the scala tympani in 1961 in two subjects, but provided no written report about this. Discussions on the intellectual property of this intervention started between House and the Doyle brothers, terminating their collaboration. In Germany, Fritz Zöllner, who learned about the experiments of Djourno and Eyries, visited them and subsequently tested electrical stimulation in two subjects. The first written report, however, came from the surgeon F. Blair Simmons and the engineer Robert White, who implanted a six-channel device into the auditory nerve of a human subject and reported on the perceptions elicited. The name "cochlear implant" appeared for the first time in a presentation by Blair Simmons subsequent to his report. At the same time, they continued to investigate the properties of electrical responses in the cat, and published papers on this topic in the early 1970s. House continued this work, this time in collaboration with the engineer Jack Urban. He implanted the next patients in 1969 and 1970. While they also used an electrode array (with several contacts), they effectively worked only with one-channel systems and used only one contact for stimulation of the auditory nerve. Their first written report appeared in 1973. Subsequently, others have joined in the efforts on the West Coast of the United States, including Robin Michelson (see Fig. 2.3), Robert Schindler, Michael M. Merzenich (who performed animal experiments), and Henri Chouard from France.

The path to a commercial device was very long. First these attempts to restore hearing were met with skepticism from the leaders in the field. Particularly, cochlear anatomists and physiologists, fascinated by the intriguing complexity of the cochlea and its function, could not believe that a device as crude as the first cochlear implant could convey any meaningful information to the brain. Graeme Clark from Melbourne, Australia, initiated cat experiments with cochlear implants, and subsequently performed implantations on human subjects in 1978. In Austria, the team around the surgeon Jan Burian and the engineers Erwin Hochmair and Ingeborg Hochmair-Desoyer developed a device and implanted the first patients around the same time. Along with the direct translational efforts, many groups around the world expanded experiments with electrical stimulation in animals to provide the optimal parameters for human application. From these developments, four major cochlear implant companies emerged: Cochlear Ltd. (Australia), MedEl Comp (Austria), Advanced Bionics (USA), and Neurelec (France; now part of Oticon Medical, Denmark). Developments of electrodes, stimulation protocols, surgical procedures, and speech encoding improved devices throughout the years. Essential discoveries were made possible by the House Ear Institute in Los Angeles, where scientists investigated outcomes of cochlear implant therapy for children and adults. The team around Robert V. Shannon has provided an exceptionally large amount of information on electric hearing. As an organizer of the biannual Conference of Implantable Auditory Prostheses since 1983, Robert Shannon has provided invaluable service to the cochlear implant field. In 1994, the continuous interleaved sampling stimulation was introduced and brought substantial boost in speech understanding, which formed the basis of all modern cochlear implant stimulation strategies. In 2013, three representatives from the community were awarded with the Lasker-DeBakey prize for the development of

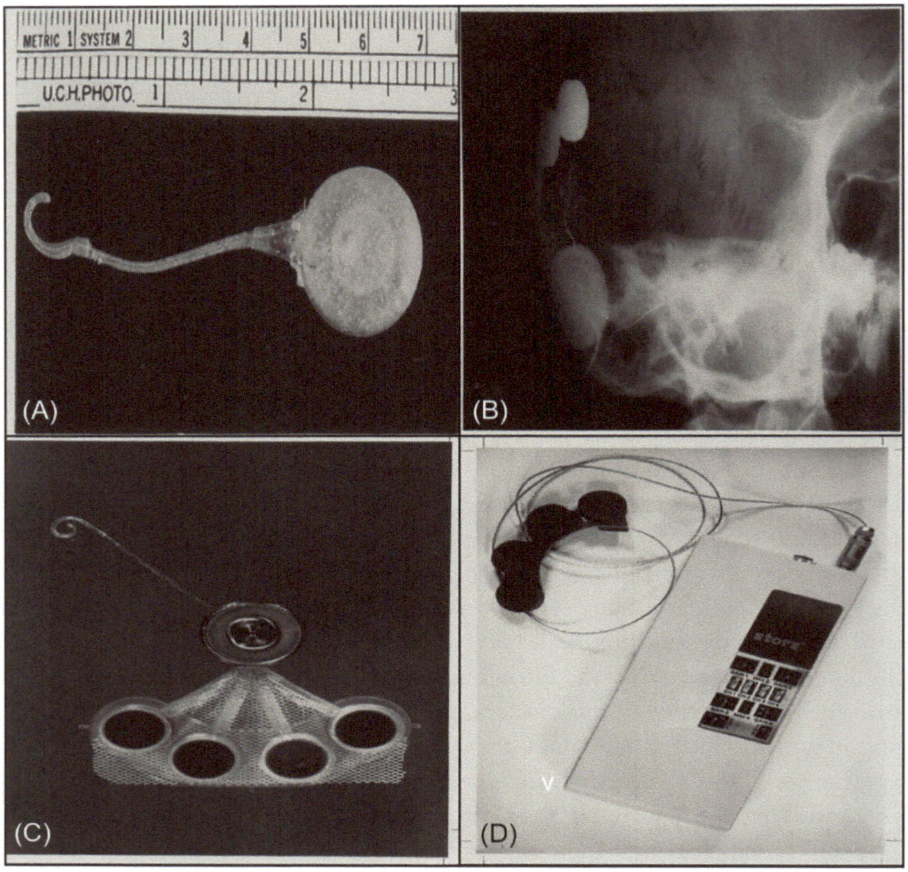

Fig. 2.3 Images of a cochlear implant developed by Michelson in 1978. (A) The electrode array that was implanted into the cochlea; (B) X-ray of the electrode array and internal electronics implanted into the head; (C) The internal electronics and electrode array; (D) The external portion of the implant. The wireless transmitter was aligned to the implanted wireless receiver in (C) to enable data and power transmission. *(Image from Eshraghi et al. (2012).)*

a multichannel cochlear implant: Graeme Clark, Ingeborg Hochmair-Desoyer, and Blake S. Wilson (Fig. 2.4). Today, ~700,000 subjects use cochlear implants in everyday life. **Chapter 11** gives further insight into this successful neuroprosthetic device.

Contemporary neuroprostheses

Today, neuroprosthetics has become an active and ambitious field of research and commercialization, and a viable competitor to pharmacological therapies. Thanks to the success of cochlear implants, there has been renewed interest in the commercial

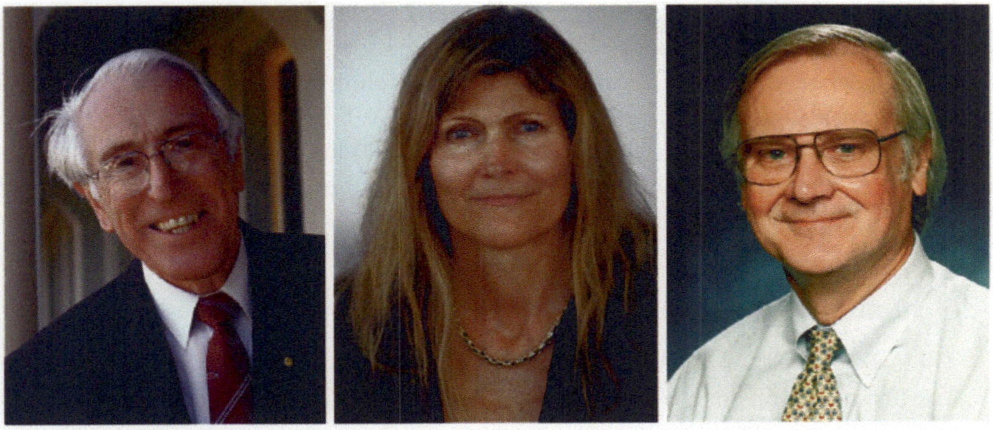

Fig. 2.4 Graeme Clark, Ingeborg Hochmair-Desoyer, and Blake S. Wilson made major contributions to the technology used in the modern multi-channel cochlear implant. *(Photo courtesy of Blake S. Wilson, with permission.)*

development of electrical stimulation for the control of peripheral sensory functions including vision, balance, touch, and pain. Simultaneously, advancements in the safety and accessibility of neurosurgery have opened the path for more sophisticated approaches in central nervous system stimulation. Today, cortical stimulation research is more oriented on less invasive approaches, where the source of the electric or magnetic field is located outside of the skull. Using coils generating large magnetic fields, cortical modulation or stimulation can be performed using a transcranial approach. Clinically available devices allow such stimulation. Magnetic stimulation is performed using dynamic fields, since static magnetic fields may synchronize neuronal activity and lead to epileptic seizures. Using such focal stimulation, functional lesions have been performed with the attempt to understand cortical function in health and disease. Recently, alternating and direct current transcranial stimulation has become popular as a method to modulate rather than stimulate the nervous system, with some conflicting opinions on efficacy. More research is needed to understand the spread of the electric field within the skull and brain and also to identify the elements that are stimulated (can be neurons or glia, or both).

A great deal of further innovation is required to extend and expand the capabilities of existing systems as well as to develop completely novel approaches. New materials and fabrication techniques will enable higher-density electronics and safer interfaces with neurons, while a greater understanding of the science behind neural stimulation will expand the breadth of applications. Neuroprosthetics is inherently multidisciplinary, requiring input from many fields of science and engineering to progress, and this can make the research at times slow and daunting. In addition, the interface of electronics and neural systems in humans raises many regulatory and ethical concerns, and it is important that they are addressed adequately (**Chapter 3** focuses on these issues). However, it should be clear from this historical overview that individual scientists, clinicians, and engineers made and continue to make substantial contributions to this field. While all scientific and technology fields are by nature collaborative, often one or a few individuals push the field substantially ahead. It may be an encouraging thought for students reading this chapter that they could be added to the list of the brilliant thinkers!

Brief summary

- The medical field of neuroprosthetics began in the mid-twentieth century.
- The first major step for the development of the field was the mapping of discreet functional brain regions using electrical current.
- Early attempts at electrical stimulation therapies followed as a consequence of difficulties with therapeutic lesioning of the brain.
- Tremor control in Parkinson's patients was one of the first uses of deep brain electrical stimulation, but it took many years for technology to enable safe and repeatable clinical translation.
- The development of the fully implantable pacemaker was a critical step that demonstrated the possibility for stable, effective, and chronically safe implantation of electrically active devices in the body.
- The cochlear implant took the basic concepts of the pacemaker and transformed them into a device suitable for neural stimulation.
- The widespread success of the cochlear implant created a popular resurgence of interest in neuroprosthetic devices.
- In the modern day, neuroprosthesis research is fast growing and active. Innovation in this field involves the development of more effective and safer materials, and translation of the technologies for the treatment of new diseases.

Key literature and further reading

Adewole, D.O., Serruya, M.D., Harris, J.P., Burrell, J.C., Petrov, D., Chen, H.I., Wolf, J.A., Cullen, D.K., 2016. The evolution of neuroprosthetic interfaces. Crit. Rev. Biomed. Eng. 44 (1-2), 123–152.

Aquilina, O., 2006. A brief history of cardiac pacing. Images Paediatr. Cardiol. 8 (2), 17–81.

Dobelle, W.H., 2000. Artificial vision for the blind by connecting a television camera to the visual cortex. ASAIO J. 46 (3), 3–9.

Eshraghi, A.A., Nazarian, R., Telischi, F.F., Rajguru, S.M., Truy, E., Gupta, C., 2012. The cochlear implant: historical aspects and future prospects. Anat. Rec. 295 (11), 1967–1980.

Feindel, W., 1977. Wilder Penfield (1891–1976): the man and his work. Neurosurgery 1 (2), 93–100.

Lewis, P.M., Rosenfeld, J.V., 2016. Electrical stimulation of the brain and the development of cortical visual prostheses: an historical perspective. Brain Res. 1630, 208–224.

Mudry, A., Mills, M., 2013. The early history of the cochlear implant: a retrospective. JAMA Otolaryngol. Head Neck Surg. 139 (5), 446–453.

Rahman, M., Murad, G.A., Mocco, J., 2009. Early history of the stereotactic apparatus in neurosurgery. Neurosurg. Focus. 27(3), E12.
Sironi, V.A., 2011. Origin and evolution of deep brain stimulation. Front. Integr. Neurosci. 5, 42.
Simmons, F.B., et al., 1965. Auditory nerve: electrical stimulation in man. Science 148 (3666), 104–106.
Wilson, B.S., Dorman, M.F., 2008. Cochlear implants: a remarkable past and a brilliant future. Hear. Res. 242, 3–21.
Zeng, F.-G., Rebscher, S., Harrison, W., Sun, X., Feng, H., 2008. Cochlear implants: system design, integration, and evaluation. IEEE Rev. Biomed. Eng. 1, 115–142.

CHAPTER 3

Ethics and technology development

This book deals with neuroprostheses; the word "prostheses" indicates that we focus on devices for medical treatment of a condition. To achieve this goal, technology is used. We do not discuss implanted devices used for changing or extending a healthy body. However, the same technology can often be used for both, generating unavoidable ethical questions. Both modern technological development and medical intervention are, after some positive and negative historical experiences, bound to strict rules based on ethical principles.

History is the teacher of today; we know from the past that scientists greatly exaggerated expectations related to brain prostheses. The cortical vision prosthesis project in the 1990s, for example, left the impression that the implanted blind subject could drive a car, with only a few dozen phosphenes. That was, of course, impossible due to the insufficient resolution of the device. Very interesting is the detailed report from one of these subjects, Jens Naumann, published as a book in 2012. It appears as if not all facts were properly disclosed to the subjects in advance; particularly left out was the immature functional state of the system. Even information on the severity of the medical intervention for implantation of the system might have been underestimated. These subjects underwent a serious neurosurgical procedure, including trephination (opening of the skull), opening of the dura mater, implantation of a grid of electrodes on the visual cortex, and fixation of a relatively large pedestal for connecting the equipment (consisting of several large boxes mounted on the belt around the hip, and connecting cables to the pedestal). The Food and Drug Administration (FDA) stopped these first implantations in the USA and so the intervention was subsequently performed in Portugal (under less strict regulatory rules). The subjects paid for this intervention out of their pockets in the expectation that this would make them see again. After the leader of the project suddenly died, the project was abandoned. Most of the implanted subjects still have the (nonfunctional) electrode array in their heads. None of them, as far as it is known, used the device for more than a few months, giving only a few of them some rudimental visual experience.

Sometimes scientists may focus too much on the most promising possibilities that new technology brings, and are too optimistic in the real assessment of the potential of the technology. Engineers, in particular, are trained to see the potentials and address problems with the attitude that all can be solved. This is the best possible attitude for an engineer, but it is a very risky attitude for a medical doctor.

Prostheses for the Brain
https://doi.org/10.1016/B978-0-12-818892-7.00010-9

Some of the devices discussed in this book have not yet reached the stage of a clinical device. In the future, professionals in this area will often be confronted with preclinical developments. Therefore this chapter discusses the ethical issues related to neuroprosthetic devices to define the present-day regulation of technological developments and clinical trials, and examines the technical development required to reach a functional product.

Ethical perspectives

There are several ethical issues related to the use of a biotechnology to replace brain functions. For a medical processional, it is the key goal of medicine to detect and replace bodily deficits by any appropriate means. Given that modern medical technology is well developed and safe, there is no question that such technology should be used to benefit the subject.

"What is conscious of its numerical identity of himself in different times is a person," as Immanuel Kant (1724–1804) defined it. An inevitable feature of a person is dignity. Dignity means that there is nothing equivalent in value to a person, that is, there cannot be a "price" for a person. A person consequently cannot be used as a purpose (means) of anything else than itself. A person is truly unique, uncountable in the ethical sense, and cannot be traded in any way. Dignity is probably the highest value in a society. Personal freedom, if not in conflict with the freedom and the needs of others, is a direct philosophical consequence of the person being conscious and having a free will. Some philosophical traditions like existentialism consequently considered freedom as the highest value that sculpts the person and based their ethical views on the concept of freedom. Therefore free decision is a high societal value, originating from the individual perspective of a person but limited by societal structure (the freedom of others).

A puristic philosophical approach is, however, difficult to transfer directly into medical practice. Medical practice is forced to take risks and balance costs to benefit. There is also a more utilitarian view of the problem; utilitarian ethics, as originally suggested by Jeremy Bentham (1748–1832) and John Stuart Mill (1806–1873), seeks to weigh individual and societal benefits in real situations that do not always allow for ideal solutions. For example, even if a therapy may be beneficial to the individual patient, if the costs are beyond what is economically feasible for the health system (the society), it becomes difficult to implement the treatment into daily routine. However, the utilitarian ethical approach must be taken with caution since it may degrade individuals to statistical units and thus interferes with the concept of individual dignity. In medical practice the concepts of human dignity and utilitarian capability must be considered together.

Ultimately, modern medical ethics must acknowledge agency to the subject who is treated. It is a personal decision whether a subject accepts a treatment or rejects it. For example, there is a large deaf community around the world, and due to historic reasons these subjects consider their way of life and their communication (by sign languages) as a personal culture that has developed over many generations. Some of them do not want treatment for their hearing loss, since they do not perceive deafness as a medical condition. Any person in a free society has the choice; medicine has to serve our needs, but if for some individuals the need is not there, there is no reason to act. This is a free decision of each person, as a subject with personal freedoms.

Sometimes the person cannot exercise his right to agency, since moral agency goes beyond free decisions by taking responsibility for the decisions. Children cannot fully assess the consequences of actions, and thus they have a limited moral agency. Children are not generally considered able to make competent decisions. Who is the right person to decide for a child when serious treatment with a brain prosthesis is indicated? This procedure may not always be reversible. Here, parents have huge responsibilities, and medicine can only support them by providing all evidence available on therapeutic options and their consequences. A deaf parent may decide against cochlear implantation, but this is not reversible later in life, with extensive consequences for the deaf child with regard to acquisition of spoken language, reading, and educational success (see **Chapter 9**). Access to balanced information is the only way of assuring *competent and responsible decisions*.

Human participants of an experimental study are persons and have a non-disposable dignity. Since it is ethically not acceptable to use a person in the above sense for achieving a goal, it is also not acceptable to use humans with the goal of developing a new prosthesis or gaining insight into brain processing. **Informed consent** is thus essential, and is only free if all relevant information has been disclosed. This issue is particularly important during introduction of new procedures in medicine. While some experimental procedures are (must be) tested in animals first in order to resolve any serious side effects and assess efficiency of the treatment, new devices eventually require human testing. It remains the responsibility of the scientist and the regulatory bodies involved to decide when to use human subjects to test technological developments. For those that are ready to participate, informed consent is strictly required. A free decision means that there are no constraints influencing the decision. Of course, decisions are in the strict sense always influenced by our memories, history, emotions, and much more. Regardless, constraints related to health status, dependence on others, and obligation toward the physician or scientist, or even to relatives, are constraints that preclude free decisions.

For these reasons, over decades the development of technology has been put into a more rigid structure that helps to guide scientists in following ethical principles. We outline these guidelines in the sections that follow.

Ethical aspects of technology development

Several key issues in development of implant technology relate to ethics. From the standpoint of technological **safety**, it is key whether the implant is *permanent* and if not, how long will it stay in the body. This will define the window in which a device can cause adverse reactions, or can partly dissolve its surface under the interaction with the body. Only *materials* to which the body does not form reactions (inert materials) are used in today's state of the art implants. Testing of longevity and functionality of the implant over time in realistic environments inform on the technological readiness for clinical transfer and the potential of successful treatment of a medical condition. This is the first key step in the development of technology.

Another ethical issue is the dependence on technology. Our society has therefore to find ways to assure, via the formation of frameworks and obligations for the industry producing these devices, a **lifetime medical and technical care** for this technology. This is a financial burden to both the medical insurance systems as well as for the participating industry. It requires a clear regulation by law for when neuroprosthetic devices will become even more abundant than they are today. Certainly, we do not want a situation in which an irreversible upgrade of a software involves the need for a subsequent operation to upgrade the hardware, which is a strategy often used in smartphones. In the context of a free market, however, it is difficult if not impossible to assign decades-long financial obligations for companies without suffocating the business.

Finally, a crucial issue is **explantation criteria** (termination criteria). When did the intervention fail? This needs definition from the beginning and is particularly important for experimental prostheses. Brain prostheses may cause bleedings, epileptic seizures, leakage of cerebrospinal fluid, infections, complications from other accompanying diseases, and so on. Acceptable side effects must be clarified in advance, as should the criteria under which the experimental procedure will be terminated. In addition, potential **complications** need to be disclosed.

Development of technology has to consider these aspects. Technology development takes place in phases, and only the final ones are ready for clinical translation. Only technology that is sufficiently well developed and thoroughly tested can be applied to human subjects. Initially developed by the National Aeronautics and Space Agency in the United States, the **technology readiness level (TRL)** classification is widely used today and describes technology development in nine subsequent steps:

TRL 1: Basic principles observed and reported. This level includes first research reports on the applicability of a certain invention; includes paper studies of the technology, mathematical formulations, design of algorithms, and principles of engineering solutions.

TRL 2: Formulation of technology concept. Essential characteristics of the application are defined and described in this phase, and tools are developed for simulation or analysis of the application.

TRL 3: Proof of concept. This level includes analytical and laboratory studies of integrated components are exercised with representative data.

TRL 4: Validation in the laboratory. Standalone prototyping is accomplished next; basic technological components are integrated to show that they work together in the laboratory. Experiments are performed with full-scale data sets.

TRL 5: Validation in a relevant environment. Laboratory investigation in the target environment for testing of safety and reliability follows.

TRL 6: Prototype demonstration. A prototype that represents the near designed configuration is used in an operational environment or laboratory with full-scale realistic problems. Limited documentation is available. Engineering feasibility has been demonstrated in actual system application.

TRL 7: Prototype for operational environment. Prototype field testing in the real environment is undertaken in this phase; most functions are available for demonstration and test. The prototype is well integrated to other systems. Limited documentation is available.

TRL 8: Actual system completed and qualified through tests. This phase marks the end of system development, it is fully integrated with operational hardware and software systems, most user documentation, training documentation, and maintenance documentation is completed. The technology has proven to work in its final form under expected conditions. All technology meets all operational requirements.

TRL 9: Technology proven through successful deployment in an operational setting. The device is fully integrated with operational hardware and software systems. All documentation is completed. Successful operational experience is provided. Sustaining engineering support is in place.

With regard to translation into practice, TRLs 7–9 are considered pre-commercialization phases with tests on living subjects: animals and subsequently humans. The visual cortical prostheses project mentioned previously suffered from maladies of new, underdeveloped technology, still hovering in TRLs 4–5, but already with tests on human subjects. Premature implementation is likely unsuccessful and leads to frustration in the subjects who undertook the procedure, and may even lead to their physical harm and eventually to a premature end of the project and the related technology. Therefore serious science must resist the temptation of premature testing.

Technology development does not stop at TRL 9; for competitive commercial products, further development in the market environment must continue. This includes continuing monitoring of defects, manufacturing problems, or side effects in the environment that have such low incidence that they cannot be determined in previous testing.

Medical technology

Biotechnology exposes implanted subjects to hazards, such as risk of the surgery and anesthesia, risk of infection, risk of damage to the target structure during implantation, risk of implant malfunction with potential further damage to the tissue, and so on. Medicine is always aimed at **balancing costs against risks and benefits** of intervention. The main medical rule is the highest standard: *Primum non nocere* (first do not harm). Whenever the benefit outweighs the risk, the medical treatment is indicated. However, this is only true for established medical treatments where hazards are known and have been evaluated with respect to severity and frequency of potential occurrence. Treatments undergoing a testing phase do not yet have firmly established hazards. Therefore, they are operating in unknown territory, partly out of the balanced risks and benefits. Termination criteria are thus an obligatory part of the design of such tests.

The **benefits** of the procedure need to be defined. What benefit can one expect in optimal and worst outcomes? In previous experimental procedures, this has often been exaggerated to the public and to the professional audience; we need to avoid this issue in the future. Medical professionals involved in testing and use of medical devices should be independent of the market and financial aspects of the products.

Firstly, medical devices are classified according to their duration of use: (1) "Transient" describes an intended continuous use <60 min; (2) "Short term" indicates use of between 60 min and 30 days; and (3) "Long term" means continuous use for more than 30 days. Regarding potential hazards, three classes of medical devices are considered:

- *Class I*: very low hazard, non-implantable devices with limited or no direct contact with the body or duration of application <60 min.
- *Class IIa*: short-term use in the body with low hazards, application into eye, intestine, or surgically prepared body openings, contact with the body less than one month.
- *Class IIb*: higher hazard, including systemic influences, contact with the body greater than one month.
- *Class III*: highest risk, long-term use with direct contact to the heart, cardiovascular system, or central nervous system (brain, meninges, and spinal cord).

Neuroprosthetic devices are considered active implantable medical devices with permanent contact with body tissue. Therefore these devices and accessories are Class III medical devices with greatest risk for the recipient.

Preclinical testing for biocompatibility of these devices is regulated by European and national laws, usually in relation to the norm ISO 10993-1 adapted also by the FDA. This norm specifies that materials and devices be tested in vitro and in vivo before use in humans to minimize or eliminate possible hazards. The in vitro tests involve testing in a dish using solutions or cell cultures, to exclude direct toxicity of the materials used in the implant on living tissue, or other relevant aspects of the implant. The in vivo testing involves use of animal models for testing the safety and efficacy of the device in the living body, allowing for study of the system's effects. DIN 10993-1 describes a decision tree (Fig. 3.1) for testing new medical devices. Involved tests should aim at (Table 3.1):

- Cytotoxicity—to exclude that the implant damages tissue directly and causes cell death.
- Delayed-type hypersensitivity and irritation—to exclude that the implant and the materials used have potential for contact sensitization.
- Local reactions—to exclude that due to the materials used the implant causes local adverse reactions that interfere with use of the implant over acute and chronic timelines.

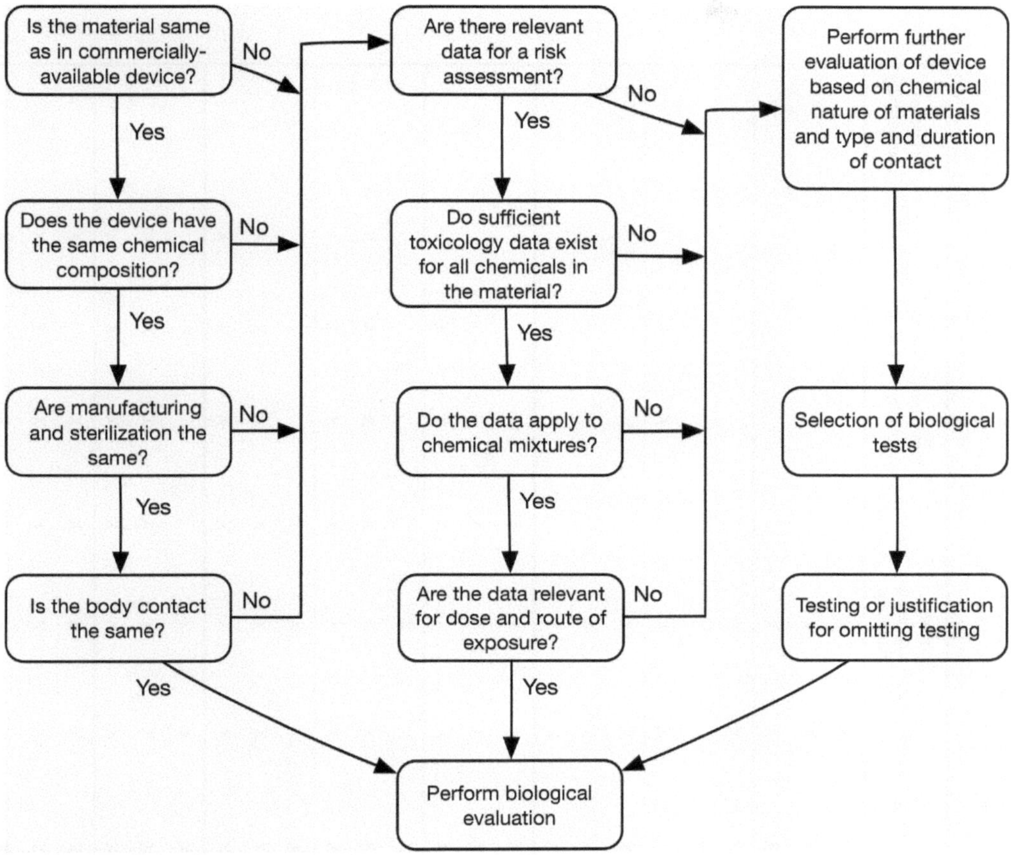

Fig. 3.1 Medical device testing decision tree based on ISO DIN 10993.

- Systemic toxicity—to exclude that the implants and the material used cause a systemic reaction both in acute and chronic use.
- Genotoxicity, reproductive toxicity, and carcinogenicity—to exclude that the materials used affect the genome or may potentially lead to development of cancer. This is particularly important for biohybrid implants that release neurotrophic substances into the tissue.
- Biodegradation—to exclude that degradation of the device, its components, and their metabolic products (intended, as in biodegradable devices, but also unintended due to long-term release of substances from the implant due to interaction with the tissue) does not lead to potentially toxic substances in concentrations problematic for the recipient.

If such preclinical steps are successful and do not indicate hazards that outweigh benefits, the next step is testing the device in humans in clinical trials.

Table 3.1 Category of device and the possible biological effects to be tested with the device.

Medical device category			Biological effect							
Category	Contact	Duration	Cytotoxicity	Sensitization	Intra-cutaneous reactivity	Acute toxicity (systemic)	Subchronic toxicity	Geno-toxicity	Implantation	Haemo-compatibility
Surface device	Skin	Limited	X	X	X					
		Prolonged	X	X	X					
		Permanent	X	X	X					
	Mucosal membrane	Limited	X	X	X					
		Prolonged	X	X	X					
		Permanent	X	X	X		X	X		
	Breached or compromised surface	Limited	X	X	X					
		Prolonged	X	X	X					
		Permanent	X	X	X		X	X		
External communicating device	Blood path, indirect	Limited	X	X	X	X				X
		Prolonged	X	X	X	X				X
		Permanent	X	X		X	X	X		X
	Tissue Bone Dentin	Limited	X	X	X					
		Prolonged	X	X	X	X	X	X	X	
		Permanent	X	X	X	X	X	X	X	
	Circulating blood	Limited	X	X	X	X				X
		Prolonged	X	X	X	X	X	X	X	X
		Permanent	X	X	X	X	X	X	X	X
Implant device	Tissue Bone	Limited	X	X	X					
		Prolonged	X	X	X	X	X	X	X	
		Permanent	X	X	X	X	X	X	X	
	Blood	Limited	X	X	X	X	X		X	X
		Prolonged	X	X	X	X	X	X	X	X
		Permanent	X	X	X	X	X	X	X	X

Contact duration: limited ~≤24 h; prolonged ~ >24 h–30 days; permanent ~>30 days. Defined in ISO DIN 10993-1.

Clinical trials have been developed for testing drugs; as a rule they require completed preclinical tests before start, and involve groups of subjects receiving the new and standard treatment or no treatment at all. In most (but not all) cases, trials are of a double-blinded design, where neither the subject nor the intervening doctor know to which group the given patient belongs. This allows for identifying frequent side effects and hazards.

Such clinical trials for pharmacological products consist of four phases:

- *Phase I, screening for safety*: A test of new biomedical intervention in a small group of subjects (ideally 20–80) for the first time in humans to evaluate safety (e.g., determine the safe dosage range, identify side effects, etc.). Sometimes, a phase 0 is also involved where first studies on the metabolism of a drug (pharmacokinetics) are performed in very few subjects
- *Phase II, establishing the preliminary efficacy* compared to placebo or another treatment: This phase determines the efficacy and further evaluates safety on a larger set of subjects (several hundred); this phase follows phase I and allows for identifying adverse effects with smaller incidence than detectable in phase I.
- *Phase III, final confirmation of efficacy and safety*: Further refinement of phase II on a larger set of subjects (depending on the indications, it can be up to several thousand). This allows for comparing the intervention to existing standard treatment and further monitoring of even rarer adverse effects. After this phase is successfully completed, the treatment is marketed.
- *Phase IV, safety post-market studies*: Includes further monitoring of the effectiveness of the treatment based on the general population and identifying side effects associated with its use.

The phases with large patient cohorts are essential in pharmacological clinical trials, since many, sometimes very serious side effects have a low incidence and thus may be overlooked in the first two phases of the clinical trial. Furthermore, the company marketing the product (drug) is in many countries required to follow further regulations; the companies need to set up a pharmacovigilance department that collects and reports side effects to the regulatory institutions.

Clinical trials for implantable devices have a modified regulation, since clinical trials with several thousands of subjects are not feasible or necessary. The effect size is usually larger with implantable devices than with drugs, and complications, if present, appear with greater incidence. Usually, clinical trials for implantable devices are conducted with few dozens of subjects. Only two phases of clinical trial (one premarket and the other post-market) are conducted. In contrast to pharmacological studies with groups of subjects receiving the new and standard or no treatment, double-blinded designs are less common in implantable Class III medical devices as placebos require a surgical intervention and are thus unethical, and efficacy is more easily identified than with pharmacological trials.

Clinical trials are co-supervised by regulatory authorities, institutional review boards (US) or ethics committees (EU). The latter are usually part of the university involved in this process, and are local. In the United States, all clinical trials are listed under clinicaltrials.gov. All medical devices used in patients must finally undergo state pre-market approval procedures; in the United States the FDA is responsible for approving medical treatments and devices. In the European Union, there is the European Medicines Agency (EMA) and national competent authorities that share the responsibilities. These institutions may ask to disclose all the material of a clinical trial to verify that all was performed according to law. Also, some clinical trials may be submitted and performed as "covered clinical studies" as a part of marketing application. For medical devices in the European Union, member state competent authorities designate notified bodies to carry out conformity assessment activities under the Medical Devices Directive or from 2021 on the newly implemented Medical Device Regulation. Notified bodies consist of separate constituent entities under national law, often regional, that are responsible (e.g., TÜV in Germany and Austria) for setting up and carrying out the necessary procedures for the assessment, designation, and notification of conformity assessment bodies, designating the products as conform to European rules (Conformite europeene approval with the "CE" mark).

If preclinical steps with implantable devices are successful and do not indicate hazards that outweigh benefits, the next step is testing the device in humans in clinical trials. Here, animal rights and human rights need to be considered together, since all testing possible on animals decreases the risk individual human participants have to bear. Clinical trials for implantable devices as a rule require completed preclinical tests and have a standard design. In the European Union,[a] for example, it starts with a **clinical investigation**, which is the systematic investigation of the device in human volunteers to assess the safety or performance of the device in a clinical trial. In implantable devices and Class III devices, a clinical investigation is required to ensure a high level of safety and performance and demonstration of compliance with general safety and performance requirements. The rules for clinical investigations should be in line with well-established international guidance in this field, such as the international standard ISO 14155 on good clinical practice for clinical investigations of medical devices for human subjects. The use of internationally accepted standards makes it easier for the results and documentation to be widely accepted, and reduces the need for doubling clinical investigations. In addition, the rules should be in line with the World Medical Association Declaration of Helsinki on Ethical Principles for Medical Research Involving Human Subjects.

When made available to market and put into service, a **post-market clinical follow-up (PMCF)** is appended. In the European Union, for example, notified bodies may require manufacturers to undertake specific PMCF studies that go beyond the scope of collected clinical data from routine examinations. A PMCF evaluation report for Class III devices and implantable devices and, if indicated, a summary of safety and clinical

[a] It is impossible to refer to all (partly different) regulatory standards in all countries; here we report the new EU regulation effective from 2021.

performance, must be updated at least annually with data from an updated clinical evaluation. Additionally the manufacturer has to set up a **risk management** system, encompassing the risks from the clinical investigation, clinical evaluation, and post-market clinical follow-up.

Regulatory processes will likely be more refined in the future; however, we should keep in mind that the new rules should not hinder the development of new devices. Optimally they should protect the subject but giving the research departments enough freedom for developing new products.

Ethical aspects for general design considerations

Neuroprostheses are devices with specific technical features that determine the benefit and risks for patients. Consequently, ethical considerations are inseparably linked to technological and medical aspects. These are in tight connection and cannot be separated. Some of the common main features that need to be taken into account for a realistic comparison of advantages and disadvantages are linked to the expected lifetime of a treatment. We discuss common weaknesses of current devices, such as consequences of different power supply concepts and lifetime limitations, in the sections that follow.

Consequences of power supply in active implants

One major aspect of neuroprosthetic devices is the interaction between technology and the human body. Technology requires a power source, and since this has a limited lifetime, replacement of the energy source becomes a medical and ethical question. Modern pacemakers can function with one battery for an extended period of time (many years). Given this circumstance and the fact that the housing of the pacemaker, including the energy source, is implanted subcutaneously and can easily, with one incision, be replaced, it is ethically acceptable to implant the whole technology into the body. However, the situation is more complex with some other devices that require complex information processing and have a different stimulation scheme and greater power consumption. To meet power requirements two main strategies exist. First, rechargeable batteries that are recharged by an inductive link can be used. However, rechargeable batteries have a limited lifetime and components containing the batteries have to be exchanged surgically after some time. Second, and an alternative strategy in these devices, is a combination of external components, worn on the body, and internal components, worn within the body (the implant). Some devices require the replacement of batteries daily and therefore, where possible, the energy source is located outside of the body to avoid the need of surgery to replace batteries. In such designs, there are two points that require consideration:

1. Transfer of energy between the external and internal part. Some older devices used direct percutaneous links that interrupt the integrity of the skin. Percutaneous links represent an open gate for infections, particularly if also crossing the dura. In the rise of

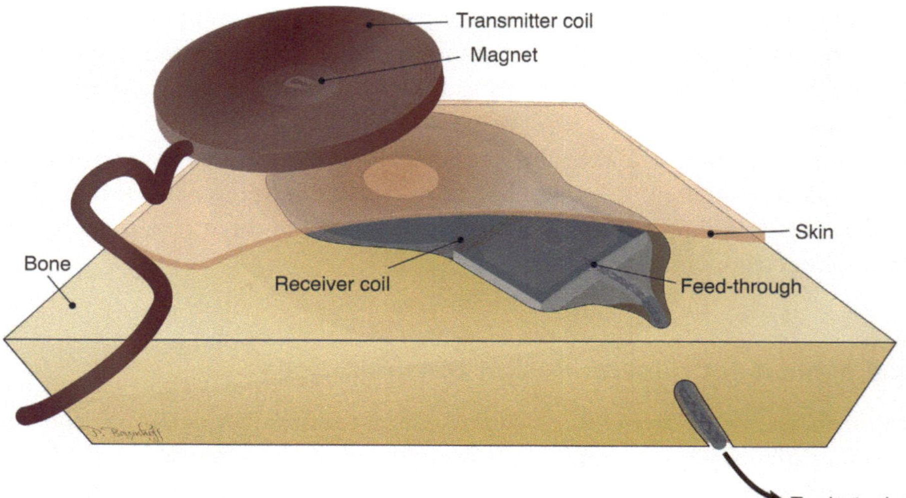

Fig. 3.2 The general design of a neuroprosthetic device as first suggested by Giles Brindley and currently used in clinical systems. Most devices avoid a percutaneous connection by use of a radio frequency transmission from a transmitter to a receiver coil. The receiver coil is placed under the skin in a fixed bed, mostly in bone. The coils "find" one another using magnets of opposite polarities placed in the center of both coils. This design allows for placing the energy source (the batteries) outside of the body, so that they can be easily replaced. However, deep brain stimulation uses more the design of a pacemaker (see **Chapter 13**).

cortical implants, Giles Brindley developed a transcutaneous connection via electromagnetic transmission. Here, integrity of the skin is preserved and both the energy and the control signals are transmitted through electromagnetic fields between a transmitter and a receiver coil (Fig. 3.2). The only issue is the fixation of the coils at a position that provides optimal energy transfer between the coils. This is usually achieved by placing two attracting magnets in the center of the coil, so that the coils automatically align and stay in position. However, the implanted magnet is subject to forces on the magnet and demagnetization in strong magnetic fields resulting in a limitation of magnetic resonance imaging (MRI) compatibility.

2. Transfer of electric signals from the well-isolated electronics in the body to the bare electric contact where stimulating charges leave the implant. Here, fluids can enter micro-leaks between the electrode and the insulating material (as a rule silicone) and can cause short circuits, or, more frequently, can infiltrate into the electronics and cause electric damage there. The critical structure is the **feedthrough** that ensures hermetic sealing of the implant housings and where wires from the electronics pass through the hermetically sealed housing to contact the electrodes of the electrode array. The distance between feedthrough and the electrodes is variable and thus the pathway between electrodes and electronics varies depending on the individual application.

Durability of the device

All devices implanted into human bodies are placed in a very unfriendly environment that is moist, warm, and has an aggressive immune system that recognizes the device as a **foreign body** (see **Chapter 8**). The main goal of the immune reaction is either to destroy and digest the foreign body or isolate it via encapsulation in a fibrous sheath. In such an aggressive environment, materials change and often lose, at least partially, their original properties.

One cardinal issue of implantable prostheses is aging of the material and the hermetic sealing of the device. The first cardiac pacemakers lost function within days.

Loss of function is often caused by:

- *Hermeticity failure (leaks).* These cause body fluids and electrolytes to enter the device resulting in short circuits in the electronics or lead wires. As already mentioned, the feedthrough is the crucial element of such devices. The housing of implanted electronics has been made of an epoxy resin (like in the first cardiac pacemakers), ceramic, and metals. The latter two are the modern standard, since resins tend to age in the body.
- *Fractures and wire breaks.* Devices, particularly those that are under mechanical stress with frequent bending of wires, will experience wire breakage. Here some materials are more resistant than others are (e.g., stainless steel several-strand braids are more resistant than platinum single-strand wire). However, choice of material is determined not only by mechanical stability but also by the ability to be welded with the platinum contact and the electrochemical compatibility of the connected materials to avoid build-up of electric potentials and corrosion. Often, to better accommodate movements and bending of the lead wires without mechanical stress to the connection with the electrode, with the feedthrough and the silicone, the wires in the lead system are bended or circled, giving them a **spiral shape** (see e.g., Fig. 11.18). This substantially improves the mechanical resistance toward bends, which is an inevitable issue during implantation surgery.
- *Corrosion of the contacts.* As we will see in following text (**Chapter 6**), when certain safety issues, such as a net charge flow in one direction, are not considered, fast corrosion and dissolution of electrodes may result. However, even when these safety issues are considered, there are oxidation/reduction chemical reactions when a metal is placed into a fluid, and these, over the long term, may partly corrode the metal. Investigation of electrodes implanted into the body document that some corrosion may be present on most contacts. In addition, after years of use, metal molecules from the elecrtode can be detected in the implanted tissue.
- *Delamination.* Delamination refers to separation of layers of materials that originally were adherent. Delamination may refer not only to laminated (multilayered) materials but also to materials made of one substance that, during aging, form layers that detach

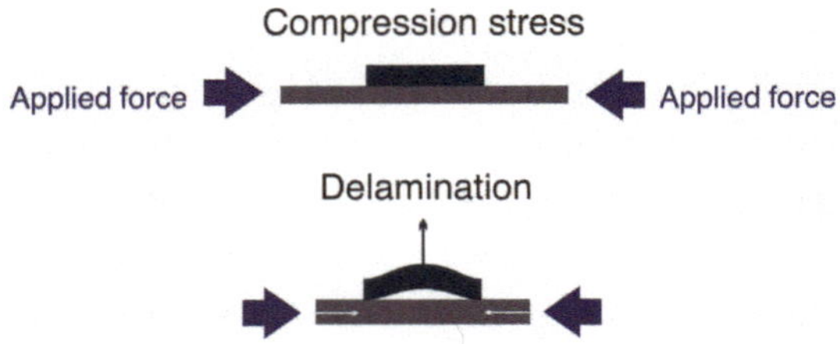

Fig. 3.3 Effect of compression stress on a layered material with adherent parts. The black drawn material differs in mechanical properties from the grey material (e.g., in the amount of compressibility). Consequently, while the materials are well adherent *(top)*, application of compression stress leads to deformation of the more flexible grey material that thickens, but the less elastic black material tends to bend and thus will detach from the grey material. The layers separate resulting in delamination.

from each other. This can be caused by inclusion of particles during the production process, which can lead to mechanical instability and fluid leakage. Delamination may result from chemical reactions that cause swelling of the material, from electrical current passing through the material leading to temperature or mechanical effects, as well as mechanical stress (Fig. 3.3).

Even after the most rigorous testing and with materials that are most resistant to bodily environment (inert materials; see **Chapter 6**), some material aging is observed and cannot be easily prevented. The implanted device is aging. The implanted neuroprostheses used clinically, however, are designed to survive in the body and remain functional over decades. To ensure this, each new device undergoes extensive testing before use. Nevertheless, in new technologies not all possible incidents can be foreseen and even the most meticulous risk analysis may miss some key issues, thus patients should be made aware of this.

One cause of device failure may also be manipulation during implantation. Surgical intervention inevitably leads to some mechanical stress to the device. If two different materials are adhering to each other (like lead wires surrounded by the silastic carrier of the electrode) and mechanical stress is applied to such a structure, the different materials will adapt differently due to different mechanical properties. Delamination is a frequently observed consequence (Fig. 3.3).

Aging tests

There is extensive experience with mechanical testing in the industry. Yet not all of these effects can be safely tested during device development. Particular issue are effects that first appear after a long time. Industrial testing includes procedures that exploit accelerated aging protocols to make such tests feasible within an acceptable time. Accelerated aging can be achieved since all chemical reactions are susceptible to temperature; the higher the temperature, the faster the kinetics of the reaction. This relation is expressed by the Arrhenius equation:

$$K = A \cdot e^{-\frac{E_a}{RT}}$$

where K is the reaction rate, T is the temperature (in Kelvin), A is a constant, E_a is the energy of activation, and R is the gas constant. Important to note is the relation of the reaction rate with the temperature, whereas the temperature is in the exponent of the equation, but also A is additionally temperature sensitive. This results in faster chemical reactions at higher temperatures. Using increased temperature, one can increase the speed of aging and thus shorten testing time. Increased temperature therefore is the means that allows accelerated aging protocols and makes some longevity tests feasible.

However, in vitro testing does not provide all the aggressive substances that exist in the living body. Although we can add cells that may adhere to the surface of the electrode, there is no functional immune system in the dish, with many aggressive enzymes that can change and degrade the electrode and the insulating material. Therefore, in vivo testing in living organisms is essential for each new device to be implanted into a human body. For example, while parylene appears stable as insulating material in vitro, it shows degenerative processes over long-term in vivo use.

All these approaches allow for minimizing patient risk. However, no medical implant is risk-free! Therefore, in the sections that follow, we also consider the ethics of using this technology for non-medical needs.

Brain implants as human "extension"?

Currently, some subjects are willing to undergo interventions to extend their capabilities in absence of true medical needs and deficits (e.g., implanted radio-frequency chips to open doors or pay bills). They are interested in implants without a medical indication. Furthermore, even with medical implants, some subjects are tempted to include function that in fact extends the body as opposed to compensates for a loss of function (why not extend hearing to ultrasound or accessing street maps directly to have a built-in world atlas that guides us through a medical implant?).

Is this an ethically acceptable application for brain implants? A related question is whether "the art of medicine" should be involved in such interventions arising beyond medical needs, and whether it is acceptable to risk medical complications due to these. Furthermore, it is the question of whether implants in the brain change not only the brain but also the person. Therefore interventions that influence the core of the human identity are less easily accepted. This can be deduced from the historic case of Jose Delgado's work, as mentioned in **Chapter 2**. Moreover, free will and the ability to decide is under question in implants that have a direct impact on perception of emotions and rational thinking. This is a matter of ongoing philosophical discussions that we cannot review conclusively in this textbook. The opinions are sharpened with the introduction of new technical possibilities and their therapeutic potential, and we must continue this discussion in the future.

The concept of the self is fluid. We easily accommodate new aspects into it. Obviously, the interaction between technology and the brain has been the focus of many novels and films. We know concepts of half human/half machine beings like **cyborgs** (e.g., the Borgs in *Star Trek*) and **androids**, which are robots with human-like traits (e.g., Data in *Star Trek*). For some of us there is an emotional difference between those two; while we have an emotional problem with the cyborgs (probably since here body integrity is compromised and this often engages feelings of disgust and rejection), we more easily accept androids.

Androids, if they have the capacity to speak, behave like persons, remember personal history, and are able to report about that, would be readily accepted as helpers and sources of information. Is a robot a person if he behaves like one? Alan Turing speculated that if a computer cannot be differentiated from a human by its behavior, then its information processing is similar to that of a human. This brings about the question what is the essence of the person, and where it is in the balance between brain as the physiological substrate and mind as the information processing entity. Emotionally, what behaves like a human tends to be treated as a human. Robots that may find application in serving, for example, elderly subjects, would be rather easy to accommodate to and would be treated as living creatures. Just a few human-like features can be enough for us to associate personhood to objects (e.g., R2D2 or BB-8 in *Star Wars*).

Technical extensions attached to the human body might in reality appear intimidating. However, over time we would likely accept such technology. Therefore it is of great importance to consider that the rejection of implant technology is sometimes based on the disruption of body integrity, something living deeply in our emotional systems over generations and developmental lines. The design of such devices is therefore key to overcoming that burden and increasing the acceptance of such technology. The aesthetic design of devices is consequently important in medical devices, particularly for acceptance of new technology.

The borders of a person and a computer appear fluid; even today we are using smartphones, iPads, and computers that extend our memory and affect our behavior significantly. We use GPS to navigate, and do other things that were not imaginable 50 years ago. Smartphones have become a part of ourselves, and we outsource skills that were essential for survival in our history, extending but also limiting our abilities. We talk to the voice behind the phone, and if they do not understand what we want, we get angry. Many friends of mine tend to argue with Siri or the voice in their GPS. Therefore the central thesis of **transhumanism**, that of an improved human augmented by technology, is closer at hand than we may think. Some philosophers (Gilbert Simondon or

Henri Bergson) consider this a natural extension of the homo faber (the working man) who develops tools, including machines, that help to achieve the next step in his development. These tools can also be understood as tools helping us to climb up the developmental line. Such views are particularly appealing in the artificial intelligence community. Is then the natural consequence a direct physical interaction between technology and the brain to augment the brain?

There is one fundamental difference between consumer electronics and neuroprosthetic devices. With consumer electronics, we are not interfering with the integrity of the body. "Reversibility" is given for all consumer electronics; if we lost all devices (or become stranded on a distant island without Internet), in principle, evolution has equipped us with all the necessary skills and we would survive without our devices or the Internet (some better, some worse). This is different for devices that are surgically hooked to our body and brains. Such technology would make us more dependent, both physically and psychically. Removal, even under full medical control, comes with medical risks and would be possible only in specialized centers.

The ethical question left is therefore whether it is acceptable to manipulate the integrity of a body and a person without medical needs, and whether it is acceptable to expose a person to risks of a medical procedure. In the ethical understanding of medical professionals, this is not justified and goes beyond the ethical standards of medical science. It violates the first medical principle to "do no harm." However, existing practice is already partly in conflict with this consideration. It applies to some forms of aesthetic surgery that in the majority of cases have no true medical indication. If a person wants a technical extension, and there is a doctor who is ready to perform the intervention, can and shall we as a society in any way interfere? Can we prohibit this even if the person knows and accepts the risks and bears the costs? Unless it does not affect others, it can be the decision of the involved individuals who are active in this process. However, even today we legally regulate substances that interfere with the ability of free decision, such as some drugs. But medical ethics may go beyond strict legal perspective and the medical profession does regulate the extent of these interventions. However, even elective surgery, if allowed, should remain the subject of the medical profession to reduce the risks to a minimum.

From the utilitarian perspective, aesthetic surgery is easily acceptable since the risks are small and the costs for society are not considerable (the patient takes the financial burden). With brain implants, however, the risks are much greater, as are the subsequent costs and dependencies. Therefore, these two types of interventions are currently not directly comparable.

Personally, we do not feel that the art of medicine should be redirected to interventions not medically indicated. However, as discussed previously, it remains questionable whether a free society should interfere with the free decisions of free citizens. Obviously, all interventions to the human body should be performed *lege artis* (complying with medical standards), and thus under medical supervision. It remains to be seen how the medical profession will react to these and similar issues in the future. Regardless, arguments that ethical regulation may slow down technological development are inappropriate.

These issues may require new standards from associations of physicians, philosophers, and ethical committees. The comprehensive discussion of these points is beyond the scope of a biomedical technology textbook and requires discussion among experts from several disciplines.

After all, developments in biomedical technology have the potential to change society significantly, for good or for bad. Utopic views of the future can be found in science fiction like the TV series *Star Trek*; however, dystopic views also exist. It remains the role of politicians and philosophers to better define the good and bad aspects of such future, and "orient" us to the directions we follow as a society. The future has great potentials and possibilities, yet we have to take care that we are not overrun by technological development faster than we can categorize it within philosophical frameworks. Only reflection, with philosophical and ethical ordering of these new, fascinating inventions into the human world, will assure the benefit and the good for all humankind.

Brief summary

- Technological development is classified into Technology Readiness Levels (TRL), and only levels 7 and greater are suitable for real tests.
- Devices used in medicine first undergo preclinical tests with animal models defined by ISO norms.
- Testing in human subjects is regulated by official institutions and involve clinical trials. To begin a clinical trial, preclinical testing is required.
- Devices used clinically must function reliably in the body over long periods of time. Hermeticity, fractures and leaks, corrosion of contacts, and aging of material are the potential causes of device failure.
- Protocols of accelerated aging help to test the long-term stability of devices.
- Many ethical questions arise during both development and clinical use of brain implants. Dignity of the individual and personal freedom in decisions are to be taken into account.
- Brain implants serving other than medical functions represent a great health risk and therefore should not be aimed at goals beyond medical treatment.

Key literature and further reading

Caldwell, R., Street, M.G., Sharma, R., Takmakov, P., Baker, B., Rieth, L., 2020. Characterization of parylene-C degradation mechanisms: in vitro reactive accelerated aging model compared to multiyear in vivo implantation. Biomaterials. 232, 119731.

Declaration of Helsinki, 2018. https://www.wma.net/policies-post/wma-declaration-of-helsinki-ethical-principles-for-medical-research-involving-human-subjects/.

Eisler, R., 2015. Kant Lexikon. Weidmansche Hildesheim.
Europa EU list of Notified Bodies, n.d.: https://ec.europa.eu/growth/tools-databases/nando/index.cfm
Food and Drug Administration: Use of International Standard ISO 10993-1, 2016. Biological evaluation of medical devices - Part 1: Evaluation and testing within a risk management process. https://www.fda.gov/media/85865/download.
Fins, J.J., Schlaepfer, T.E., Nuttin, B., Kubu, C.S., Galert, T., Sturm, V., Merkel, R., Mayberg, H.S., 2011. Ethical guidance for the management of conflicts of interest for researchers, engineers and clinicians engaged in the development of therapeutic deep brain stimulation. J. Neural Eng 8, 033001.
Gillett, G., 2006. Cyborgs and moral identity. J. Med. Ethics 32, 79–83.
ISO 14155:2020, 2020. Clinical investigation of medical devices for human subjects – good clinical practice.
ISO 10993:2009(E), 2009. Biological evaluation of medical devices.
Naumann, J., 2012. Search for Paradise. Lighting Source UK Ltd., Xlibris, Milton Keynes, UK.
Nadol, J.B., O'Malley, J.T., Burgess, B.J., Galler, D., 2014. Cellular immunologic responses to cochlear implantation in the human. Hear. Res. 318, 11–17.
Nuttin, B., Wu, H., Mayberg, H., Hariz, M., Gabriëls, L., Galert, T., Merkel, R., Kubu, C., Vilela-Filho, O., Matthews, K., Taira, T., Lozano, A.M., Schechtmann, G., Doshi, P., Broggi, G., Régis, J., Alkhani, A., Sun, B., Eljamel, S., Schulder, M., Kaplitt, M., et al., 2014. Consensus on guidelines for stereotactic neurosurgery for psychiatric disorders. J. Neurol. Neurosurg. Psychiatry 85, 1003–1008.
Rabins, P., Appleby, B.S., Brandt, J., DeLong, M.R., Dunn, L.B., Gabriëls, L., Greenberg, B.D., Haber, S.N., Holtzheimer, P.E., Mari, Z., Mayberg, H.S., McCann, E., Mink, S.P., Rasmussen, S., Schlaepfer, T.E., Vawter, D.E., Vitek, J.L., Walkup, J., Mathews, D.J., 2009. Scientific and ethical issues related to deep brain stimulation for disorders of mood, behavior, and thought. Arch. Gen. Psychiatry 66, 931–937.
Regulation (EU), 2017. 2017/745 of the European Parliament and of the Council of 5 April 2017 on medical devices, amending Directive 2001/83/EC, Regulation (EC) No 178/2002 and Regulation (EC) No 1223/2009 and repealing Council Directives 90/385/EEC and 93/42/EEC. https://eur-lex.europa.eu/legal-content/EN/TXT/?uri=CELEX:32017R0745.

PART 2

Principles

CHAPTER 4

Neuronal excitation

The blueprint of living tissue consists of a principal component, the cell, a structure enclosed by a membrane that allows for the differentiation of the space within (*intracellular space*) and the space beyond, the *extracellular space.* A cell usually contains a nucleus that stores genetic information and the cytosol (the remaining space within the cell) with many *organelles* (subcellular structures serving a variety of functions, including oxygenation, production of proteins, digestion, energy production, etc.). Cells of the nervous system are called neurons and have a distinct morphology with several characteristic features that may substantially vary. The brain itself contains approximately 10^{11} such *neurons*, but also other cells (*glia*) that support the neurons in their function.

Neurons (Fig. 4.1) generally have a neuronal body (*soma*), a morphologically variable *dendritic tree*, and one "output" fiber (*axon*). Neurons are surrounded by an extracellular matrix (*neuropil*) and glia or Schwann cells. Glial and Schwann cells have important function for the neurons; they are the source of *myelin*, an insulation layer on the axon (and sometimes dendrites) important for propagation of excitation (see below). Neurons primarily serve the function of processing electrical signals with the goal of information processing.

Glial cells have a variety of functions, including protection of the tissue from infection and nutrition (e.g., they convey immune response, are a biological barrier with nutritional function, and so on). In principle, in the central nervous system three types of glial cells exist, with slightly different functions: *astrocytes*, *oligodendrocytes*, and *microglia*. While astrocytes have important functions for regulating the ion content of extracellular space surrounding neurons, form the brain-blood barrier, oligodendrocytes form myelin sheath in the central nervous system and the microglia primarily serve immune functions. For more details on these aspects, we refer the reader to neuroscience textbooks.

Neurons, as all cells in the human body, are enclosed by a membrane. This membrane is composed of a phospholipid bilayer (Fig. 4.2) with interposed proteins. These proteins form channels that connect the inside with the outside of the cell and can transport particles (ions and other molecules) in and out of the cell. The membrane is *semipermeable* in the sense that water can normally move freely through the membrane by making use of specialized water channels (*aquaporins*). Large water-soluble molecules cannot pass the cell membrane and require specialized molecular transport mechanisms to enter the cell. Lipophilic substances that do not dissolve in water but do dissolve in fats, on the other hand, can penetrate through the phospholipid membrane even in absence of specialized

Prostheses for the Brain
https://doi.org/10.1016/B978-0-12-818892-7.00003-1

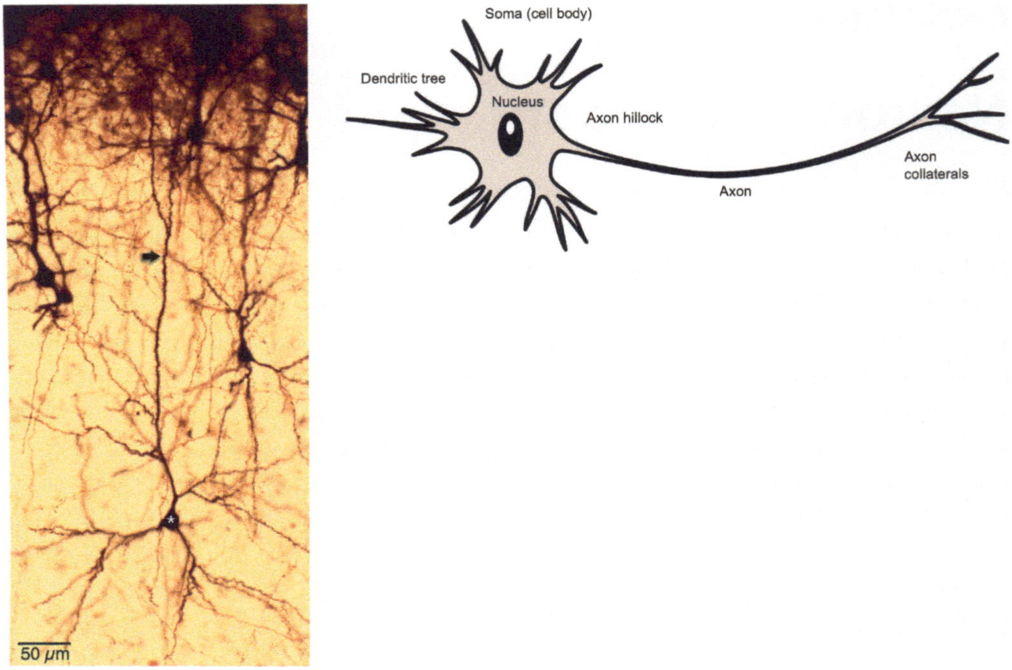

Fig. 4.1 A pyramidal neuron from the auditory cortex of a cat (Golgi staining). A neuron has a distinct morphology with a small cell body (soma, *marked by the asterisk*) and a tree of very thin peripheral branches called dendrites *(arrow)*. Another distinct type of branch is the single output element, the axon; it is usually one of the thinnest branches and is characterized by specific composition of the neuronal membrane. A simplified sketch of the neurons is shown on the top right. Neurons can have different morphologies; some have only one or two dendrites, while some have extensive branchings and many tiny protrusions called dendritic spines. In others, no spines are found.

transporting systems. Therefore, for example, the cell membrane does not impose a barrier for some hormones.

There are ionic channels in the cellular membrane that are open under normal conditions most of the time. Through these, some ions and small molecules can enter and exit the cell. Usually, a channel is designed to allow the passage of only one or very few molecules or ions; channels are *selective*. One part of the channel, the *gate*, blocks the passage of other molecules and allows the passage of only one (or few) ions. Constantly open channels include the aforementioned *aquaporins* that allow the passage of water from and into a cell, and *leakage potassium channels*. Other ions can also pass in small amounts through the neuronal membrane, but the conductivity for these ions is much less than for potassium.

Active ionic pumps in the neuronal membrane move particles in and out of the cell while using cellular energy stored in a highly energetic molecule (adenosine triphosphate; ATP). The most abundant ionic pump is the Na^+/K^+ pump (in fact it is an enzyme called Na^+/K^+ *ATPase*) that moves, by use of energy released from an ATP molecule, three

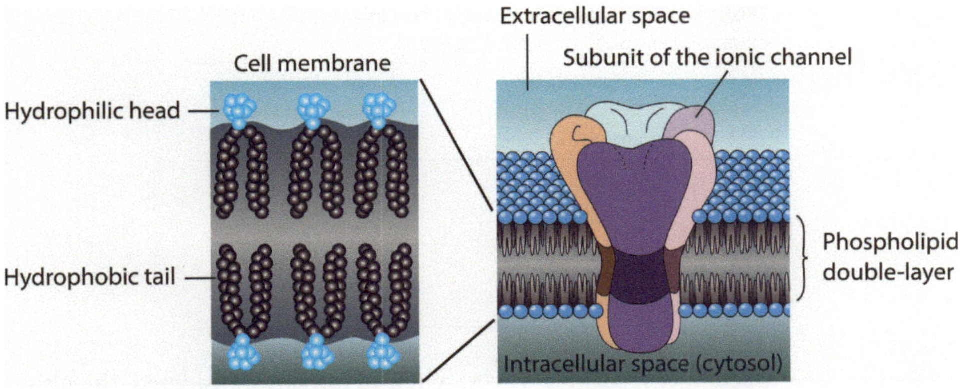

Fig. 4.2 *Left*: A neuronal membrane consists of a bilayer of phospholipids. They orient their hydrophobic (insoluble in water) parts towards each other so that their hydrophilic (soluble in water) parts orient on one side towards the cytosol and on the other side towards the extracellular space. Although the bilayer membrane is a flexible, fluid structure, it isolates the intracellular from the extracellular space for hydrophilic substances. To allow communication from inside to outside, the membrane contains different transportation systems. The most important in the present context are channels *(right panel)*. They consist of several protein parts (subunits) that bind together and form a channel. Usually, the channel is selective for one type of molecule that it can permit to pass the membrane. For details, see Bear et al. (2015).

molecules of sodium out of the cell and two molecules of potassium into the cell. As both these ions carry one positive charge (they are cations), moving three positive charges out and two in causes a net positive charge outflow; this pump is *electrogenic* (generates a membrane potential with more positive charge on the outside of the cell).

Existence of non-permeable molecules on both sides of the (semipermeable) cell membrane causes *osmotic pressure*; higher concentrations of free molecules on one side of the membrane cause the movement of water into this compartment. A substantial increase in water content of the cell can lead to its damage. For this reason, the transport of molecules through the membrane is strictly regulated. Furthermore, proteins inside the cell, under physiological conditions and normal acidity, exist in the form of negatively charged anions (concentration of 100–150 mmol/L) and are an additional cause of charge imbalance across the membrane. Due to this, achieving equilibrium in both charge and concentration across the cell membrane is impossible; as osmotic changes can destroy the cell, electric unbalance is the only possible option for the living organism to reach a steady state.

The ultimate consequence of these processes is the negative charge of the cell's inside (*cytoplasm*) relative to the extracellular space and an uneven distribution of ions across the cell membrane (Table 4.1). Neurons have a *resting (membrane) potential* of −70 to −80 mV (inside the cell). The distribution of ions in the intracellular and the extracellular space is consequently different. Potassium is more abundant in the cell, whereas sodium is more

Table 4.1 Ionic concentrations in the intracellular and extracellular space of typical neurons.

	Intracellular concentration (mmol/L)	Extracellular concentration (mmol/L)
Na^+	8–30	145
K^+	100–155	4.4
Ca^{2+}	<0.001	1.25
Cl^-	4–30	117
HCO_3^-	8–15	27

abundant in the extracellular space. However, when all ions are considered, the ultimate difference in concentration between positive and negative ions responsible for the resting potential is very small (in the range of μmol/L). Remember that one mol of charged molecules carries a large charge (defined by the Faraday constant), so that large potentials can result already from a few excessive charged particles. Due to the generated electric field, the movement of ions is stopped and an equilibrium is achieved (**Chapter 10**).

The resting potential is one essential prerequisite for neuronal information processing. By making use of the changes in membrane potential it is possible to code information. If an ionic channel in the neuronal membrane opens, additional ions can flow out from or into the neuron. Two driving forces for ionic movement exist: the *concentration gradient* and the *electrical gradient*. After an ionic channel has been opened, the given ion will flow along the concentration gradient, equalizing the concentrations on both sides of the membrane. However, this movement will be affected by the membrane potential. Ions will preferentially flow into the compartment of opposite charge. These two gradients can be in the same or opposite direction. They may cancel each other out and prevent any net movement of ions. To be able to assess the ionic flow through the membrane, the combination of both gradients needs to be considered, which is called the *electrochemical gradient*.

For each ion there will be a membrane potential at which the inward and outward movement of the ion will be equal and the net movement will be zero. This potential is called *equilibrium potential* and is specific for the given ion (Table 4.2). It can be computed by the Nernst equation (Box 4.1). However, the membrane contains several different

Table 4.2 Equilibrium potentials for the three most important ions.

	Equilibrium potential
Potassium	−80 mV
Sodium	+55 mV
Chloride	−70 mV

Box 4.1: Equilibrium potential

The diffusion of substances, under the assumption of a steady state, can be quantified using Fick's law of diffusion for the given concentration gradient Δc, the barrier (e.g., a membrane) of area A, and the transported amount of substance J:

$$\frac{J_{diff}}{A} = P \cdot \Delta c \left[\frac{mol}{s \cdot m^2}\right]$$

Here, P is the permeability of the barrier (in m/s). For large molecules (for which the barrier is less permeable and P is smaller) the diffusion across the membrane will be low, whereas for small molecules the diffusion will be higher. Biological membranes are more permeable for gases like CO_2, O_2, and N_2 as well as substances that are dissolved in lipids (hydrophilic substances like some hormones or alcohol), so even though these molecules can be larger, they easily pass.

Two elements determine the net driving force for charged particles: the electric field (the existing potential) and the concentration gradient. The ions that can easily diffuse through the membrane (mainly K^+ and Cl^-) will achieve a dynamic equilibrium state known as the Gibbs-Donnan equilibrium:

$$\frac{[K^+]_{in}}{[K^+]_{out}} = \frac{[Cl^-]_{out}}{[Cl^-]_{in}}$$

However, there is a deviation from this equilibrium state that is caused by non-diffusible but charged proteins. These are mainly present in the cell and mean that the preceding equation does not hold for living cells, although the ratios are not very different.

There is a way to calculate the transmembrane potential at which the inflow and the outflow of the given ion will reach an equilibrium, known as the equilibrium potential for that ion. Assuming a difference in concentrations across the membrane, the stored energy is the consequence of the concentration gradient ($c_{out} - c_{in}$); however, it is proportional to the logarithm of those concentrations:

$$W \approx \ln(c_{out}) - \ln(c_{in}) = \ln\left(\frac{c_{out}}{c_{in}}\right)$$

There are, however, two missing elements; this logarithm relates to energy proportional of the gas constant R (that relates energy to mol of a substance). This is also dependent on temperature T; the higher the temperature, the more energy is stored in the concentration gradient. Thus, in total, the energy per amount of substance stored in such a concentration gradient is

$$W = R \cdot T \cdot \ln\left(\frac{c_{out}}{c_{in}}\right)$$

The other form of energy stored in the system is the electrical energy (per mol substance). It is the consequence of membrane potential (i.e., the instantaneous potential gradient through the membrane) and is proportional to the potential gradient and the (potentially) resulting current of this:

$$W = z \cdot F \cdot (E_{out} - E_{in})$$

Continued

Box 4.1: Equilibrium potential—cont'd

In this equation, z is the valence of the ion and F is the Faraday constant. Faraday constant relates *charge* to *substance amount* and equals the Avogadro constant (the number of particles in one mol of a substance) multiplied by the elementary charge of one particle. W thus results in energy per mol substance.

As the energy from the chemical gradient and the electrical gradient in the equilibrium state have to be equal, we can write:

$$R \cdot T \cdot \ln\left(\frac{c_{out}}{c_{in}}\right) = z \cdot F \cdot (E_{out} - E_{in})$$

$$E_{eq} = E_{out} - E_{in} = \frac{R \cdot T}{z \cdot F} \ln\left(\frac{c_{out}}{c_{in}}\right)$$

The last formula is the Nernst equation. It can be used to calculate the equilibrium potentials given in Table 3.1.

Interestingly, the potassium equilibrium potential for different potassium concentrations is very close to the resting potential of neuronal membranes in the given condition, deviating only at more negative values of resting potential (from ~ -60 mV), where the Nernst equation predicts an even more negative value than the actual membrane potential. This deviation is caused by the membrane also being conductive for other ions that are not considered in the Nernst equation. The Goldman-Hodgkin-Katz equation includes other important ions:

$$E_m = \frac{R \cdot T}{F} \cdot \ln\left(\frac{p_{K^+} \cdot [K^+]_{out} + p_{Na^+} \cdot [Na^+]_{out} + p_{Cl^-} \cdot [Cl^-]_{in}}{p_{K^+} \cdot [K^+]_{in} + p_{Na^+} \cdot [Na^+]_{in} + p_{Cl^-} \cdot [Cl^-]_{out}}\right)$$

This equation is derived from the Nernst equation. Valence is missing, since all ions have a valence of $z=1$. For chloride, the nominator and denominator are reversed to account for the negative charge of the ion.

The main permeabilities for a resting neuronal membrane are:

	Permeability (cm/s)
H_2O	1.2×10^{-2}
Cl^-	1.1×10^{-10}
K^+	6.0×10^{-11}
Na^+	1.0×10^{-12}

ionic channels with non-zero conductivities (although with less permeability than that of potassium channels). In other words, the membrane in the resting state is actually slightly permeable to the ions given in Table 4.1. As such, the resting transmembrane potential, although close to the equilibrium potential of potassium, slightly deviates from it.

To predict the resting transmembrane potential exactly, the Goldman-Hodgkin-Katz equation is used to extend the original Nernst equation (Box 4.1).

The difference of the membrane and equilibrium potential is the electrochemical force driving the ions in the given condition. If the membrane potential is $-80\,\text{mV}$ and a sodium channel becomes opened, sodium flows into the cell (along both the concentration gradient and the electrical gradient), theoretically until the membrane potential equals the sodium equilibrium potential. In reality, the channel shuts off before this condition is reached; this is the consequence of the channel physiology that is sensitive to the membrane potential. The change in transmembrane potential of the cell closes this channel again and stops the electrical processes. The original permeability of the membrane is thus restored and the cell returns to the original resting potential (however, other channels support this return; see below).

The process of discharging the membrane potential by ionic flow through the membrane is called *depolarization*. The opposite process, the decrease of the membrane potential to more negative values, is called *hyperpolarization*. As will be shown, a sufficiently large depolarization can sometimes lead to a pulsatile discharge of the neuron called ***action potential***.

From an electrochemical point of view, the neuronal membrane can be approximated by a resistor-capacitor (RC) circuit where these two elements are arranged in parallel. The electrical properties of the tissue can be well approximated by the equivalent circuitry, so that electrical properties of a dendrite may be modeled by the circuitry shown in Fig. 4.3. Although this is not a perfect approximation (e.g., ions are not as mobile as electrons in metals and consequently the precise timing of events may slightly differ), it represents a good model for further considerations. In absence of action potentials, such a model can approximate the propagation of depolarization along the membrane, including the effects of the membrane on the spatio-temporal properties of the depolarization.

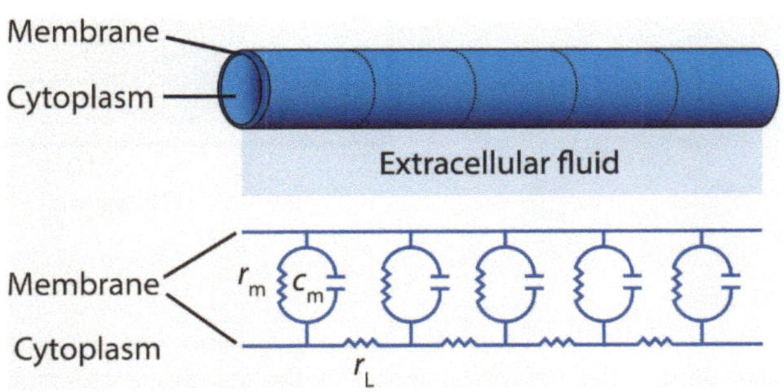

Fig. 4.3 Equivalent circuitry for a portion of the dendrite. The extracellular space is large and has a low resistance. The resistance of the neuronal membrane (r_m) is high due to a small number of open (leakage) ionic channels at rest. The resistance of the fluid inside the cell, the cytoplasm (r_L), is low, but higher than the resistance of the extracellular space due to the much smaller volume.

Neuronal excitation

Neurons form complex neuronal networks that together form an information-processing unit. To achieve this goal, information has to be propagated from one cell to another. A specialized structure has evolved to serve this function: the synapse (Fig. 4.4). The synapse is a polar (directed) structure with propagation from the presynaptic to the postsynaptic neuron, but not vice versa. In the presynaptic neuron, a substance, the *neurotransmitter*, is produced and stored in vesicles to be released on demand. Once released, the neurotransmitter diffuses through the tiny synaptic cleft to the membrane of the postsynaptic neuron. The neurotransmitter is the ligand for the *ligand-gated ionic channels* at the membrane of the postsynaptic neuron. These ionic channels allow transformation of chemical signals into electrical signals. The ligand binds to the extracellular binding side of the channel. The channel opens for a few milliseconds and causes an ionic flow through the neuronal membrane.

As such, ligand-gated channels open after the neurotransmitter is released and generate a *postsynaptic potential* (Fig. 4.4). The postsynaptic potential has an amplitude of a few mV and typically lasts about 10–20 ms. If the ligand-gated channel is selective for sodium, the transmembrane potential becomes more positive and the postsynaptic neuron depolarizes (resulting in an *exitatory postsynaptic potential; EPSP*). If the channel is selective for potassium or chloride, it hyperpolarizes the membrane (or "locks" the membrane more near

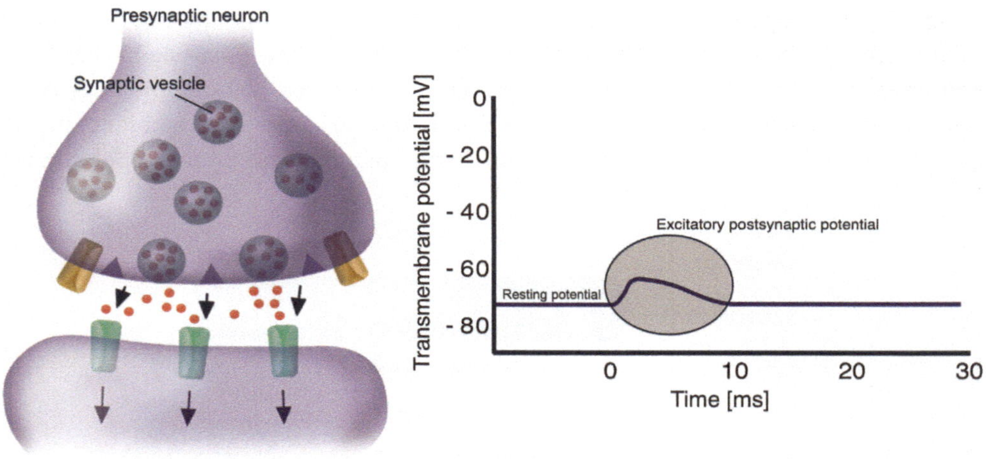

Fig. 4.4 A synapse: the contact between the presynaptic and postsynaptic neuron *(left)*. The presynaptic neuron synthetizes the neurotransmitter in the soma and stores it in vesicles that are transported to the synaptic contact along the axon. It is released after the membrane of the presynaptic neuron has been depolarized. It diffuses through the synaptic cleft to the postsynaptic membrane and binds to ligand-gated channels. *Right*: An excitatory postsynaptic potential is a decrease in transmembrane potential of a few mV, lasting a few ms.

the resting potential, which is in fact very close to the equilibrium potential of potassium). An *inhibitory postsynaptic potential (IPSP)* results. There are many different types of neurotransmitters (e.g., glutamate, GABA, dopamine, serotonin, etc.) that can be selective for different types of ligand-gated channels. By this, the neuronal network can control whether certain synaptic connections are *excitatory* or *inhibitory*.

The membrane at different spots of the neuron is different. For example, *fast voltage-sensitive sodium channels* are found at particularly high density in the axonal membrane and less so on dendrites. When the potential reaches the axon hillock (the initial segment of the axon where voltage-sensitive sodium channels are abundant), these ion channels open. If sufficient depolarization is reached (a *threshold*), this depolarization further opens the channels in a self-propagating sequence (opening some of the channels causes further depolarization, which opens additional sodium channels to further depolarize the membrane, etc.). This is comparable to a spark igniting a whole barrel of explosive powder by igniting an exponentially rising cascade of particles.

Such self-propagating depolarization terminates by another voltage-sensitive process of these channels. Additional to the fast opening and closing of the channel by transmembrane potential, sodium channels may **inactivate** due to plugging of the intracellular side of the channel by a spherical structure connected to the channel (a kind of "plug"). When the transmembrane potential reaches positive values (thus reverses the initially negatively charged inner surface of the membrane) it triggers this inactivation process in voltage-sensitive sodium channels. The channel in the inactive state cannot convey any ion flow. Only after the membrane has been repolarized back to the resting potential for a certain period of time (typically milliseconds) the plug is removed, and the channel is thus ready to reopen again. The inactivation thus conveys a kind of a molecular memory trace of a preceding states of the channel.

Consequently, the voltage-sensitive sodium channel can attain *three discreet states*: *opened*, *closed*, and *inactivated*.

While inactivation is initiated by large depolarization reaching values close to 0 mV, at rest approximately 30% of the sodium channels are also in the inactivated state. While this is normally of no functional impact due to the presence of the remaining 70% active channels, further hyperpolarization can remove this inactivation and make the membrane even more excitable than normal. When the neuron has been hyperpolarized for some time, return to the resting potential makes the membrane more excitable by removing the inactivation block of the normally 30% inactivated channels. This is the consequence of the fast opening and closing channel kinetics on one hand, but much slower activation/inactivation kinetics on the other hand; thus, the channel is ready to be opened quickly, but the activation state changes only slowly. Consequently, even if the cell after a period of hyperpolarization returns only back to the resting potential, the neuron may still generate a few action potentials due to this effect (a phenomenon called **postinhibitory rebound**).

Additional to sodium channels, at depolarized states of the membrane a specific group of potassium channels (called *delayed rectifiers*) start opening. They open after a fraction of a millisecond (are "delayed") and cause an outflow of potassium that then forces the transmembrane potential to become more negative again (due to the negative equilibrium potential for potassium) and by that *repolarize* the membrane back to the resting level. The consequence of these events in concert is a pulse-like depolarization called an *action potential* (Fig. 4.5).

The action potential is not explainable from the equivalent circuit-like behavior of the neuronal membrane shown in Fig. 4.3. To make action potentials possible, the membrane has to be equipped with fast voltage-gated sodium channels. Membranes containing these are sometimes called active to differentiate them from the passive membrane characterized by the equivalent RC circuit described previously. Voltage-gated sodium channels open whenever the membrane of the neuron is depolarized by some amount below the resting potential (as a rule 5–10 mVs). They augment the existing depolarization by an additional inflow of sodium into the cell.

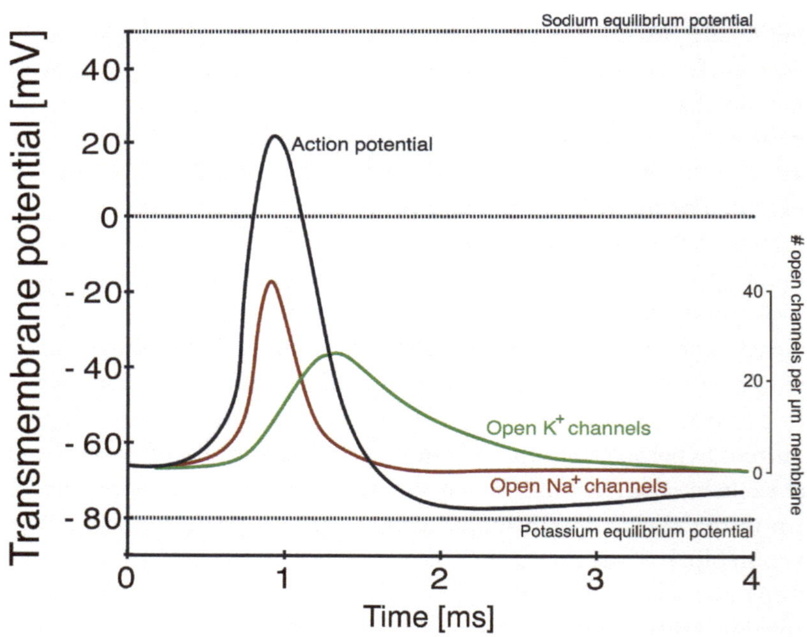

Fig. 4.5 When a glass micropipette is inserted into excited axons, pulse-like depolarizations can be recorded (black trace). These are called action potentials. They last ~1 ms and have a steep depolarizing and a shallower repolarizing flank. Action potential involves a number of channels (sodium and potassium, brown and green trace).

As only a limited number of molecules move in and out of the cell during the action potential (per 1 μm^2 membrane several hundred molecules), this process can repeat in fast sequence. The phase characterized by the inactivation of the majority of sodium channels is called the *refractory period*. In the refractory period, action potentials cannot be induced (*absolute refractory phase*). Fortunately, the absolute refractory period lasts only ~1–2 ms. The existence of some remaining open potassium channels (delayed rectifiers) can lessen the excitation a bit even after the absolute refractory phase. This stage, characterized by terminated inactivation yet opened delayed rectifiers is called the *relative refractory phase*. In the relative refractory phase action potentials can be elicited, but at a smaller amplitude. As can be concluded from Fig. 4.5, both refractory phases cover only a period of a couple of ms after the onset of an action potential. They are key in preventing action potentials traveling along the axon from constantly generating back-propagating action potentials. Since the membrane of neurons that had an action potential is refractory, they typically propagate along the membrane only in one direction (towards the synapse).

Restoration of ionic concentrations is achieved by active ion transport via Na^+/K^+ ATPase and passive diffusion (in the case of potassium). As only a limited number of ions physically pass the membrane during an action potential (few hundred per μm^2), they have no significant influence in ionic concentrations (the changes are <5 μmol/L, while the overall concentrations are, depending on the ion and compartment, from a few mmol/L to ca. 150 mmol/L, see Table 4.1). Effects on intracellular concentrations can be of significance only if excitation is strong and long lasting.

Note that minute changes in concentration, hardly measurable, can cause large effects on electric potentials!

Propagation of excitation

Neuronal excitation can propagate as an active or passive process. *Passive (electrotonic) propagation* along the neuronal membrane in the absence of fast voltage-sensitive sodium channels follows the rule of equivalent circuits as described previously. Due to the inherent leaky nature of the membrane (r_m in Fig. 4.3), part of the ions that entered the cytosol escape again. This is due to the action of the leaky K^+ channels. Consequently, the amplitude of the depolarization (e.g., excitatory postsynaptic potentials) decreases with distance from the synapse (Fig. 4.6). However, the propagation is very fast since it does not require any channel openings or other slower membrane processes.

If many synapses are active at the same time (or within a short time window), the signals add up and may generate large summated postsynaptic potentials. These may be sufficient to generate an action potential (at the axon hillock) and thus an active neuronal excitation. The summation thus takes place in space over the dendritic field of the neuron (*spatial summation*) and in time, where even one repetitively activated synapse may sum up into large postsynaptic potentials (*temporal summation*). This latter is

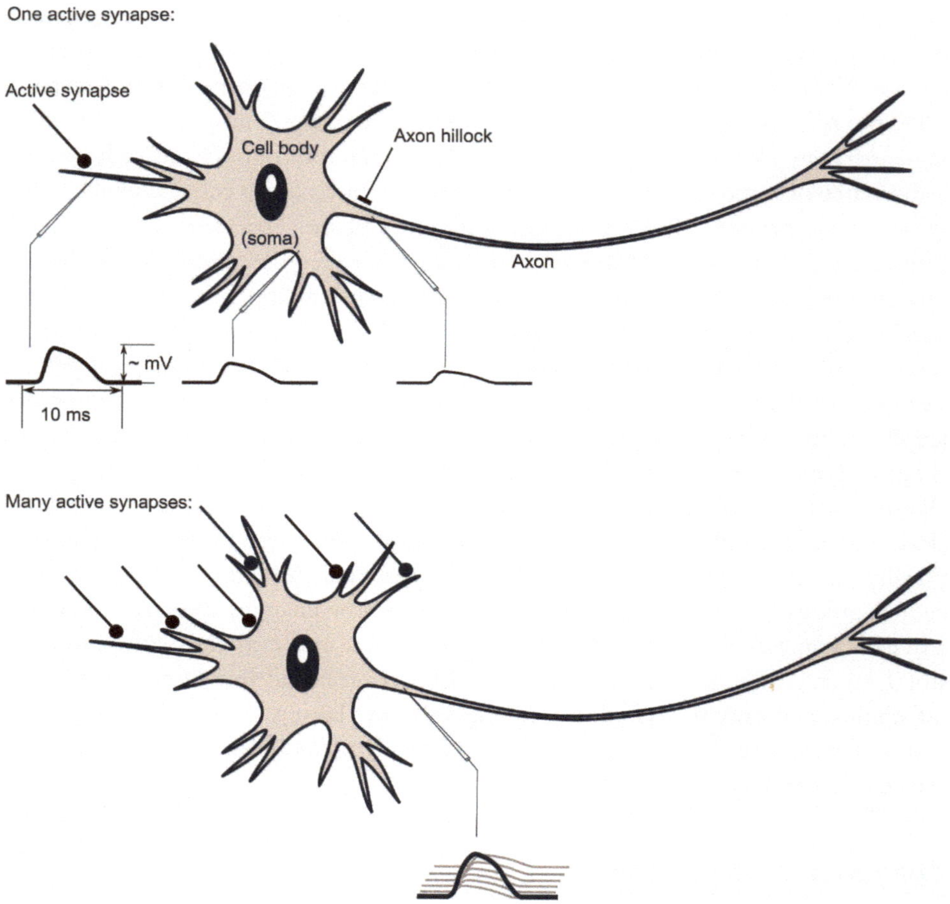

Fig. 4.6 *Top*: If one excitatory synapse of the neuron becomes activated, a change in the transmembrane potential from resting (i.e., −80 mV) to more positive values is generated (inset); this is called postsynaptic potential. This typically lasts one to tens of ms and has an amplitude of a few mV. Due to the passive properties of the dendritic tree, the postsynaptic potential propagates towards the axon, but with decreasing amplitude. This is due to the leaky properties of the neuronal membrane. *Below*: If many synapses are active, the postsynaptic potentials sum up in time and over space (the dendritic tree). This may be sufficient to cause a strong depolarization at the axon hillock. That in turn can activate fast voltage-gated sodium channels in such a number that an action potential results.

possible since postsynaptic potentials last ~10 ms or more, and are thus much longer than action potentials. Summation in time is thus possible even if synaptic activity is not perfectly synchronous. As a rule, both temporal and spatial summation are necessary to initiate an action potential in most neurons. The relative importance of temporal and spatial summation for the initiation of an action potential helps to fine-tune the information-processing properties of the neuron.

In the presence of voltage-sensitive ion channels, additional to the passive propagation of potentials, the transmembrane potential can be further affected by opening of these channels. They can either further reduce the potential or increase it, depending on which channel is opened. There is a large multiplicity of ionic channels that are voltage-gated, and different neurons have different compositions of these channels. Additional to sodium and potassium channels, they include calcium channels that initiate a large inward current due to the concentration gradient of calcium (its near absence in cytosol) and its double charge. These may increase or decrease the amplitude of the passively propagated potential.

This type of propagation of potentials is *active propagation*. It is observed in cases when the membrane has a sufficient concentration of fast voltage-gated sodium channels to generate action potentials. Once an action potential is generated at one spot of the membrane, it will propagate to the neighboring spot by passive propagation (the **local current** or "*strömchen*"). If in the neighboring section enough sodium channels are present to generate action potentials, an action potential will occur there, too. This way, section by section, the action potential travels along the membrane. As the amplitude of the action potential is always determined by the sodium channels, it will not shrink over time (and space); the propagation is without decrement. Using this mechanism, excitation can be propagated over very large distances along axons. Some neurons (e.g., motor neurons of the spinal cord, or axons constituting the vagus nerve) can reach lengths greater than 1 m. With passive propagation, over such long distances the depolarization would lose too much amplitude and would thus cease along the axon. This is called the "all or none" rule; this type of excitation is a binary process, either generating an action potential or not.

Propagation of excitation along a fiber depends on the membrane parameters, particularly the specific capacitance and the resistance. Typical values are given in Table 4.3. The inner resistance of neurons is much less than the resistance of the neuronal membrane. The resistance of extracellular space is also less than the resistance of intracellular space due to the greater volume of the extracellular space. To assess the propagation of excitation along an axon, the specific resistance and capacitance (per μm^2 of the membrane) have to be considered together with the size of the membrane. The surface of the membrane increases proportionally to the diameter of the axon. A larger surface of the

Table 4.3 Typical physiological values of neuronal membranes.

Parameter	Typical value
R_m	1–100 $k\Omega/cm^2$
R_L	50–200 Ω/cm
C	1 $\mu F/cm^2$

membrane results in a smaller resistance of the membrane r_m (the axon's surface area is proportional to its diameter) and a lower longitudinal resistance of the axon r_L (the section area of the axon is directly proportional to the square of the radius multiplied by π). The capacitance is directly proportional to the surface of the membrane and thus also to the diameter of the axon.

Thus, fiber diameter affects the conduction properties of the fiber. Another property that affects the conduction along the axon is myelination. Myelin consists of layers of glial (Schwann) cell membranes that surround the neuronal axon. During development, some axons are wrapped up by additional layers of the membrane that condense in what is called the myelin sheath (Fig. 4.7). The myelin sheath has a high resistance; ions cannot pass it. Consequently, ionic channels redistribute along the myelinated axon towards myelin-free portions called nodes of Ranvier. These nodes are located at places where a region covered by myelin from one Schwann cell ends and another takes over. The density of fast sodium channels is consequently high at the node and low at internodal segments.

The consequence of such an arrangement is that the local currents can no longer flow locally, but rather have to pass the whole internodal distance. As r_m is high in the internodal region, and due to the absence of fast sodium channels in this region, the current has to reach the next node of Ranvier to allow the propagation of action potentials to

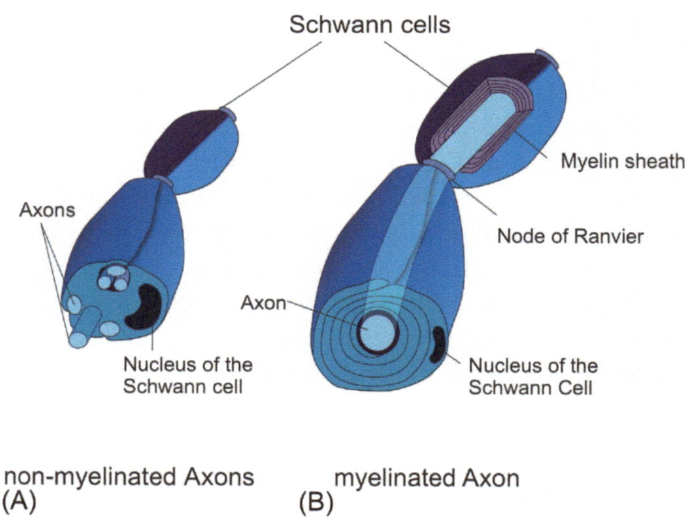

Fig. 4.7 Two types of axons: unmyelinated axons of a peripheral nerve wrapped in one layer of a Schwann cell membrane (A) and a myelinated peripheral axon wrapped in several layers of neuronal membrane of the Schwann cell (B). This onion-type sheath has strong insulating properties and therefore significantly affects currents passing through the membrane. In the central nervous system, the function of Schwann cells is performed by glial cells.

continue. This carries a significant advantage; as the passive local currents do not require gating of voltage-sensitive channels, they travel faster than an action potential that requires many channels to open and close. Thus, the speed of propagation of the action potential is accelerated by the presence of myelin. As the action potential "jumps" from one node to the next, this conduction is called "saltatory conduction." The existence of this mechanism can increase the propagation velocity of action potentials from a few m/s to 120 m/s.

The rules of excitability with relation to the diameter of the fiber are valid also for myelinated fibers. In fact, the conduction velocity is directly proportional to the diameter in myelinated fibers. As an approximation,

$$v \sim 6 * d,$$

where v is the velocity of action potential propagation in (m/s) and d is the diameter of the axon in (μm). Thicker axons thus propagate action potentials faster.

Finally, the density of the fast voltage-sensitive sodium currents determine the speed of depolarization and consequently the temporal and spatial electrical gradient on neighboring portions of the membrane. The more of these channels are present in the membrane, the lower the excitation threshold and the faster the propagation of the action potential along the neuronal membrane.

In total, four parameters define the propagation velocity:

1. Diameter of the fiber affecting r_L and r_m
2. Myelination (further affecting r_m and causing saltatory conduction)
3. Density of the voltage-sensitive channels
4. Temperature. The lower the temperature, the lower the propagation velocity. This effect relates to the Nernst equation and its consequences.

Propagation of action potentials is in principle bidirectional. However, under physiological conditions, the neuron is a polar structure; it receives input excitation at the synaptic contacts and relays this with decrement to the place of action potential generation, from where it travels along the membrane (through the axon) to the presynaptic contact. The synapse relays electrical information from presynaptic to postsynaptic element. Although the action potential can passively back-propagate to the soma, within the axon the refractory period prevents the initiation of backward-traveling action potentials. In consequence, back-propagation only exists at the passive membrane. Exception is non-physiological (e.g., electrical or optogenetic) stimulation that can be initiated at an artificial point of the neuron, such as in the middle of the axon. Since no action potentials have traveled to this point yet, no portion of the membrane is in the refractory period and the action potential can travel from the point of artificial excitation in both directions: in the "normal" direction to the synapse (**orthodromic**), but also in the opposite direction to the soma (**antidromic**).

Dynamic properties of the neuronal membranes: Time and length constants

Not all changes in electric fields within or outside the neuronal membrane cause a depolarization. This is related to the fact that the neuronal membrane is leaky and balances the extracellular and intracellular potential to achieve a constant transmembrane potential. Thus, putting the whole organism on a static potential (slow charging of the body) does not cause excitation. Excitation results only when transmembrane potential is changed. For this, the intracellular or the extracellular potential has to change differentially. That can be achieved by an isolated change of the intracellular or the extracellular potential that is sufficiently fast to achieve a significant change in transmembrane potential that the membrane cannot counterbalance by the leakage ionic channels. The transmembrane potential activates voltage-gated ionic channels. But how fast does this change have to be?

To investigate this, one can induce a step-like change either in the intracellular compartment or in the extracellular compartment, and investigate the change in the transmembrane potential. Due to the "low-pass" filtering property of the equivalent RC circuit, the step-like change will be transformed into a smooth change in the transmembrane current, as shown in Fig. 4.8. The effect can be quantified using the time constant of the membrane, being $\tau = r_m.C$.

This explains why a slow increase in intracellular potential (e.g., by application of a very small current) may not activate the voltage-sensitive channels at all; at the rate the charges are introduced into the cell they can also escape through the leakage channels. In consequence, there is no significant membrane potential shift and by that no excitation of the cell.

To determine a measure of the time constant of the neuronal membrane, strength-duration relations are used. For both intracellular and extracellular charge application, pulsed electrical signals are used and the threshold current for action potential initiation is plotted as a function of the duration of the pulse. Example of the strength-duration curve is shown in Fig. 4.9. On this curve, the threshold current (to initiate an action potential) for an infinite duration of the pulse is called the *rheobase*. At double the value of the rheobase, the strength-duration curve determines the *chronaxie*. This value is used as a measure of the time constant of the neuron. The chronaxie is between 100 and 300 μs for myelinated axons, 700 and 2000 μs for unmyelinated axons, and 10 and 22 ms for cell bodies of neurons. These data demonstrate that cell bodies are, as a rule, leakier and thus less excitable (mainly because of the higher capacitance of the soma).

Finally, as previously mentioned, in myelinated fibers the local currents need to reach neighboring nodes of Ranvier to allow propagation of excitation. The extent of decrease in the depolarization along the membrane is characterized by the length constant λ (Fig. 4.10). In addition, this constant is dependent on the membrane electrical properties.

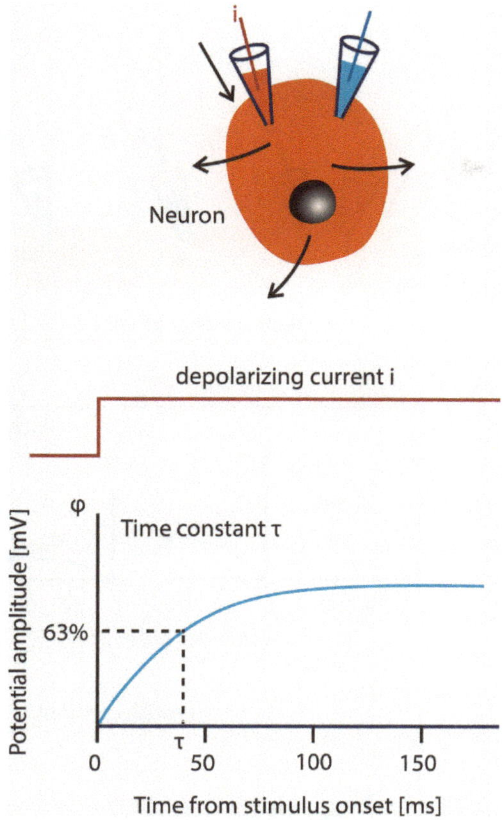

Fig. 4.8 Effects of a step-like depolarizing current applied into the cell. The transmembrane potential increases slowly, as parts of the applied charges are counterbalanced by ions escaping the cell through leakage channels and the capacitance of the membrane. The slower increase in membrane potential can be approximated by an exponential function with the exponent including a time constant τ (the time when 63% of the maximum potential is achieved, see (Schmidt and Unsicker, 2003)). The time constant thus defines the "sluggishness" of the membrane in consequence to a depolarizing (or hyperpolarizing) pulse. It is the consequence of the r_m and the C of the cell membrane ($\tau = r_m \cdot C$).

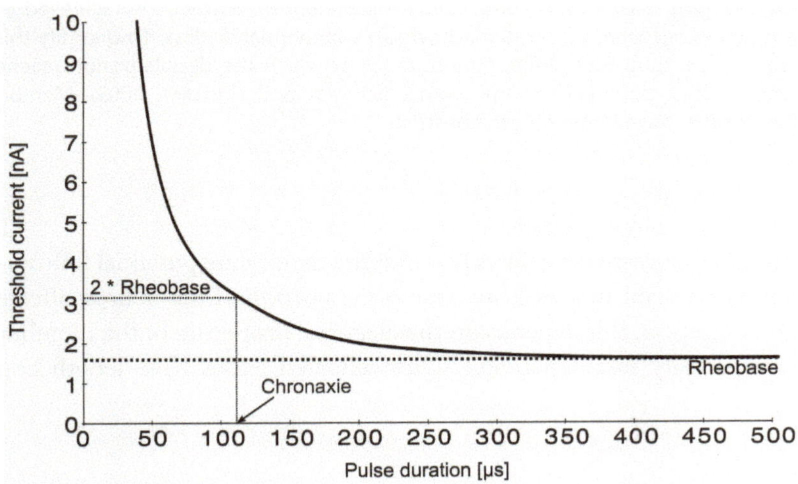

Fig. 4.9 A strength-duration curve for intracellular stimulation. The curve shows a chronaxie of ~120μs. Similar chronaxies are also obtained for extracellular stimulation, albeit with higher currents (in μA). Myelination shifts the curve to smaller chronaxies.

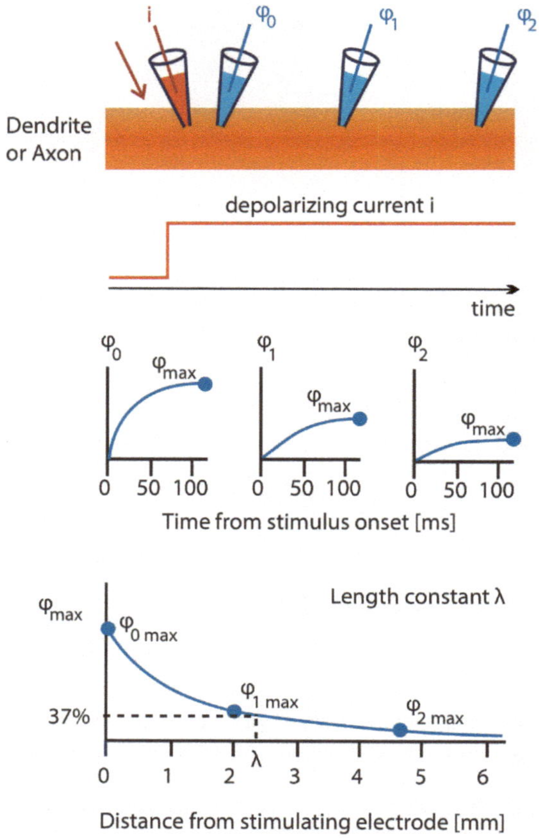

Fig. 4.10 A depolarization induced in a fiber spreads passively over a distance with decrement. The stimulus is shown in *red* below the fiber. The potential is measured at three positions along the stimulated dendrite. At each position, the potential changes over time according to time constant, but reaches a different maximum potential φ_{max} *(middle panel). Bottom*: The achieved φ_{max}, when plotted as a function of recording position, shows an exponential decline. To quantify this behavior a length constant λ is used that defines the distance at which the depolarization reached 37% of the maximum induced potential change (comp. Schmidt and Unsicker, 2003). Membranes with higher r_m and lower r_L have larger length constants.

Whereas the time constant defines how fast the membrane potential follows the stimulus, the length constant defines how large is the portion of the neuron affected by the induced depolarization; this depends on the electrical properties of the membrane. Both constants are partially interdependent. Unmyelinated axons have length constants of 2–5 mm.

Thresholds in excitation

Individual neurons function as an integrator of inputs; the activation of the presynaptic neuron ultimately causes postsynaptic potentials that sum up at the passive membrane of the postsynaptic neuron. However, as these propagate along the passive membrane, their amplitudes decrease due to the leaky nature of the passive membrane (Fig. 4.10). At the point where the axon originates (called the "action potential initiation zone" or "trigger zone"), the voltage-gated channels are found in large numbers. If the depolarization is sufficient at this point to generate an action potential, this will be propagated along the axonal membrane to the presynaptic elements. Thus, the neuron is a leaky integrator of inputs, whereas the temporal and spatial properties are defined by the time and the length constants of the neuronal membrane. A significant portion of the charge injected into a neuron may exit the stimulated cell and may therefore not be effective. This also has implications for neuroprosthetic stimulation.

The excitation threshold itself as well as the synaptic efficacy can change over time in response to a repeated stimulus. It is assumed that these processes underlie the ability for learning (see **Chapter 9**). However, not all synapses learn similarly fast. Synapses located in the peripheral nervous system or connecting sensory organs to the brain as a rule are highly active, must be very reliable, and therefore do not undergo plastic changes. Synapses in the central nervous system, particularly the cerebral cortex, are more plastic and change with learning.

For the present context of brain prostheses, the temporal and spatial constraints for excitation are of essential importance. The properties make clear that a constant electrical field that does not change in time or space does not induce neuronal excitation. In such a steady state, the membrane will keep its constant transmembrane potential given by the concentrations of ions on both sides of the membrane. Only if the electrical field around the neuron can induce a change in transmembrane potential sufficient to generate action potentials, excitation results. For this, gradients in time and space are required that are steeper than the membrane constants. **Chapter 6** examines these in detail.

The neurons as described above form macroscopic structures: nerves, neuronal ganglia, the spinal cord, and the brain. They are embedded in structures that provide protection, nutrition, and oxygen. These macroscopic structures are the eventual targets for neuroprosthetic intervention.

Macroanatomy of the nervous system

The nervous system on the macroscopic level consists of two anatomic components: the peripheral nervous system and the central nervous system. The **peripheral nervous system** (PNS) consists of groups of neurons arranged in groups into ganglia and connected via the axons of neurons bundled into nerves. Ganglia and nerves are not simply a group of neurons or axons; they are additionally supplied with energy and oxygen by vessels (vasa nervorum) and embedded in connective tissue (epineurium and perineurium) so that the nerve cells have the required conditions for their survival and appropriate function (see **Chapter 14**). They are located throughout the body and provide both input to the brain as well as control signals for the muscles throughout the body.

The **central nervous system** (CNS) has two main components: the spinal cord and the brain. They contain a large number of neurons and are found within protective bony structures (the vertebral column and the skull), embedded in a fluid (liquor cerebrospinalis) that provides further protection from mechanical injury. The brain and spinal cord are covered by three layers of tissue. The first is the **pia mater**, which is in intimate contact with the surface of the brain and spinal cord. The next layer, the **arachnoid**, consists mainly of vessels and attaches to the pia and thus to the surface of the brain. The vessels penetrate into the brain and provide energy and oxygen for the neurons. The **dura mater** is the last layer, the outer layer that is normally not directly attached to the arachnoid, separated from it by the liquor and sparsely connected by vessels bridging the arachnoid and the dura. Dura mater is the outer layer that seals the liquor cerebrospinalis-filled space from the rest of the body and thus provides mechanical and immune protection. All interventions that open dura mater are more susceptible to brain or spinal cord infection. Therefore surgeons avoid opening the dura if possible.

The PNS and CNS, among other things, also differ in non-neuronal composition. In the CNS the glia provides the scaffold for the neuronal structures, whereas in the PNS it is Schwann cells that structure, protect, and shield neurons from their surroundings.

Brief summary

- The (trans)membrane potential is the electrical potential difference between the inside and the outside of the cell.
- The membrane potential results from the differing ionic compositions of the inside and the outside of the cell.
- The membrane potential is determined by the permeabilities of the cell membrane to ions and the activity of electrogenic ion pumps.
- Electrically, the membrane of the cell can be approximated by an RC circuit.
- The permeability can be changed by opening or closing ionic channels.
- An action potential is a series of membrane permeability changes induced by the initial changes of the transmembrane potential that create a rapid depolarization of the membrane followed by a repolarization to the resting transmembrane potential.
- Length and time constants determine the electrical behavior of the cell membrane.

Key literature and further reading

Barrett, K., Barman, S., Yuan, J., Brooks, H., 2019. Ganong's Review of Medical Physiology. McGraw-Hill Education/Medical.
Bear, M.F., Paradiso, M.A., Connors, B.W., 2015. Neuroscience. Wolters Kluwer, Philadelphia/Baltimore/New York/London.
Hall, J.E., 2015. Guyton and Hall Textbook of Medical Physiology, 13th ed. Saunders.
Hille, B., 2001. Ion Channels of Excitable Membranes. Sinauer Associates, Inc., Sunderland, Mass
Klinke, R., Paper, H.-C., Silbernagl, S., 2005. Physiologie. Georg Thieme Verlag, Stuttgart/New York.
Malmivuo, J., Plonsey, R., 1995. Bioelectromagnetism. Oxford University Press, New York/Oxford.
Schmidt, R.F., Unsicker, K., 2003. Lehrbuch der Vorklinik. Deutscher Ärzte-Verlag.

CHAPTER 5

Electrode-tissue interface

To stimulate neurons artificially, the first task is to create an electric field. Such electric fields lead to current flow in the tissue and can in principle activate voltage-sensitive channels in the membrane of neurons. In this sense, the electric fields are the natural stimulus for excitable neuronal membranes, depolarizing, or hyperpolarizing neurons. Stimulation electrodes are devices used to generate electrical fields in tissue. To stimulate excitable tissue effectively, electrodes need to be placed close to the target tissue. This implicates that they often need to be inserted into living tissue or placed in direct contact with its surface.

Physically, electric current is the movement of electric charge in space. Electric field (difference in electric potential) is the driving force of this movement. Depending on the material, different movable electric charges are responsible for the current. In a metal the electrons are freely movable. They can easily travel along potential gradients depending on electrical resistance. A metal wire itself is not physically changed by the current, since electrons that move away in the metal are replaced by electrons supplied by the electric source. Thus no physical or chemical changes are observed in metal wires even during long-term current stimulation (provided that the temperature remains stable). The relation between voltage and current is expressed by Ohm's law, which states that current equals voltage divided by material resistance ($I = U/R$). **Resistance** depends on the availability of the electrons in the material and their free movement. In case of a wire, the latter is defined by the cross-sectional area (the larger the area, the smaller the resistance), the length of the wire, and the material. However, when using alternating current of different frequencies, the resistance is highly dependent on frequency as well. Therefore, the term **impedance** has been introduced that reflects the frequency dependence of resistance. To take this property into account, a complex number for impedance is used to describe its frequency dependence.

There are two possible ways to generate an electric stimulus: constant current and constant voltage sources (Box 5.1). A **constant voltage source** keeps the voltage at the outlet of the source constant. An electric outlet at home is such a voltage source; it keeps a constant voltage (in Europe 240 V, in USA 110 V). If one short-circuits a voltage source (e.g., by directly connecting the terminals of the outlet with a conductor), current starts to flow between the terminals. Yet, despite the low resistance of the short circuit and the charge flow through it, the voltage source "tries" to maintain the voltage at the set value (e.g., 240 V) irrespective of the load (resistance) connected to it. This

Prostheses for the Brain
https://doi.org/10.1016/B978-0-12-818892-7.00004-3

BOX 5.1: Current and voltage source

Electric stimulation for neuroprosthetics requires full control of current. Since the source of electric fields is a voltage source that controls voltage, but not current, constant current requires modification of the circuitry providing the electric energy.

To understand the circuitry behind this requires an explanation of the concept of internal resistance. The internal resistance of a device (R_i) secures safe function when using a range of load resistances. The view of the electric source therefore includes not only the source of voltage but also the internal resistance:

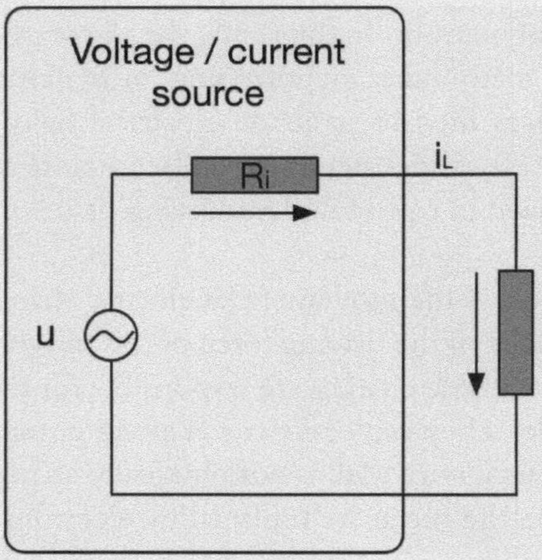

When the poles of the electric source are connected by a resistance (load resistance R_L), this resistance leads to a current i_L (load current) that is the consequence of the voltage of the source and Ohm's law. However, we need to consider the internal resistance and its relation to the load resistance:

$$i_L = \frac{u}{R_i + R_L}$$

The internal resistance of the voltage source determines how the current changes when the load of the source changes. If the internal resistance is low ($R_i \ll R_L$), the denominator of the above equation will be mainly determined by the load resistance and thus the current will change with changing load resistance. This is typical for a voltage source.

If the internal resistance is very high ($R_i \gg R_L$), the resulting load current is mainly dependent on R_i, since in the denominator of the above equation the R_L will be negligible compared to R_i. Thus, selection of u and R_i can determine how the current changes with the load resistance. In cases with very high R_i, the load current will be less dependent on R_L and thus will be relatively constant. This is what is called a passive current source. Of course, the given source of voltage must deliver the high voltage u required to generate the requested i_L in spite of the high R_i.

BOX 5.1: Current and voltage source—CONT'D

However, another approach is to actively regulate the current. In this case, there is a small differential amplifier and a small resistance R_M in series of R_i inside the current source. This measures the voltage at the known R_M and provides feedback to the voltage source.

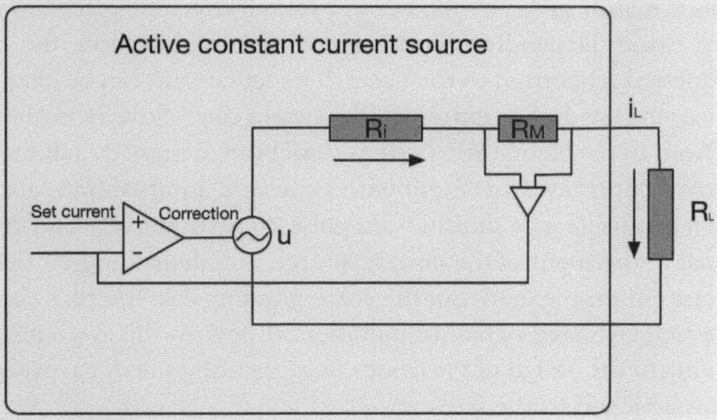

If one registers the load current i_L deviating from the set current, the feedback can increase the voltage u to provide the required current and by that keep the current at the constant set current. A precondition for this is a fast (as a rule nanosecond) feedback. In this constellation it is meaningful if R_i is very large and R_M very small (negligible) compared to R_L. Other, more complex, forms of active current control are possible but not discussed here.

results in very high current if the attached resistance is low; $R = 1\,\Omega$ (metal wire) would lead to 240 A if the voltage was to be kept constant at 240 V. This is a gigantic current! The electric fuses used for the whole household usually supply at most 25–36 A. If they are fast enough, they will disconnect before the high current increases the temperature of the conductor so that it melts. Consequently, as we were taught as children, it is not a good idea to short-circuit such a voltage source. The best "resting" condition of a voltage source is the high-resistance open-circuit, with no current between the terminals.

The **constant current source**, on the other hand, controls the current and keeps it constant while regulating the voltage (within available power compliance limits). Like the set voltage in the voltage source, there is a set current in the current source. The current source "tries" to supply this current irrespective of the load resistance. In contrast to the voltage source, the terminals of the current source with non-zero set current can be kept short-circuited in resting condition. Of course, then current will constantly flow between the terminals. However, when the terminals are open, the current source will increase the voltage to its absolute upper limit in an "attempt" to drive the required set current through the infinite resistance at the output. Current sources, if open-circuited, can develop voltages of many hundred volts. This can lead to current overshoot when connected to a device, and the high voltage may cause damage in the device or tissue.

These two sources of electrical power are thus fundamentally different. In everyday life, we only experience constant voltage sources. However, for neuronal stimulation, constant current sources are the appropriate choice. As will be made clearer later in the chapter, this is mainly given by the current source controlling the amount of charge delivered to the tissue. Depending on the needs of the application, the current source supplies the requested set current to the tissue. The set current can be changed over time depending on varying needs. For example, the current can follow a sinusoidal function or a pulsatile function. In the laboratory, current sources are designed such that their current output can follow a control voltage input with a constant input-output relation. This way one can program a signal (e.g., a sinusoid or a pulse on a computer), send the corresponding voltage signal to the input of the current source, and depending on the amplitude of the signal, the current source sends out the corresponding current, thus copying the time function of the input voltage signal. In commercial devices this is preprogrammed and changed according to the design of the device (e.g., by using the signal processing strategy of the stimulator attached to the implant).

The water hose analogy

The behavior of electrical stimulation can be approximated using an analogy of watering plants with a water hose (Fig. 5.1). We are all familiar with this system, and we are well aware what happens if there is low pressure in the system (the tap is not sufficiently open) or what happens when somebody steps on the hose. In this analogy the plants are the neurons, the water molecules are the charges that stimulate the neurons, the water pressure is voltage, the tube diameter is inverse to electrical resistance (i.e., larger tube diameter means less resistance), and the rate of water flow is the current. The goal is to deliver a steady flow of water to the plant.

If the diameter of the hose is restricted (resistance is increased), the water pressure before the narrowing increases (voltage increases) and the water flow (charge delivered, i.e., current) decreases.

A voltage source corresponds to a watering system that is regulated by water pressure in the tap. Thus, a decrease of the diameter of the tubing results in an increase in the pressure before the narrowing, which decreases the pressure gradient between the tap and the narrowing, thus decreasing water flow. The consequence is less water coming out of the hose. If the end of the hose corresponds to the interface of the electrode to the tissue, then under this situation the resistance change will affect how much charge (water) will leave the hose and enter the tissue. Monitoring water pressure in the hose (i.e., voltage in the lead wire) does not inform us about how much water exits the tubing.

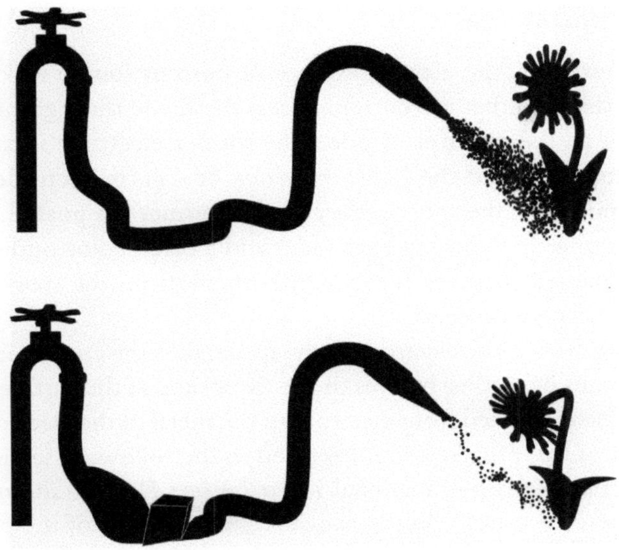

Fig. 5.1 The water hose analogy. Shown is the tap delivering the water, corresponding to a voltage source. It provides constant water pressure delivering water drops (charges) to the plants (neurons). When the hose is blocked (below, example of high resistance), the constant pressure in the tap is not sufficient to deliver the same amount of water (charges) and thus the neurons cannot be excited. Only a current source, controlling (securing) constant water flow through the tap can compensate for the partial blockage.

A much better way to guarantee a steady flow would be to control the volume of water exiting the tap in a given time interval (current or charge over time), since this volume cannot evaporate within the hose and thus must reach the plants (tissue). This would guarantee the same amount of water dispensed to the plant in the given time, as the flow of water through the tap gives information about how much water has exited the hose. This, in the analogy, provides much more reliable information on the potential excitation of the neurons around the electrode tip and, most importantly, is independent on the changes of electrode resistance (hose diameter or opening). Whenever the hose narrows, such system has to increase the pressure to provide the same amount of water exiting the tap in the given time. By increasing the pressure, it can still dispense the same volume of water to the plants even though the hose is narrowed. Thus, delivered water is best guaranteed by controlling the water flow.

Our own water hose in the garden does not control water flow; it rather guarantees the same pressure (ca. 2.5 bars in Germany) and thus better corresponds to the operation of a constant voltage source that controls the pressure and not the water flow. Such a system is simple but blind to leaks or constrictions in the tubing. In the case of a garden, this is unimportant, but in the case of an implanted electrical device, the equivalent could be problematic.

Electrode configurations

For stimulation purposes, the electric voltage or current source is connected to two electrodes in the tissue so that the current enters the tissue through one electrode and returns back through the other electrode. The former electrode is called the *stimulation* or *working* electrode, and the latter the *return* or *counter* electrode. To better differentiate the terminals of the source, they are sometimes designated with a red color outlet (for connecting the working electrode) and a black color outlet (for the return electrode). The charged particles consequently move from the working electrode to the return electrode or vice versa.

However, there are no free electrons in the tissue, thus the current in the tissue is not mediated by electrons but rather by ions in the tissue, and at the surface of the electrode the current has to be converted from electrons in the metal of the electrode to ions in the tissue. The details of this processes are described in the following section.

Current flow may be one-directional *(direct current; DC)* or alternating *(alternating current; AC)*. "One-directional" flow means that one terminal of the power source has a positive polarity and the other has a negative polarity (therefore the terminals are sometimes also designated by "+" and "−"). Since in the tissue the positive electrode attracts negative charges, it is called an *anode*. Correspondingly, the negative electrode attracts positive charges and is therefore called the *cathode*. In alternating current, however, this property changes over time and each anode is from time to time a cathode and vice versa. The terms *working* and *return* electrode are then only of terminological importance, since in alternating current stimulation the direction of particle movement changes over time. However, for didactic reasons we stick to these terms. If one electrode is placed close to the target neuron ("working") and the other far away from the target tissue ("return"), as is often the case, the terminology fits the function well for AC stimulation as well, since only the electrode close to the target can stimulate. As you will see later, the anodic and cathodic components stimulate in a fundamentally different way, and in AC stimulation, the effects achieved therefore may change throughout the stimulus cycle.

If the working electrode is close to the target neuron and the return electrode is placed far away from the target, as in the preceding example, the resulting electrical field is very broad and many neurons neighboring the target neuron may also be activated. This *stimulation configuration* is called *monopolar* (details in **Chapter 7**), as only one electrode (a single pole, a monopole) is really affecting the target structure. However, sometimes a more focused stimulation is required. In that case, the electrodes are placed close to each other and the electrical field develops mainly in the region between the electrodes. The achieved current density between the electrodes is high, and the current spread is small. Such a configuration is called *bipolar*, as both electrodes (two poles) stimulate. There are further possibilities to shape the electrical field. It has been proposed that *current focusing* may be achieved by splitting the electrical field into two return electrodes, so that 50% of the current flows toward one electrode and 50% toward the other electrode. Such configuration is called *tripolar* or *multipolar* (if more return electrodes are involved; see **Chapters 7 and 11**).

As some ionic channels of the neuronal membrane are voltage sensitive, a constant voltage source might be considered the right choice for a stimulation device at first sight. However, the electrical properties of the electrode contact complicate the consideration and prevent the proper control of the amount of excitation achieved in the tissue. To understand this, we need to dive into the details of the electrochemical processes at the electrode-tissue interface and into current conduction in the tissue. In the sections that follow we explain the basic terms; **Chapter 10** provides detailed insight for those readers who are more familiar with chemical and physical concepts.

Current conduction in electrolytes

In principle, to excite neurons, the aim is generating a potential difference across the neuronal membrane (i.e., the goal is to affect the transmembrane potential). Thus what we need to change is either the extracellular or the intracellular potential, or both in opposite directions. At first glance the easiest approach may appear to directly apply voltage into the cell (into the cytosol), by controlling the transmembrane potential from the site with the smallest volume. Due to the small intracellular volume, we might achieve the largest effect with the least power. In experimental studies on animals, this is possible; however, in neuroprosthetic devices such an approach is not feasible. Over time, the penetrating electrode damages the stimulated cell. Furthermore, the electrodes are intricate, and to activate a large number of neurons, as is the case in most applications, one would need many microelectrodes. This is pragmatically not possible.

It is much easier to place the electrode in the extracellular space (outside of the neuron). However, the effect on the transmembrane potential is more widespread (distant neurons can be affected as well) and less predictable, since the charge will flow into the extracellular space that is larger than the intracellular space and has a complex geometry. Both the intracellular and the extracellular space are from the electrical point of view an *electrolyte* (i.e., an electrically conductive medium due to the presence of charged molecules or ions). As we have learned in **Chapter 4**, the neuronal membrane itself is leaky. A part of the electrical charges supplied to the extracellular space will thus also penetrate into the cell through leakage channels (Fig. 5.2), while the other part (the majority) will stay outside of the cell. The complex and numerous charge transfer processes (leakage channels, ionic pumps, etc.) through neuronal membrane (as discussed in **Chapter 4**) tend to keep a constant transmembrane potential irrespective of the absolute extracellular potential. Thus the effect of extracellularly applied electric fields is not straightforwardly transferred to excitation of neurons, and a common approach is to aim at abrupt changes of the potential in time, faster than the temporal behavior of neurons described by their time function (**Chapter 4**). Furthermore, it is important to

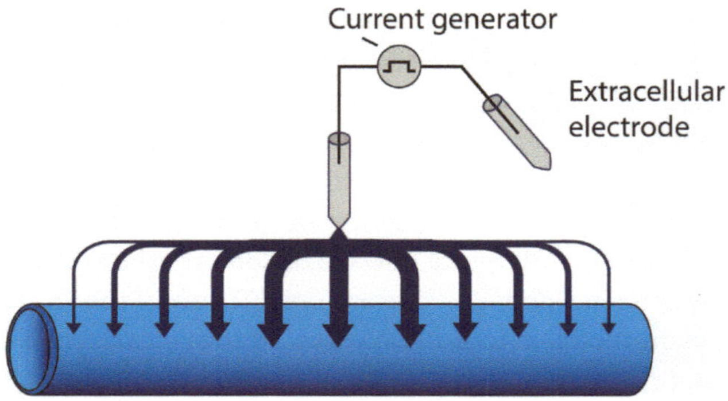

Fig. 5.2 Stimulation of a neuronal fiber with extracellular electrodes. The electrical field spreads preferentially in the extracellular space, however, the neuronal membrane is leaky and the current enters the cytosol as well. The essential aspect for neuronal excitation is how much transmembrane potential change this stimulation achieved. For this, the membrane time constant (**Chapter 4**) is essential.

consider that the resistance of the electrode-tissue interface changes over time due to tissue reactions to the electrode (**Chapter 8**). This is another reason why voltage sources are not appropriate in neuroprostheses, since the voltage at the electrode is not directly informative about the charge delivered into the tissue, and thus the electric potential in the tissue.

Despite the aforementioned disadvantages, the extracellular space is at present used for placement of the stimulation electrodes in neuroprosthetic applications. This is also the consequence of the processes at the electrode surface, which we discuss later in this chapter. Another reason is that electrical stimulation may lead to damage of the tissue, too, and this safety limit is lower for electrodes with small contact size and thus high current densities. We discuss this issue in detail in **Chapter 6**. However, this is another reason why intracellular chronic stimulation is not clinically feasible.

Electrode-electrolyte reactions

Present-day stimulators all use metal electrodes to deliver electric fields into the tissue. As mentioned previously, the charge responsible for current in metals is carried by free electrons that are supplied by the current source. In the tissue there are different mobile charged particles present: ions in a dissolved state (e.g., sodium, potassium, chloride, calcium, hydrogen, bicarbonates and other salts in ionized state, large organic molecules that are polarized and also may carry charge, etc.). In such an electrolyte, the electrical field causes physical movement of these charged molecules and ions that are transported from one place to the other, generating the current. Since they move, their concentrations are affected by the current; they may be removed from one electrode and transported to the other electrode. Of course this is very dependent on their mobility, given also by their size (smaller molecules with lower mass or size tend to be more mobile).[a] This also means that their contribution to the electrical current may differ.

Electric fields thus may shift the ionic concentrations in the electrolyte. Consequently, the electrolyte concentration changes under the influence of an electrical field.

The situation is even more complicated; when placing a metal into the electrolyte, the electrode material will lose/gain electrons or undergo a chemical reduction/oxidation (redox) reaction. These reactions may cause free electrons (from the metal) to enter the solution, reacting with components in the electrolyte or alternatively, the entry of metal cations into the solution (i.e., the metal is dissolved). In the former case, the metal becomes positively charged, and a substance from the electrolyte binds the free electron and becomes more negatively charged. In the latter case, the metal will become negative. A consequence is that the electrode is no longer electrically neutral relative to the electrolyte, but shows an electric potential soon after the metal has been immersed into the solution. In the following text, we will call such potential of the metal in the electrolyte, in absence of externally supplied current, the **electrochemical electrode potential**. Since the electrode potential (and the electric field resulting from it) is the consequence of the electrochemical process (loss of charged particles), the development of the electrode potential will reduce further loss of charged particles (that have opposite polarity). Thus the electrode potential counterbalances and stops the electrochemical processes generating it by abandoning the transfer of further charges through the electrode-electrolyte border. Since the charge carried by one molecule represents a strong physical force generating a relatively large voltage, small amounts of chemical changes will be sufficient to generate an electrode potential. An "electro-chemical equilibrium" is achieved when the electric potential stops the movement of charges across the electrode-tissue interface (the chemical reaction). As small amounts of substances can affect the electrode potential due to adhering molecules and impurities, the electrode potential is unstable and may fluctuate over time, particularly during initial period after immersion of the metal into the electrolyte.

It is impossible to measure the electrode potential of one material alone; the electrode potential can only be determined with reference to another electrode. In the optimal case this should be an electrode that does not develop an electrode potential itself (otherwise the measurement includes the electrode potentials of both the measurement and the reference electrodes). Since all electrodes have some electrode potential, a standard has been introduced; electrode potentials are always measured with reference to the *standard hydrogen electrode (SHE,* see **Chapter 10***).* This is essentially a platinum black

[a] Electric field has been used to separate and identify chemical components from a mixture using the technique of electrophoresis. The substances are placed in a conductive gel and a homogeneous (direct current; DC) electric field is applied to electrically attract the charged molecules to a specific place. How far they travel in the given gel provides information about their size and composition.

electrode (**Chapter 6**) placed in an acid-standardized environment with a saturation hydrogen concentration. Electrode potentials are important to know, since they affect the stimulation behavior and can become a source of undesired currents, particularly if two different metals in the body of a recipient develop different potentials. This may lead to DC currents and subsequently to pain generated by stimulation of neurons conveying pain signals. Such DC currents remove charge from the electrode and thus the chemical reactions described in this chapter continue, eventually leading to corrosion or dissolution of the metals, with additional complications resulting from that.

Different potentials on metals immersed in an electrolyte are also used beneficially in daily life. Based on reactions between metal and electrolyte and the different electrical potentials resulting from this process (depending on the metal and the electrolyte), chemical batteries (so-called *galvanic elements*) have been developed. Such batteries include different chemical processes in each half-cell, resulting in potential difference between the half-cells. The chemical process on each of them does not stop if the + and − terminals of the battery are connected and the electrons can transfer from one to the other terminal until the electrodes are entirely consumed. This enables the use of the battery as a voltage source.

The electrode double layer

The electrode potential has consequences for the surface of the electrode. Water molecules have a strong electrical dipole moment. Consequently, they orientate under the influence of the electrode potential so that their dipole adapts relative to the polarity of the electrode surface. This orientation is an extremely fast process and quickly results in a layer of water molecules attached to the electrode surface. It is followed by the (slower) movement of charged ions (to a different extent, ions are surrounded by water molecules, i.e., they are hydrated[b]) toward the electrode, attracted by the electric field caused by the electrode potential. At physiological concentrations, such chemical reactions result in a **Helmholtz-Debye double layer** (bilayer) at the surface of the charged electrode (Fig. 5.3). The first layer of the double-layer is the consequence of the fast orientation of water molecules; this layer is adsorbed to the metal surface and may additionally include ions from the electrolyte or products of the chemical reaction between the metal and the electrolyte. The second layer consists of ions that are more or less concentrated than they are in the overall solution (called *excess* and *deficiency ions*, respectively). This layer is much more mobile, since it is only attracted by electrical forces (under the influence of thermal motion). The layers may quickly change if the electrode potential is changed. The water dipoles may turn 180 degrees and the ions may be released or additionally attracted.

[b] E.g., sodium is a highly hydrated ion, whereas potassium is less hydrated.

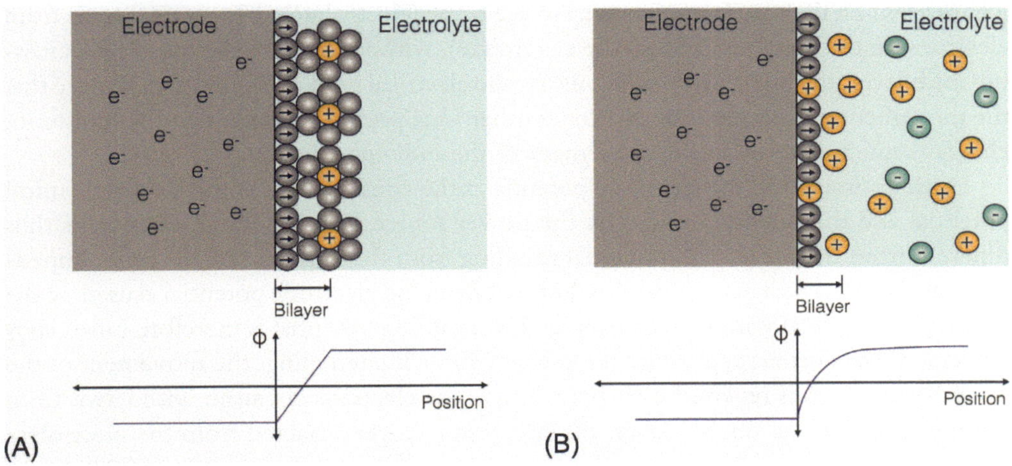

Fig. 5.3 The metal electrode-electrolyte boundary is usually characterized by chemical reactions with the consequent buildup of a double layer of water molecules and ions of the electrolyte. When measuring the electrical potential across the barrier, one may register a change of potential through the bilayer over a distance of the dimension of few molecules. (A) The original Helmholtz model with linear change in potential over the electrode-electrolyte interface. (B) At low concentrations the situation is better described by the Gouy-Chapman model, with nonlinear change in potential across the barrier and bigger bilayer dimension. This model also includes dependence of bilayer thickness on concentration of the electrolyte. For details, see **Chapter 10**.

The bilayer at the surface of an electrode can electrically be considered as a charged capacitor. The capacitor consists of two conductive plates and a non-conductive dielectric. In this analogy, one plate represents the charged metal, and the other plate represents the second layer of the bilayer (the excess and deficiency ions layer). The electric current that is applied via the lead wire can charge and discharge this capacitor. There is no exchange of material between the plates of the capacitor (the dielectric between the plates is not conductive). Therefore, transfer of current is indirect; changing the charge on one plate of the capacitor sets charges on the other plate free or attracts new ones, generating a current there. This is the concept of *capacitive (displacement) currents*. Let us now assume that the electrode potential that has built up is positive. If now the electrode is connected to a power source,[c] further electrons arrive at the metal side of the double layer. They reduce the electrode potential and thus the electrical field that is generated in the electrolyte. Consequently, some of the ions that form the second, mobile layer of the double-layer become free and detach from the bilayer. They represent a physical current that is delivered to the tissue. This effect transfers the current from the electrode into the electrolyte, but does not include transfer of material between the metal and the electrolyte.

[c] The reactions described here are in fact identical for a voltage or a current source.

The current on the way from the metal to the tissue (electrolyte) changes its carriers from electrons (in the metal) to ions (in the electrolyte), without any particles physically crossing the bilayer; the bilayer is crossed only by the electrical field. It is important to note that the movement of ions repulses or attracts other ions, and so on, such that the transfer of charge is much faster than the movement of the individual ions.

During stimulation the electrode potential is the consequence of the electrochemical potential and the potential added by the power source. The resulting potential is thus different from the theoretical potential resulting from the current and electrode impedance (as Ohm's law dictates), but also different from the electrode potential caused by the contact of the metal with the electrolyte. The resulting potential is therefore called *overpotential*. If the current applied by the power source is alternating, the movement of the electrons and ions is reversed over time, and as the electrons are again withdrawn from the metal side of the double-layer, the negative ions get attracted from the electrolyte again; the overpotential reverses polarity.

Electrodes forming a Helmholtz-Debye bilayer have the disadvantage of electric instability; the bilayer can be easily disturbed by many influences. Two electrodes of the same material, when connected, may show fluctuating non-zero voltage. This is particularly the case with zinc and platinum that have the tendency for the greatest electrical instability. The electrical instability may come from local processes but also *chemical contamination* with other substances that even in smallest concentrations may generate a galvanic element and cause currents to flow between the two contacts. In clinical applications the presence of two differently composed materials in the tissue is a serious complication with side effects (e.g., pain). Therefore, purity of materials is key in any medical application.[d]

In practical application and using several electrodes, different electrode potentials may thus result in DC current flowing between electrodes. This might cause stimulation of neurons, but also could corrode the electrodes. To prevent build-up of different potentials on different electrodes of the implant, causing unwanted currents between different electrodes, the standard approach is to short the unused electrodes together and connect them with the casing of the pulse generators. (N.B. There is of course no ground lead in the active, moving human subject.)

The bilayer can become unstable also due to local effects like *mechanical influences* (e.g., convection or movement), or due to *biological and chemical reactions* (e.g., those caused by inflammation). These may seriously affect the electrode function. Mechanical movement affects the bilayer, causing noise in the recordings or, with stimulation electrodes, is a source of instability in the resistance and its frequency characteristics.

[d] In experimental neuroscience with recording electrodes, this may manifest as fluctuating noise. It has been a rule to short-circuit the working and reference contacts from time to time to eliminate this effect and obtain cleaner signals.

Mechanical effects cause the well-known movement artifacts in recording from behaving subjects. Unfortunately, these occur in the frequency range that is of interest for the recorded signals, too, and are therefore a serious complication. One potential work-around is the use of **recessed electrodes** with conductive electrode gels connecting skin and the electrode. The bilayer is then formed by the contact of the gel and the electrode and not the electrode and the body. Also all chemical processes will then take place between the gel and the electrode. The gel forms a conductive flexible bridge to the tissue where recording would otherwise take place; it reduces the mechanical consequences of movement, given that the gel is highly flexible and to some extent can maintain a good conductive contact even if the tissue surface is subject to movement. This ensures that the bilayer, developed between the electrode and the gel, is displaced from the moving surface and thus is much less affected by movement. Placing filter paper soaked in an electrolyte between the electrode and the surface of the recorded tissue (skin) may also alleviate movement artifacts by the same principle. Artifact-free recording has been of key importance (e.g., in aeronautics). However, these techniques for reduced movement artifacts cannot be directly applied to microelectrodes.

Electrodes that with stimulation behave like an ideal capacitor, that is, there is no charge transfer across the bilayer (or, in the electric model, across the dielectric of the capacitor), are called **polarized electrodes**. These electrodes show only capacitive (displacement) currents. The term polarized comes from the fact that stimulation current solely increases (or decreases) the voltage across the plates of the capacitor (there is no current between the plates of the capacitor), and thus polarizes the capacitor. Electrodes that lead to physical charge transfer between the electrode and the electrolyte (thus, current flows through the dielectric of the capacitor) are **non-polarized electrodes**. However, as we show later, ideal polarized and non-polarized electrodes are only theoretical concepts; electrodes used in reality have their properties somewhere in between these theoretical extremes.

Electric models of the double layer

To better understand the consequence of bilayer formation, and to be able to make quantitative predictions about the behavior of the polarized electrodes, scientists have developed electrical models of the electrode-tissue interface. Numerous historic studies concentrated on the electrical properties of the electrode-tissue interface. These models have been confirmed by comparing them to the real behavior of electrodes. Using such models, it is possible to analyze the electrical behavior of the stimulation device and the electrode in one circuit diagram.

The outcome of these studies is the equivalent circuit for polarized electrodes (Fig. 5.4). The metal resistance of the wires connecting the electrode to the current source,

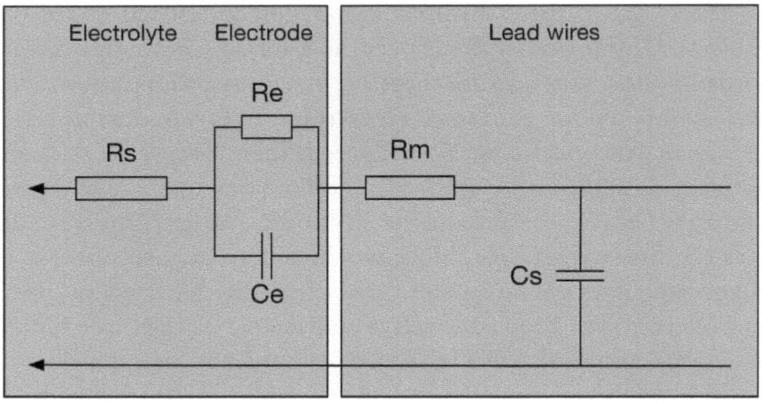

Fig. 5.4 Equivalent circuit for a recording or stimulation electrode. R_s, series resistance; R_e, leakage resistance; R_m, metal resistance; C_e, capacitance of the bilayer; C_s, capacitance of lead wires.

designated R_m in Fig. 5.4, is very low and will not be considered further. The remaining resistances called **leakage resistance** (R_e) and **series resistance** (R_s) are important particularly for polarized electrodes. The capacitance of the connecting lead wires and the insulating materials (C_s) becomes important for small high-frequency signals and relatively long lead wires, particularly in polarized electrodes. This is of lesser importance for the present subject and will not be considered in further detail here.

The parallel capacitor C_e and resistor R_e represent the electrical properties of the double-layer. As mentioned in **Chapter 4**, the circuit consisting of a resistance and capacitance is called an *RC circuit*. Technically, the series and the leakage resistance are required to explain the electrical behavior of the electrode-tissue interface. Under direct current stimulation, some current can pass through the electrode which a capacitor alone would not allow. That would require the leakage resistor to be in parallel. Furthermore, with alternating current stimulation at very high frequencies, the resistance is not zero (as would be predicted by a capacitor alone), implicating the need for a series resistance. In total, two resistors are needed, one in series and one in parallel to the capacitance of the double-layer (C_e). For direct current stimulation, the summed resistance of both leakage and series resistance becomes important; for very high frequency stimulation the capacitance acts as a short-circuit and only the series resistance is important.

A crucial property of the electrode is the capacitance. It acts as an infinite resistor for direct current stimulation (that cannot pass the capacitor) and short-circuits at high frequencies. Due to the existence of the capacitor in the model (i.e., the bilayer in reality), the behavior of the electrode contact is dependent on the frequency of the signals (Fig. 5.5). The maximum resistance reached at low frequencies (direct currents) is due to the sum of series and leakage resistance (for direct currents, the capacitor isolates), whereas the asymptote at high frequencies is defined by series resistance alone (for high

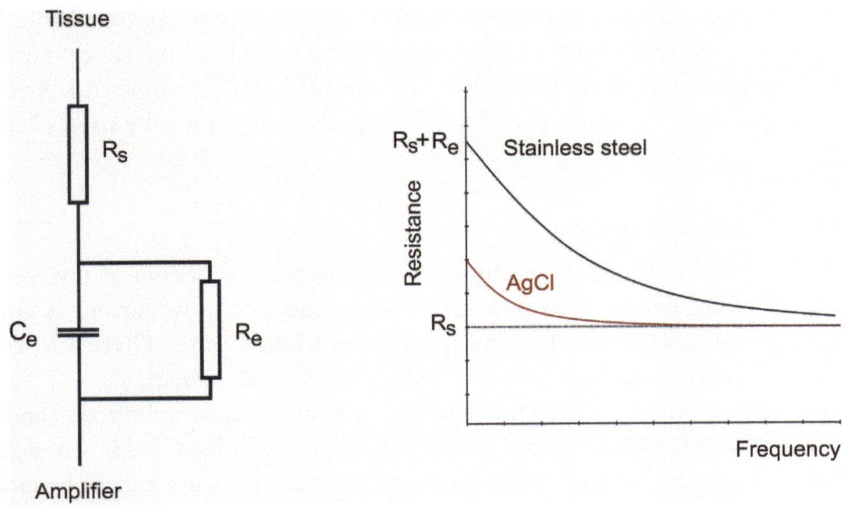

Fig. 5.5 Tissue-electrode interface of a polarized electrode. Series (R_s) and leakage (R_e) resistance in the equivalent circuit and their influence on the frequency response in a stainless steel electrode. In *brown*, a silver chloride electrode is shown with lower impedance but same size.

frequencies, the capacitor is a short-circuit bypassing the leakage resistance). The capacitance of the electrode also means that the stimulating electrical field will be shaped in the frequency domain at the electrode/electrolyte interface.

The ideal polarized electrode has an infinite leakage (R_e) resistance and therefore cannot conduct direct currents at all (at 0 Hz resistance would be infinite in the plot in Fig. 5.5 for such materials). The ideal non-polarized electrode, on the other hand, has a zero leakage (R_e) resistance (no bilayer, therefore the capacitance is short-cut) and therefore flat frequency characteristics. Pragmatically, all electrodes lie somewhere between these idealized cases depending on the material of the electrode.

"Ideal" non-polarized electrodes are rare; one example is silver electrodes placed in silver ion solution. The silver ions in the electrolyte serve as electron recipients. Unfortunately, silver ions are toxic and therefore these electrodes cannot be used in tissue. A common highly (but not ideal) non-polarized electrode is a *silver/silver chloride* (Ag/AgCl) electrode. Here a layer of silver chloride is deposited on the surface of the silver electrode, and this acts as a recipient of the electrons. The advantage of this sandwich electrode is that chloride is one of the naturally occurring components of extracellular fluid. Deposition of silver chloride on silver electrodes, *chloridization* of the electrodes, can be achieved through DC current as electrodeposition, or much slower by simply immersing the electrodes into a solution containing chloride ions. Chloridization substantially decreases the impedance of the electrode and flattens the frequency dependence of impedance, moving the electrode into the non-polarized region of electrodes. The electrode potential of this electrode compared to a SHE is small but measurable. While these electrodes are ideal for recording, silver is essentially toxic and degrades over time when used for stimulation. Therefore Ag/AgCl electrodes are usable only for acute stimulation purposes, but cannot be used chronically in the tissue.

Crossing the double layer

After we have learned about the complex electrochemical processes at the electrode–electrolyte interface, we need to return to the question of how current is conveyed through the bilayer and discuss it using the acquired knowledge. There are two ways for the current to cross the barrier from metal to electrolyte (tissue):

(i) By redistribution of ions within the solution, without any chemical reaction and charge transfer between the electrode and the electrolyte. As mentioned, this is very similar to a capacitor where the dielectric between the plates of the capacitor cannot be crossed by charges physically, but the electric field can cross it and cause charges to move. In other words, in the tissue-electrode interface the electrical field generated by the electrode causes some ions in the solution to redistribute. Such processes are called **non-Faradaic reactions.**

(ii) By crossing of electrons through the electrode-electrolyte barrier. Such processes are called **Faradaic reactions**. In the electric model, the current flows here through the leakage resistance only and bypasses the capacitor. As will be shown, Faradaic reactions are observed in non-polarized electrodes and in polarized electrodes at higher currents.[e]

It is key to differentiate these two alternatives, since the ultimate consequence of Faradaic reactions can be an oxidation or reduction of substances in the solution and of the electrode. This can be harmful for the tissue, as discussed in the next chapter.

Brief summary

- Artificial electrical stimulation is performed using current sources.
- Metal electrodes polarize in the tissue, generating an electrochemical double-layer and an electrode potential.
- The double layer can be modeled by an electrical capacitor.
- The electrode-electrolyte barrier corresponds to an RC circuit.
- Ideal polarized and non-polarized electrodes are theoretical concepts, but all electrodes share some form of polarized and non-polarized properties.
- Electrons can cross the electrode-electrolyte barrier through leakage resistance.

[e] However, the ideal polarized electrode with infinite leakage resistance cannot show any Faradaic reaction and thus is a purely capacitive electrode.

Key literature and further reading

Cogan, S.F., 2008. Neural stimulation and recording electrodes. Annu. Rev. Biomed. Eng. 10, 275–309.

Cogan, S.F., Garrett, D.J., Green, R.A., 2016. Electrochemical principles of safe current injection. In: Shepherd, R.K. (Ed.), Neurobionics. John Wiley & Sons, Inc., Hoboken, New Jersey, pp. 55–88.

Geddes, L.A., Baker, L.E., 1989. Principles of Applied Biomedical Instrumentation. John Wiley & Sons, Inc., Hoboken, NJ.

Horch, K.W., Gurpeet, D.S., 2004. Neuroprosthetics: Theory and Practice. World Scientific Publishing Co., Singapore.

Kandel, E.R., Schartz, J.H., Jessel, T.M., Siegelbaum, S.A., Hudspeth, A.J., 2012. Principles of Neural Science. McGraw-Hill Education Ltd., New York.

Merrill, D.R., 2010. The electrochemistry of charge injection at the electrode/tissue interface. In: Zhou, D., Greenbaum, E. (Eds.), Implantable Prostheses 2: Techniques and Engineering Approaches. Springer Verlag, pp. 86–135.

CHAPTER 6

Artificial electrical stimulation: Principles, efficacy, and safety

Electric fields surround an electric charge and are characterized by the existence of force generated by the electric charge. The consequence of the force is the movement of other charged particles within the field. In **Chapter 5** we already introduced the problem of charge delivery into the tissue. An electric field that is generated by a voltage source can change the extracellular potential of the neurons and in turn activate ionic channels. A problem with a voltage source from the view of neuroprosthetic is the lack of control of the effect size; the voltage source maintains a constant voltage at the electrode, that is, before the Helmholtz-Debye bilayer, and not behind it (in the electrolyte and the tissue). The measured voltage therefore does not reflect the voltage in the tissue, but rather only the potential of the electrode. Electrode impedance changes, like those caused by forming the double layer or by tissue reaction to the implant and the implantation (**Chapter 8**), thus affect the electric field in the tissue substantially. In case of a voltage source (Box 5.1), if the load resistance and the capacitance vary (due to impedance changes of the electrode), given the voltage is constant, it follows from Ohm's law that the current will vary and the amount of charge delivered to the tissue will vary correspondingly. The previous chapter more extensively summarized the reasons why current sources are the optimal choice for neuroprosthetic applications. This chapter describes the consequences of this choice.

Charge, current, and thresholds

Current source stimulation delivers a stimulus independent of impedance. However, with sinusoidal currents, perceptual thresholds systematically vary with stimulus frequency (Fig. 6.1). This can be explained by the delivered charge that decreases with increasing frequency (the area under the curve, i.e., the integral of the sinusoidal function, decreases with increasing frequency). The theoretical consideration would predict a doubling in perceptual thresholds with doubling frequency (6 dB per octave[a]), but in fact such functions slightly deviate from this prediction and increase less steeply (ca. 4 dB/octave). This is due to the leakiness of the neuronal membrane; not all charge delivered to the tissue can cause excitation (see strength-duration curves in **Chapter 4**, Fig. 4.9).

[a] Octave corresponds to doubling of frequency.

Prostheses for the Brain
https://doi.org/10.1016/B978-0-12-818892-7.00008-0

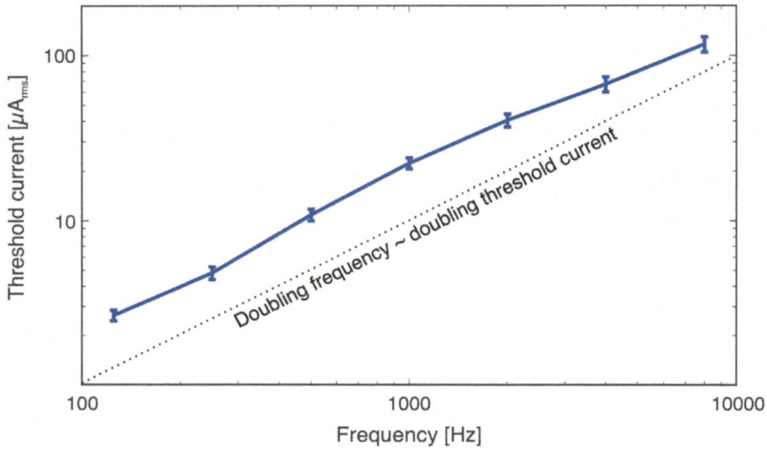

Fig. 6.1 Perceptual threshold currents approximately double with doubling frequency. This is the consequence of the charge delivered and is observed in all forms of electrical stimulation and in all neuronal targets. This example is cat orientation reflex thresholds with cochlear implant stimulation using sinusoidal currents. Shown are means with standard error (10 cats; Kral et al., 2013). Similar effects are also observed with pulsatile stimulation (see **Chapter 11**).

As explained in **Chapter 5**, the ability of electric current to stimulate neurons is dependent on the temporal properties of the neuronal membrane that are in turn dependent on the membrane time constant. From this point of view, the properties of the stimulation current must consider this temporal behavior of neurons.

If the current changes are slow, the ions in the intracellular and extracellular space have enough time to rearrange through the leakage channels, and the responsiveness will be less (this occurs below the frequency range shown in Fig. 6.1). They will reach an equilibrium reflected by the Nernst and Goldman-Hodgkin-Katz equations. The extracellular potential will increase (or decrease, depending on the direction of the stimulation current), but the intracellular potential will change accordingly, with a near-constant transmembrane potential. That will preclude the opening of voltage-sensitive channels. The process is called *accommodation* and is further discussed in **Chapter 7**. Therefore the changes in the time function of the stimulating current must be large and fast enough to make an effect on excitation.

Pulsatile stimulation with steep current changes at onset and offset of the pulse is therefore a good and efficient alternative for sinusoidal charge-balanced stimulation. It is used in all modern conventional devices. Using pulsatile stimulation, interleaved multi-electrode stimulation is possible without electrical interference of one stimulus on the other.

With pulsatile stimulation, energetic efficiency of stimulation is highest if the pulse duration is similar to the chronaxie of the target neurons. For both shorter and longer pulses, stimulation becomes less efficient either due to the open leak channels of the neuronal membrane or due to capacitive effects. For practical reasons (e.g., high-frequency multichannel stimulation), energetically less efficient approaches have been used. The relation of efficiency and chronaxie may be used to stimulate one target neuron compared to another, provided they have different chronaxies. This way a given pulse duration may target primarily those neurons that have a similar chronaxie and thus increase the specificity of the electrical stimulus.

The relationship shown in Fig. 6.1 has to be considered when using alternating current of different frequencies for stimulation and when variable pulse duration is used (which has similar effects as increasing the period of a sinusoidal stimulus). The relationship therefore represents an important general property of electrostimulation.

Materials for electrostimulation

Neural prosthetics are often expected to remain functional in the body for many years or decades and are in close contact with particularly fragile tissues. Therefore, they have stringent *biocompatibility* requirements. Animal studies have investigated tissue reaction in response to chronic implantation of electrodes (Table 6.1). Some metals induced significantly greater reaction to the electrode following chronic implantation compared to single acute puncture into the brain with the same electrode material; usually, after

Table 6.1 Review of metal properties for chronic electrostimulation.

Metal	Toxicity	Biostability	Electrode potential (V)
Aluminum	Toxic	Low	−1.66
Copper	Toxic	Low	0.34
Gold	Biocompatible	High	1.45
Iron	Toxic	Low	−0.44
Molybdenum	Reactive	Low	−0.15
Platinum/Platinum-iridium	Biocompatible	High	1.20
Platinum black (platinized platinum)	Reactive	Low	1.20
Silver	Toxic	Low	0.80
Silver chloride	Toxic	Low	0.22
Stainless steel	Biocompatible	Low	from −0.10 to −0.44[b]
Tantalum	Reactive	High	−0.60
Tungsten	Biocompatible	High	−0.58
Titanium	Biocompatible	High	−1.63
Zinc	Biocompatible	Low	−0.76

Toxicity refers to the property of causing local or systemic damage. "Toxic" represents such a reaction, "Reactive" refers here to local tissue reaction like gliosis, and "Biocompatible" means that the material does not cause any reaction beyond the implantation trauma. "Biostability" refers to degradation of the material in the body. Electrode potentials were measured at 25°C, 101,325 Pa, and 1 mol solution against a standard hydrogen electrode.

chronic stimulation these were encapsulated by scar (glial) tissue. This *foreign body reaction*, is caused by the immune system and glia after recognizing a foreign body in the brain (**Chapter 8**). The glial scar can create a "dead zone" that raises impedances and stimulation thresholds. *Toxic effects* are intense reactions involving considerable cell death. Less intense are *reactive effects*, referring to a local connective tissue reaction after passive implantation. Reactivity is considered absent if normal nervous tissue is observed within a certain distance (usually dozens of micrometers) from the electrode. However, different authors use different criteria and terms to refer to brain reaction to prosthetic devices. Another important factor to consider is *biostability*. Here we use it to denote if the material itself will degrade by the reaction of the body to its presence. Reactive and toxic materials are not suitable for chronic electro-stimulation, but they may be usable for acute studies.

Stainless steel,[b] while used in some short-term medical applications (e.g., bone screws) for example, is known to undergo chemical reactions over longer periods of time in the body. Stainless steel material therefore needs to be removed after months of use. Furthermore, current stimulation may lead to accelerated corrosion of stainless steel. Platinum, when electroplated with platinum microparticles, shows dramatically greater electrode capacitance than untreated platinum. Electroplating to increase surface area at the microscopic level also causes increased light absorption so that the surface turns black. As such, this material is known as *platinum black* and was designed by chemists to allow high chemical reactivity of the platinum due to enlarged surface. The high capacitance of platinum black is a favorable property, as it increases the range of currents that can be delivered as capacitive currents. The material, despite this property, is unfortunately not chronically biostable; the loose platinum particles at the plated surface are easily wiped off and released into the tissue. Platinum ions are toxic. Therefore platinum black is not suitable for stimulation purposes.[c] Aside from metal electrodes, other materials have also been used in physiology. For example, carbon or graphite (which are highly conductive) have also been used as recording electrodes due to their low noise, particularly as microelectrodes in multi-barrel electrodes. They are not suitable as chronically implanted stimulating electrodes because they decompose under electric stimulation.

So far, *gold*, *platinum*, *titanium*, and *tungsten* are the only materials proven biostable for stimulation applications.

In summary, the metal used for neuroprosthetic devices should be *biocompatible* in the sense that the material alone does not evoke a significant response in the surrounding

[b] The exact chemical composition of stainless steel depends on the fabrication process and can vary. Therefore, both electrode potential and other properties differ in different publications.

[c] Nanoporous platinum has recently been tested as an alternative to increase the capacitance but preserve the connection of the platinum molecules with the platinum contact. This substance is also black but does not have loose particles at the surface.

tissue or the body that would indicate it being toxic. Table 6.1 summarizes the key properties of the most common metals in prosthetics.

Other essential aspects for electrostimulation are the electrochemical reactions occurring on the surface of a metal electrode. They strongly depend on the metal itself and the composition of the electrolyte. Depending on these properties, the electrode potentials vary. Electrode potentials are important for charge transfer into the tissue and the capacity of currents delivered via capacitive effects. For recording electrodes, particularly if low-frequency signals have to be measured, the polarization of the electrode is an important confounding factor.

Silver chloride (AgCl) has a low electrode potential. One particular advantage of this material is the abundance of chloride ions in the tissue that attach to the surface of silver and generate an electrode-tissue interface consisting of a layer of silver, and a layer of silver chloride surrounded by chloride. This sandwich structure allows small electrode potentials, and is sometimes considered a highly non-polarizing material. Additionally, due to this structure, the electrical instability of the electrode-tissue interface mentioned in **Chapter 5** and expressed in fluctuations of the electrode potentials are extremely small for Ag/AgCl electrodes (only 0.2 mV under optimal conditions). This small electrode potential also reflects the fact that, considering the equivalent RC circuit (Fig. 5.4), capacitance plays less of a role in the properties of the Ag/AgCl electrode. In consequence, when using the same material for the working and the reference electrode, Ag/AgCl is an excellent material for recording biopotentials. Unfortunately, Ag/AgCl is toxic in long-term use and therefore not available for clinical neuroprosthetic applications. Furthermore, when stimulation is considered, the low electrode potential also means that the capacitance of the bilayer is low and that has disadvantageous consequences for capacitive stimulation. This is an example of why ideal recording electrodes are not necessarily optimal stimulation electrodes and vice versa.

Another complication arising indirectly from polarization and electrode potentials is related to the measurement of electrode impedances. This is important for checking the integrity of the devices in clinical applications (**Chapter 8**), for which a reference electrode is required. Neither a "standard hydrogen electrode" nor Ag/AgCl counter electrodes are a possible practical choice. A larger surface area of the counter electrode (at least ten times larger than the working electrode) may diminish its influence on the overall measured impedance. Therefore, in some applications, the housing of the implanted device is used as the counter electrode to determine electrode impedances. The housing of many stimulation devices (pacemakers and neuroprostheses) is made of titanium, whereas the electrodes are made of platinum. In itself, this configuration with two different metals would constitute a galvanic element with DC potential differences generated between housing and electrodes. However, titanium has the peculiar property that it quickly oxidizes and generates an electrically insulating layer on the surface of the casing (called *passivation*). By that, the casing is isolated from the tissue and DC current is minimal with titanium. (Covering the casing with a thin layer of platinum is an alternative solution.)

Additional to the biocompatibility of the metal itself, biocompatibility of the insulating materials in medical applications needs to be considered. A substantial part of the body's reaction to the electrode can be the consequence of the insulating material. Previous studies have proven the biocompatibility of silicone, Teflon (with high purity only!), alumina ceramic, polyethylene, and polypropylene. However, Teflon may slightly increase in volume over time and is not suitable in applications where mechanical stress is imposed on the implanted device (particles can be released into the tissue and cause inflammation). A material frequently used in medicine, Dacron, is strictly speaking also not biostable over very long periods of time (years). It is important to note that inert materials are required for insulating the lead wires connecting the electrode to the current source. These insulations are most frequently made of silicone, but in some cases they are made of Teflon or parylene. The latter material, while having the advantage of being able to make a thin surface coating, is not perfectly stable over a long time and may show cracks and become degraded in living tissue.

Faradaic charge transfer

With increasing current and duration of the electric stimulation, additional possible reactions on the electrode surface (*faradaic effects*) also need to be considered. With longer duration of current flow, such as in direct current stimulation, faradaic chemical reactions are in fact an unavoidable consequence. In general, these reactions are the result of electrons leaving the electrode surface and entering the tissue due to the stimulating electrical current.

The reactions caused by the release of electrons from the electrode can be reversible or irreversible. Reversible reactions can be effectively and completely reversed if the stimulus polarity reverses; then all substances return to their original state. Reversible reactions, provided no toxic products appear, do not represent a problem for stimulation. If the stimulation is balanced between positive and negative currents (i.e., there are no direct current components involved), the electrons that left the electrode during one phase can return back in the other phase.

Depending on the electrode material and the electrolyte, different types of chemical reactions may take place at the electrode surface with faradaic charge transfer. Because of the present focus on biocompatible materials, we consider only materials suitable for electrical stimulation (active electrodes). With respect to material and reversible faradaic reactions, iridium oxide and platinum are the materials used for stimulation electrodes. Examples of reversible reactions with platinum include *oxide formation*

$$H_2O + Pt \rightarrow PtO + 2H^+ + 2e^-$$

$$Ir + 2\,H_2O \rightarrow Ir(OH)_2 + 2\,H^+ + 2\,e^-$$

or metal hydrogen complex formation (*H-atom-plating*)

$$Pt + e^- + H^+ \rightarrow Pt - H$$

$$Pt + H_2O + e^- \rightarrow Pt - H + OH^-$$

For these reversible reactions under charge-balanced AC stimulation, the products of these reactions are reversed before they can diffuse into the electrolyte and cause damage. However, if they remain in the electrolyte for a sufficient time, diffusion may alter the concentrations next to the electrode. For example, the accumulation of H^+ may lead to pH changes of larger magnitude in the electrolyte. Such pH changes have adverse consequences that can alter the function of or damage the tissue.

Irreversible reactions, on the other hand, are a problem since they permanently change the materials of the electrode and the electrolyte, leading to decomposition (dissolution) of the electrode over time. Delamination (splitting of the electrode into layers as described in **Chapter 3**) can also occur in iridium oxide. These reactions can create products that are highly reactive (like oxygen radicals) or become irreversible because a part of the products leaves the solution (e.g., when forming a gas). Reversible reactions can become irreversible (e.g., in situations when one product is removed from the solution and is no longer available for the reverse chemical process, as can happen if there is fluid flow around the electrode). While often the pathophysiology of tissue damage has not been clarified mechanistically, it is assumed that some electrochemical products (e.g., oxygen radicals) that result from irreversible reactions can accumulate over time, and eventually become toxic for the tissue.

At the cathode in the irreversible case, electrons may be transferred from the electrode to the electrolyte (tissue). Consequently, water reduction may appear, with *hydrogen gas formation* (in blue)

$$2\,H_2O + 2e^- \rightarrow H_2 + 2\,OH^-$$

This reaction is irreversible since the hydrogen is a gas that leaves the solution if present in sufficient concentration (that is no longer soluble). It can become toxic for the tissue due to the alkaline product; again, the amount makes the difference. In case of existing iron (Fe^{3+}) or copper ions (Cu^{2+}) in the solution, these can also become reduced (can gain electrons). In the case of copper, this leads to metal deposition on the electrode ($Cu^{2+} + 2\,e^- \rightarrow Cu$). Finally, reduction of platinum- or iridium-oxides in the solution can take place. However, short current pulses may release only a small amount of hydrogen that remains dissolved in the fluid and thus stay reversible (particularly if it does not diffuse out of the Helmholtz-Debye bilayer).

For the anode (the positively charged electrode), a set of irreversible oxidation processes can take place, the most important being the *oxidation of water*:

$$2\,H_2O \rightarrow O_2 + 4H^+ + 4e^-$$

This process is irreversible due to the appearance of a gas that leaves the solution (but again can still remain reversible if only small amounts of oxygen are produced that stay dissolved in the solution/tissue). Furthermore, the reaction is toxic due to acidification of the tissue and appearance of highly reactive electrons and protons. Oxygen in an acidic environment can also form H_2O_2, which is highly toxic for tissue. Another anodic irreversible reaction is the *corrosion of platinum electrodes* by the generation of stable platinum complexes:

$$Pt + 4\,Cl^- \rightarrow [PtCl_4]^{2-} + 2\,e^-$$

Finally, gas generation is also possible at the anode due to *oxidation of chloride ions*:

$$2\,Cl^- \rightarrow Cl_2 + 2\,e^-$$

Here the reaction may be irreversible due to the escape of chloride gas from the solution. Chloride itself can have toxic effects in tissue.

If the anode is made of iron, a *dissolution of the electrode* can additionally take place, since the resulting iron ions are soluble:

$$Fe \rightarrow Fe^{2+} + 2\,e^-$$

These reactions may limit the use of a certain material for stimulation, and more importantly set technical limits for stimulation with a given material. Reactions typically start occurring from voltages of $\pm$1–2 V with platinum electrodes where a "*water window*" is exceeded (reactions involving water hydrolysis, i.e., oxide formation and oxidation of water); O_2 and platinum oxide (PtO) are the first typical products. PtO is typically reduced back to Pt when present in the tissue.

It is important to note that loss of electrons from the electrode itself does not directly affect the electrode and does not chemically change it, since the source of the electrons is the current source and every lost electron will be replaced from the current source. Rather, electrode corrosion requires a chemical reaction at the electrode like those mentioned here. As previously discussed, remaining free electrons in the solution may bind to other substances and make them reactive, and this can damage tissue as well.

AC/DC stimulation

The electrical stimulation mode is important for preventing harmful effects at the electrode surface. Direct current stimulation will pass the bilayer (and thus bypass the capacitor in the electric model through the leakage resistance) and transport charged particles in one or the other direction depending on their charge. Due to this, the concentrations at the electrodes accumulate over time and cause irreversible damage to both electrodes and the tissue. Such reactions are well known, and neuroscience has been using them for many decades to document the position of a recording microelectrode. A few μA of DC current for *15s* is already sufficient to leave histologically observable tissue damage.

John C. Lilly (1915–2001) was the first to propose the use of charge-balanced electrical stimulation. Using alternating currents, the effects on the tissue in one phase of the stimulus could be reversed in the other phase and thus damage to the target structure caused by the electrical stimulation was minimized. It is clear that alternating currents can best exploit the capacitive charge stored in the double-layer and can make best use of reversible faradaic effects to safely transfer charge to the tissue.

Charge-balancing means that the time structure of the positive and negative areas is balanced; the stimulus has exactly the same time integrals during positive and negative currents. In other words, the amount of positive charge transferred is exactly the same as the amount of negative charges transferred. This sounds obvious, but it is not, as tiny amounts of charge imbalance during stimulation can sum up over time to significant chemical effect. The simplest way to achieve charge balance is to insert a capacitor between the current source and the electrode. By doing so, each direct current component is filtered out by the high-pass properties of the capacitor. The problem with this approach is the size minimization in clinical applications, as the capacitor requires some space. Other less-secure options include short-circuiting the electrodes that are in a non-active state to the casing of the implants.

In summary, a desirable stimulation electrode material should:

- be biocompatible (i.e., should not be toxic for tissue or be degraded by reactions of the body to the material),
- have a high capacitance, allowing safe injection of charge into tissue even with a small electrode surface area,
- only generate reversible faradaic reactions at high charge densities (and irreversible reactions at even higher densities),
- only generate products of reversible faradaic reactions that are non-toxic.

Safety limits

There are two main factors that require consideration with respect to safety limits: (1) reversibility of the faradaic reactions and (2) the toxicity of the products that result from faradaic reactions. Some materials can generate products that are very toxic, but some products are less toxic and therefore the tissue can tolerate greater concentrations. Nonetheless, all non-reversible faradaic reactions cause corrosion of the electrode material, and this is an effect to avoid in practical applications to ensure long-term stability of the electrodes.

Thresholds at which these occur are very material dependent and not directly related to each other. Thus some materials might have the potential to generate very toxic products (like platinum), but at such high current levels that are never reached in practical applications, and thus are safe. On the other hand, even non-toxic products can become a problem, as the corresponding reactions corrode the electrode and change the electrolyte. Thus, if irreversible reactions occur at low current, even if non-toxic, it prevents the use of that material for chronic stimulation.

One possibility is to prevent any charge transfer between electrode and tissue and exploit **capacitive effects**. This means that it is only the capacitance of the surface bilayer that is charged and discharged and that generates currents in the tissue. Current only leaves the electrode through the capacitance and none through the leakage resistance. The dielectric of the capacitor is unchanged. Using such *capacitive electrodes* provides sufficient current for stimulation if the electrode has a very large surface area.[d] Practically, the stimulation thresholds are near the upper limit of the sole capacitive effects in the vast majority of applications. Thus, even if using biocompatible materials and using charge-balanced stimulation (e.g., charge-balanced pulses), faradaic reactions cannot be avoided in practical applications. The capacitance of the electrodes is based on a layer of water molecules; by the short distance of the bilayer ($\sim$1 nm at physiologic concentrations) the corresponding capacitance is high (10–20 $\mu F/cm^2$). Currents can destroy the bilayer, leading to a **dielectric breakdown**. Due to the small size of the bilayer, the breakdown occurs already at current densities of 3 $\mu C/cm^2$. At dielectric breakdown, the dielectric becomes conductive, the capacitance is lost, and faradaic (chemical) reactions are the ultimate consequence. This is thus the moment when the capacitance of the bilayer is overcome and the leakage resistance becomes the decisive factor in stimulation. With some materials (e.g., tantalum pentoxide) much higher limits for dielectric breakdown have been reported than for platinum. These therefore function as capacitive electrodes and have the advantage that their faradaic reactions are limited. However, tantalum has not yet found a clinical application.

If faradaic reactions are confined to the bilayer and do not corrode the electrode or generate highly reactive products, these faradaic reactions are reversible and do not damage the tissue. Tissue damage is thus dependent on the amount of current passed through the bilayer and the maximum **charge delivery capacity** of the material, defined as a sum of all reactions that contribute to charge transfer on the electrode. One simple quantification of the charge delivery capacity of a material is to apply current until a certain safe voltage (e.g., 1 V) at the electrode is reached, and then determine the amount of charge that passed through the electrode area.[e] The more charge that is possible to pass through the electrode, the greater the charge delivery capacity.

[d] For this reason, increasing the surface of the electrodes is a safe way of increasing the delivery of charges to the tissue. Many research attempts therefore concentrate on increasing the area of the electrode by nanostructuring.

[e] More exact measurements of charge delivery capacity are possible with voltammetry; see **Chapter 8**.

Materials with high charge delivery capacity (iridium oxide, tantalum pentoxide, and platinum) are more suitable for electrodes since they allow effective charge transfer at operating conditions that do not approach the safety limit. Some biocompatible materials have a low charge delivery capacity and therefore their operational range for electric stimulation is narrow as safety limits are close to response thresholds. Stainless steel has a lower charge delivery capacity additional to low biostability and is therefore also not used for chronic stimulation. In some applications, alloys like Elgiloy (nickel-cobalt alloy) or cobalt-nickel-chromium-molybdenum alloys have been tested as electrode materials (Elgiloy has been also used as a cheap alternative to platinum in pacemaker electrodes). The low charge delivery capacity makes these materials not optimal for neural stimulation purposes.

Further essential variables for safety are:

- diffusion rate (how fast does the product of the faradaic reaction diffuse away from the bilayer and so potentially interact with the tissue),
- stimulation parameters (particularly the phase duration in pulsatile stimulation that determines how much time is left for the products to cause reactions),
- in case of gases the gas partial pressure and solubility coefficient of the given gas in the given condition, and
- stimulation rate (how many pulses per second are applied to one electrode, which may limit the reversibility).

With increasing current, the effects on the electrode surface may thus turn from non-faradaic capacitive (safe) effects through reversible faradaic effects (potentially unsafe) to irreversible faradaic (unsafe) effects (Fig. 6.2). The transition from reversible to irreversible effects can happen due to longer phase duration, faster pulse repetition rates, or greater current. The main goal of safety is to limit faradaic effects to reversible ones and guarantee charge balance during stimulation. As the exact limits for these effects are not clear for all combinations of stimulus characteristics, extracellular tissue composition, electrode materials, and geometries (which combined is nearly an infinite space), conservative approaches are needed to prevent harm in patients.

The preceding considerations lead to the concept of safety limits with electrical stimulation. In the following section, we focus on the material that is at present used in the vast majority of clinically implanted neuroprosthetic devices: platinum.

The limits of reversible reactions for platinum electrodes have been investigated experimentally in studies across several different laboratories. Consistently, the studies observed damaging effects of currents as a function of charge density; in other words, over a certain charge per area of the electrode, damaging effects became apparent. Tissue damage was further dependent on the type of the contact and overall charge delivered. Fig. 6.3 compiles the results of several studies. From this figure, it is obvious that with increasing charge density a greater probability of tissue damage can be observed. However, it also suggests that there is a relation between the charge density limit and the

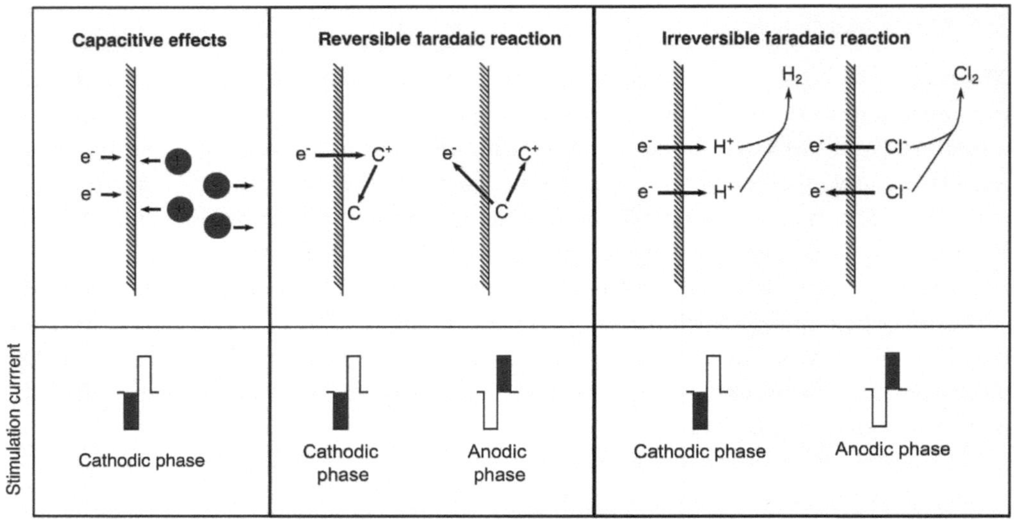

Fig. 6.2 Faradaic vs. non-faradaic charge transfer. *Left*: During the cathodic phase of a stimulus, electrons in the electrode attract positive and repel negative charges in the electrolyte. This mechanism causes current flow through the tissue in absence of a charge transfer between electrode and electrolyte. *Middle*: With faradaic effects, electrons may cross the boundary of the electrode and enter the electrolyte, where they react with cations (C). If these stay in close proximity of the electrode, during the following anodic phase on the same electrode, the electrons may reenter the electrode, with no net long-term material transfer. *Right*: If the reaction leads to fugitive products (like gases, as in the case of H_2), the products escape during the cathodic phase, are not available for the anodic phase, and the reaction is irreversible. In the anodic phase, another irreversible reaction can take place. In this case, both the material of the electrode as well as the electrolyte change over time, leading to corrosion of the electrode (here cathode) or deposition of material from the electrolyte (here anode). *(Figure based on Merrill, 2010, redrawn and extended.)*

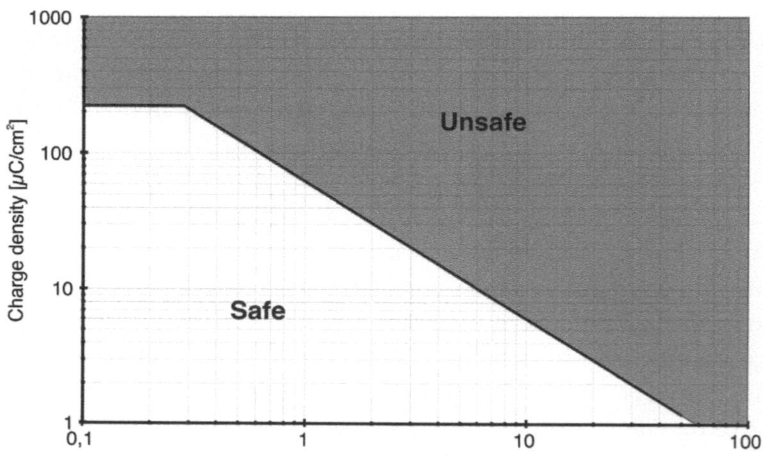

Fig. 6.3 Meta-analysis of safety studies performed on animals from different groups and using different platinum electrodes, compiled by Merrill et al. (2005) and Cogan et al. (2016). The *blue line* divides the assumed unsafe and safe region, here assuming the border of the Shannon formula by $k = 1.85$.

absolute charge delivered. The more absolute charge is delivered through the electrode, the lower the maximum safe charge density. This relation has been also questioned by some studies and remains the topic of ongoing research.

A *charge density safety limit* varies in the literature, with reversible faradaic reactions occurring from $5\,\mu C/cm^2$/phase. For cathodic stimulation a current density safety limit of $\sim J_{thr} = 100$–$150\,\mu C/cm^2$/phase has been reported. For anodic stimulation, it was even lower at $\sim J_{thr} = 50\,\mu C/cm^2$/phase. However, as discussed, the details of the pulse shape (phase duration) and repetition rate need to be taken into account. Commercial systems typically use very short phase durations ($<100\,\mu s$) and therefore even a higher limit of up to 200–$400\,\mu C/cm^2$/phase is still considered safe. Between 200 and $400\,\mu C/cm^2$ some corrosion and damage can already occur.

In practical applications it is necessary to relate the safety threshold to the excitation threshold and determine whether the safety threshold may be reached within the working range of the device. The consequence of this may be limiting the current below safety threshold or otherwise producing larger electrodes (increasing the surface area and thus safety thresholds). With regard to excitation thresholds usually observed, safety thresholds may be reached even in practical applications. For computing the radius of a round (circular) electrode for safe stimulation (r), the knowledge on the pulse duration (t), maximum required current (I), and the assumed charge density safety threshold (J_{thr}) is required. The critical diameter for circular electrodes can be computed from

$$J_{thr} = \frac{Q}{A} = \frac{I \cdot t}{\pi \cdot r^2} \Rightarrow r = \sqrt{\frac{I \cdot t}{\pi \cdot J_{thr}}}$$

Here we assume a circular electrode contact. More generally, technical literature often uses the term **geometric surface area** to describe the area used for stimulation. Complicating factors include delay between positive and negative phases of the biphasic pulse (*interphase delay or gap*) and the overall charge delivered over time (thus pulse repetition rate). These further influence safety of stimulation.

The safety limit is further affected by the actual shape of the electrode contact. The charge density equations assume a uniform electrode surface. Sharp edges of the electrodes may lead to current densities that are beyond the safety limit even though the overall charge density (charge/area) did not reach the safety limit yet. For these reasons, the active electrodes usually have a shape without edges and some companies indent the electrode contact in the silicone carrier (Fig. 6.4). As such, all edges are covered and the current density above the electrode is more homogeneous. This also helps to limit the mechanical damage to adjacent tissues. Nonetheless, even in a recessed contact the current density is higher at the sides than at the center of the contact due to geometry of the electric field, as documented in experimental and modeling studies. Thus probability of adverse reactions are most likely at the sides of the contact, and corrosion is also observed

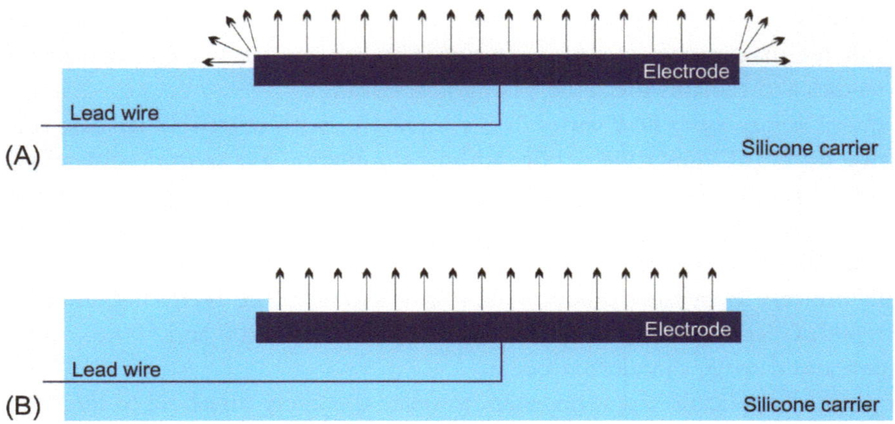

Fig. 6.4 Current density is dependent on the geometry of the electrode. (A) In case of an electrode placed on the top of the carrier the sharp edges of the electrode lead to high current densities around them. This may cause water hydrolysis or other faradaic reactions that can damage the tissue. (B) To prevent these effects, sharp edges are eliminated and the electrode contact is placed inside the silicone so that the sharp edges are covered and do not provide the source of currents into the tissue. This is a recessed contact design.

preferentially there. Most studies quantify only mean current or charge density for an electrode, and therefore this may be an underestimation for some regions of the contact.

We want to emphasize that a brief presentation of electric pulses may not lead to tissue damage even if they are slightly above the safety limit, particularly if the electrode is not in direct contact with neurons. However, small effects accumulate and prolonged stimulation protocols with fast repetition rates of the stimulus may still lead to observable damage. Therefore, testing requires estimation of the charge density and exposure time.

Not all possible parameter combinations have been investigated with respect to their safety thresholds. Safety limits ensure that no damage occurs during the expected operating lifespan of the device, not that such a device is permanently safe. Thus it is important to recognize that a "safe" device used outside of its normal operating limits, including its operational lifetime, can become unsafe.

For practical applications, Robert Shannon defined the "Shannon formula" for the dividing line between safe and unsafe region with respect to charge density and charge in Fig. 6.3 by

$$\log\left(\frac{Q}{A}\right) = k - \log(Q)$$

where A is the electrode area in cm^2, Q is the charge in μC/phase, and Q/A is the corresponding charge density. Fig. 6.3 shows the border for $k = 1.85$ (depending on the study, the critical value is between 1.75 and 1.9). The charge density $>\sim 215\,\mu C/cm^2$

in the plot is assumed to lead to damage even at small charges, therefore the border of the unsafe region deviates from the line defined by the Shannon formula. This has to be considered with respect to the working range of the electrodes: the usual excitation threshold reached with large stimulation electrodes is between 4 and 40 nC/phase and between 2 and 50 μC/cm^2. The outcome of this is that often safety considerations can limit the usable stimulation range.

To better appreciate the difference of threshold for faradaic reaction and safety limit, Fig. 6.5 provides an estimation of these boundaries for a clinical application: the cochlear implant electrode contact. As the data show, most of the stimulation in practical conditions are performed within the range of reversible faradaic reactions.

Finally, since maximum charge capacity of the materials differ, *safety limits differ for different metals*. For example, gold has lower maximum charge delivery capacity than platinum, whereas iridium oxide has a much higher charge delivery capacity. Therefore gold is not an ideal material for electrical stimulation, despite being biologically inert, as it has much lower safety limits.

Microelectrodes

Microelectrodes used for stimulation are usually penetrating electrodes with a surface area of <10,000 μm^2, usually < 2000 μm^2. For such small electrodes the safety limit is even closer to the stimulation thresholds. These electrodes are produced from iridium and not

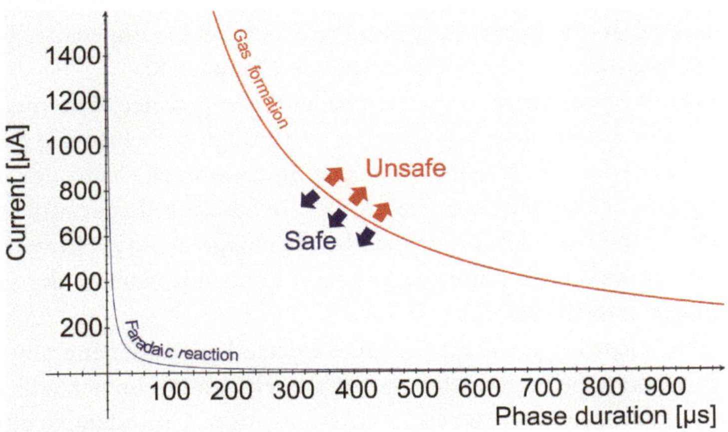

Fig. 6.5 Relationship between safety limit and faradaic reaction limit for a human cochlear implant with platinum electrode size of 0.0007 cm^2. Assumed gas formation limit was 400 μC/cm^2 and faradaic reaction threshold was 5 μC/cm^2. True capacitive effects are discernible only for short pulses and small currents, since for many combinations neuronal thresholds are already in the faradaic range. Infinite phase duration corresponds to DC stimulation that is unsafe even with minimal currents. The safety border is also influenced by the pulse repetition rate.

platinum, and consequently the safety limits are higher than for platinum. Thresholds for neuronal excitation are reached near 1 nC/phase in microelectrodes. Tissue damage is observed between 40 and 60 nC/phase (2–3 mC/cm^2) for Ir-based electrodes. While such electrodes tolerate more charge before making lesions, the size of the electrode and the thresholds with these electrodes require consideration. The range between stimulation threshold and lesion threshold (safety limit) may be more limiting than with macroelectrodes.

Electrode surface and electrode impedance

The electrode surface is thus crucial for the both stimulation and recording electrodes. The functional state of the electrode surface can be considered using raster electron microscopy, but this is only possible in vitro (i.e., in the dish). If a neuroprosthetic device is implanted in a subject, the surface of the electrode cannot be visualized. However, its condition can be assessed using electrode impedance. As shown in Fig. 5.5, the resistance is dependent on the frequency of the stimulus and falls with increasing frequency, whereas the logarithm of the resistance is linearly related to log frequency. In other words, knowing the resistance at two sufficiently different frequencies allows for a reliable estimate of the resistance at all frequencies.[f]

Many animal studies have shown that the electrode impedance is dependent on the surrounding tissue, too. The more the electrode is encapsulated by fibrous tissue, the greater the impedance. All material deposited on the surface of the electrode that has a greater resistivity than the extracellular fluid will increase the impedance by decreasing the effective stimulation area of the electrode (see **Chapter 8**).

The larger the effective surface area, the smaller the impedance. This means that, for a current source to be able to pass a given current through the electrode contact, larger electrodes do not need to increase the voltage as much as small electrodes. This reduces the energy demands of the stimulator electronics. In addition, larger surface areas allow safer stimulation, as the safety limit is defined by the charge density. However, very large electrodes can introduce surface irregularities and so do not increase the safety limit as much as one might naively assume.

In conclusion, a low impedance and a large electrode size are generally desirable for stimulation. However, increasing the size of the electrode contact will increase the current spread, which defocuses the electrical stimulation. Considerable effort has been put into the attempt to increase the effective size without expanding the size of the contact. This is possible by microstructuring the electrode surface. However, this

[f] There is only one exception: a deviation of this relation can be observed in kHz region of the curve; however, the deviation is rather small and will not be considered now.

may then introduce current density irregularities and be more susceptible to corrosion. It should be clear from the preceding discussion that electrode design in neural prosthetics is about balancing multiple opposing factors to achieve an optimized design for the specific application.

Other surface materials

In conclusion, although metals do allow for the delivery of electrical current into tissue, they cause many difficulties at the electrode-tissue interface that need to be considered for safe and effective chronic stimulation. Research in recent years has focused on conditioning the electrode surface. Increasing the area of the electrode contact, for example, by micro- or nanostructuring, helps to reduce the above problems by increasing the size of the electrode surface without changing the electrode geometry. Platinum nanostructuring has been successfully used to reduce electrode impedance. Iridium electrodes have a particularly large surface. Furthermore, use of new materials for the connecting wires may bring new, more flexible, and less traumatic materials in the future.

Nanostructures and nanomaterials in particular bring additional problems in practical applications; the small structures may be released to the body and cross biological barriers with ease. They might consequently accumulate in some distant organs, including the liver and kidneys. The concern is that they might cause immune reactions, initiate autoimmune processes, and subsequently damage healthy organs. Therefore, safety testing in nanomaterials will be the quest for applied research in the next decades.

Another option is to cover the surface of existing electrodes with materials based on conductive polymers. Poly(3,4-ethylen-edioxythiphene) (PEDOT) has been used to cover the surface of electrodes, substantially decreasing electrode impedance and increasing charge capacity. However, these substances are not yet being used in clinical practice due to stability issues and the use of very aggressive solvents during production. Similarly, coating with carbon nanotubes is an option for decreasing impedance and increasing capacitance. The issue again is that nanomaterials, when released from the contacts, distribute throughout the body easily. Therefore, more research is required to find out how these new materials may be clinically used.

Brief summary

- Constant current sources deliver charge to the tissue in a controlled way, independent of potential impedance changes.
- Electrical stimulation generates faradaic and non-faradaic effects at the electrode surface.
- Faradaic effects at low currents do not necessarily generate tissue damage if full reversibility is given.

- In absence of reversibility, faradaic effects are toxic for the tissue.
- The threshold for irreversible faradaic effects is increased by using AC charge-balanced stimulation.
- There are only a few biocompatible metals that safely avoid irreversible reactions that are suitable for neuronal stimulation. These include platinum and platinum-iridium alloys.
- Pulsatile charge-balanced stimulation with platinum contacts is used in most commercial stimulating electrodes.

Key literature and further reading

Brummer, S.B., Robblee, L.S., Hambrecht, F.T., 1983. Criteria for selecting electrodes for electrical stimulation: theoretical and practical considerations. Ann. N. Y. Acad. Sci. 405, 159–171.

Brummer, S.B., Turner, M.J., 1977a. Electrical stimulation with Pt electrodes: I-a method for determination of "real" electrode areas. I.E.E.E. Trans. Biomed. Eng. 24, 436–439.

Brummer, S.B., Turner, M.J., 1977b. Electrical stimulation with Pt electrodes: II-estimation of maximum surface redox (theoretical non-gassing) limits. I.E.E.E. Trans. Biomed. Eng. 24, 440–443.

Brummer, S.B., Turner, M.J., 1977c. Electrochemical considerations for safe electrical stimulation of the nervous system with platinum electrodes. I.E.E.E. Trans. Biomed. Eng. 24, 59–63.

Cogan, S.F., 2008. Neural stimulation and recording electrodes. Annu. Rev. Biomed. Eng. 10, 275–309.

Cogan, S.F., Garrett, D.J., Green, R.A., 2016. Electrochemical principles of safe current injection. In: Shephed, R.K. (Ed.), Neurobionics. John Willey & Sons, Hoboken, New Jersey, pp. 55–88.

Geddes, L.A., Baker, L.E., 1989. Principles of Applied Biomedical Instrumentation. Wiley & Sons, Inc., Hoboken, NJ.

Grill, W.M., 2005. Safety considerations for deep brain stimulation: review and analysis. Expert Rev. Med. Devices 2, 409–420.

Hadjinicolaou, A.E., Leung, R.T., Garrett, D.J., Ganesan, K., Fox, K., Nayagam, D.A., Shivdasani, M.N., Meffin, H., Ibbotson, M.R., Prawer, S., O'Brien, B.J., 2012. Electrical stimulation of retinal ganglion cells with diamond and the development of an all diamond retinal prosthesis. Biomaterials 33, 5812–5820.

Horch, K.W., Gurpeet, D.S., 2004. Neuroprosthetics: Theory and Practice. World Scientific Publishing Co., Singapore.

Kelliher, E.M., Rose, T.L., 1987. Evaluation of charge injection properties of thin film redox materials for use as neural stimulation electrodes. MRS Online Proc. Libr. Arch. 110, 23. https://doi.org/10.1557/PROC-110-23.

Kral, A., Hubka, P., Heid, S., Tillein, J., 2013. Single-sided deafness leads to unilateral aural preference within an early sensitive period. Brain 136, 180–193.

Merrill, D.R., Bikson, M., Jefferys, J.G., 2005. Electrical stimulation of excitable tissue: design of efficacious and safe protocols. J. Neurosci. Methods 141, 171–198.

Merrill, D.R., 2010. The electrochemistry of charge injection at the electrode/tissue interface. In: Zhou, D., Greenbaum, E. (Eds.), Implantable Prostheses 2: Techniques and Engineering Approaches. Springer Verlag, pp. 86–135.

Rose, T.L., Robblee, L.S., 1990. Electrical stimulation with Pt electrodes. VIII. Electro-chemically safe charge injection limits with 0.2 ms pulses. I.E.E.E. Trans. Biomed. Eng. 37, 1118–1120.

Robblee, L.S., McHardy, J., Agnew, W.F., Bullara, L.A., 1983. Electrical stimulation with Pt electrodes. VII. Dissolution of Pt electrodes during electrical stimulation of the cat cerebral cortex. J. Neurosci. Methods 9, 301–308.

Robblee, L.S., McHardy, J., Marston, J.M., Brummer, S.B., 1980. Electrical stimulation with Pt electrodes. V. The effect of protein on Pt dissolution. Biomaterials 1, 135–139.

Shepherd, R.K., Carter, P., Enke, Y.L., Wise, A.K., Fallon, J.B., 2019. Chronic intracochlear electrical stimulation at high charge densities results in platinum dissolution but not neural loss or functional changes in vivo. J. Neural. Eng. 16, 026009.
Shepherd, R.K., Villalobos, J., Burns, O., Nayagam, D.A.X., 2018. The development of neural stimulators: a review of preclinical safety and efficacy studies. J. Neural Eng. 15, 041004.
Sidambe, A.T., 2014. Biocompatibility of advanced manufactured titanium implants—a review. Materials (Basel) 7, 8168–8188.
Stieglitz, T., 2004. Electrode materials for recording and stimulation. In: Horch, K.W., Gurpeet, D.S. (Eds.), Neuroprosthetics: Theory and Practice. World Scientific Publishing Co., Singapore, pp. 475–516.

CHAPTER 7

Stimulation rules

The effects of electrical stimulation on excitable tissue depend not only on the proximity of the excitable cells but also on the (1) mutual geometric relation of the electrical fields and the excitable elements, (2) previous history of excitation, and (3) the signal form. In this chapter, we discuss these influencing factors in more detail.

The goal of artificial stimulation is to depolarize the excitable cells sufficiently to initiate an action potential. The action potential then travels along the neuronal pathways and the signal is transferred across synapses and to other neurons in the brain, ultimately leading to perception and/or motor action.

Imagine a neuron as described in **Chapter 4**, with its complex anatomy, isolated in a small dish. How do we have to place the working and return electrode to use the electric field to stimulate the neuron most effectively? In other words, what characteristics of the electrical field affect the excitation threshold? Neurons in the brain are not homogeneous with respect to size, morphology, and ionic composition of the intracellular fluids and neuronal membranes. Therefore, particular characteristics of the target structure need to be taken into account as well. We will limit the text to the description of the rules believed to be generally applicable to common implementations of neuroprostheses. We will address the specific aspects of the different brain structures that can be stimulated in the "Applications" section of this book (Chapters 11–16).

Geometry of the electric field and the neurons

The electric field generated by stimulating electrodes is determined by two main factors:
- position of the working and return electrode,
- impedance of the tissue.

Position of the working and return electrode

As mentioned in **Chapter 6**, placement of one of the stimulating electrodes close to the target cell and the counter electrodes at a large distance from it (e.g., in another structure of the body) results in a **monopolar configuration** (Fig. 7.1). If the structure where the working electrode is positioned is electrically homogeneous, the resulting electrical field will have a circular shape as in the two-dimensional example or a globe shape in three dimensions. Isopotential planes are formed by the sets of locations in space with the same electric potential. They will also be arranged in a series of spheres. The current vectors

Prostheses for the Brain
https://doi.org/10.1016/B978-0-12-818892-7.00002-X

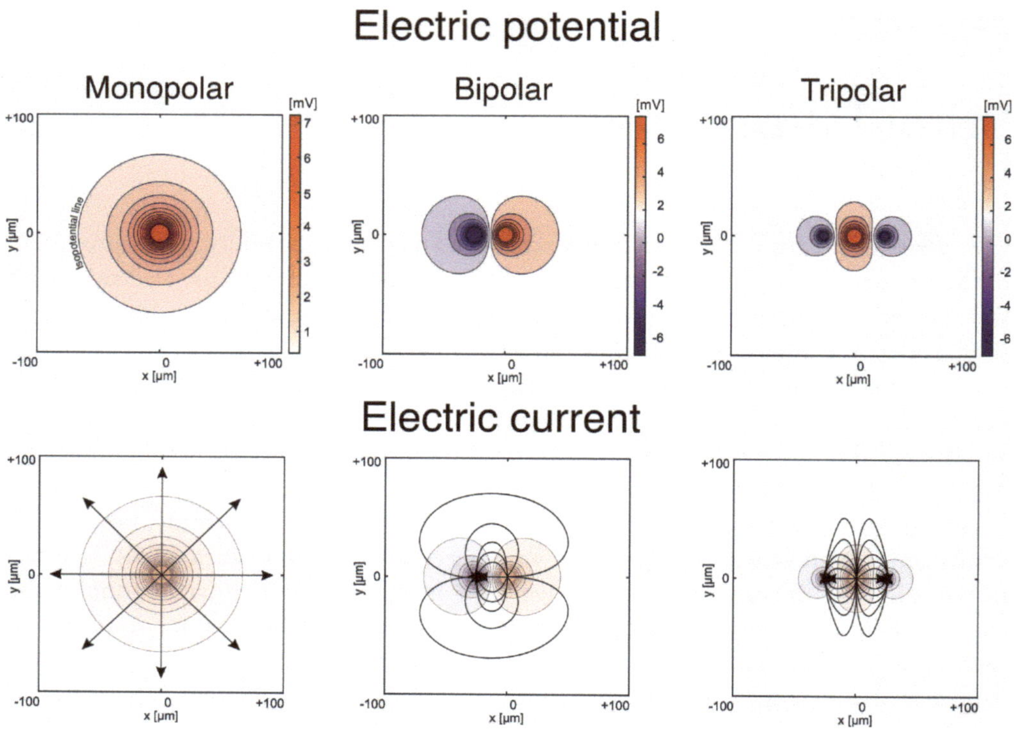

Fig. 7.1 Potential distribution in idealized conditions of a 2D infinite homogeneous brain tissue (complex permitivity of 30 kF/m) caused by a current of 100 µA by a circular electrode with the diameter of 7 µm. *Black circles* connect positions with same potential (isopotential lines) and *black arrows* show examples of the current flow (that is between positions with different potentials and are in principle perpendicular to the isopotential lines). Current flows between different potentials in space, thus along an isopotential line the current is zero. Shown are monopolar, bipolar, and tripolar configurations. In the monopolar configuration *(left panel)* the return electrode is infinitely far. Monopolar configuration results in large symmetric electric fields that spread out circularly. In the bipolar configuration *(middle panel)* with assumed interelectrode distance of 25 µm, the electric field has a limited expansion and the isopotential lines are dense in the space between the electrodes, where current density is highest and the majority of current flows. Thus, bipolar configuration focuses the currents in between the working and return electrode, however, the electric field becomes asymmetric. In tripolar configuration *(right panel)*, the field is even more focused. Below are the current vectors plotted on the potential field for each configuration as *black arrows*. *(Modeling from the PhD thesis of Dr. G. Quass, Institute of Audio-NeuroTechnology, Hannover, Germany.)*

(the direction of current flow) will be radially arranged from the stimulating electrode, perpendicularly cutting the isopotential planes.

Moving the return electrode closer to the working electrode will change this field (**bipolar configuration**; Fig. 7.1): the isopotential lines will approach the return electrode and the electric field, which will no longer be circular. The isopotential lines will thus become densely packed between the stimulation and return electrodes. Since current flows between positions with different potentials, current vectors will deviate from the radial shape observed in the monopolar configuration and will organize toward the return electrode in the bipolar configuration. The resulting electrical field of each electrode will become asymmetric. While in a monopolar configuration the idealized electric field will have a radial arrangement of the currents around the working electrode, in the bipolar configuration the electric current will concentrate at the positions where the working and the return electrode are closest (i.e., between them). However, some weaker current will also be observed at other positions, including those that are opposite to the electrodes. Thus, placement of the stimulating electrodes will extensively shape the electrical field and can help to focus the electrical field to a certain region in space (the region between the active electrodes).

Such focusing of the electrical field limits the spread of the current. If the excitable cells are not located between the working and return electrodes (within the current path), less current will reach them than in the monopolar configuration. Unfortunately, adding another electrode to shape the electric field complicates the situation, as this additional electrode is not a passive return for current; it will also excite neurons. Furthermore, stimulation is usually performed using linear electrode arrays such as in cochlear implants or deep brain stimulation implants. In these arrays, there is no excitable tissue directly between the active electrodes; rather, they are located to the side of the linear array, with the non-conductive body of the array located between the active contacts. As current cannot pass through such non-conducting element, the electric field and the current distribution will be shaped by the insulating elements. Bipolar stimulation limits the spread of the resulting electrical field at a cost: most currents flow very close to the surface of the electrode body, and are unlikely to reach many neurons. Consequently, excitation becomes less effective with bipolar stimulation, and threshold currents typically rise when configuration changes from monopolar to bipolar. Finally, the return electrode will stimulate neurons, and thus one stimulation site will be replaced by two stimulation sites, partly counterbalancing the reduced spread of excitation.

Using a technique of beam forming this disadvantage may be partly overcome. Optimally, an electric field in the form of a laser-like beam would be ideal for selection of individual cells within a tissue. However, such focusing has not yet been possible. Some focusing has been achieved using a **tripolar configuration** (Fig. 7.1, Fig. 11.10). Here, the return electrode of the bipolar configuration is split into two electrode contacts flanking the working electrode. Half of the current then flows to one neighboring contact, and half of the current to the other neighboring contact. Due to the current being shared between the two return electrodes, their stimulating effect is lessened. Distributing the current to two or more return electrodes has the effect that currents near the working electrode can be kept above the excitation threshold, while those in the return electrodes will stay below the threshold. This configuration further eliminates the asymmetry in the polarity of the electric field observed with bipolar stimulation. However, a significant portion of the current may still flow along the electrode carrier and may hit only a few neurons. The consequent effect is intermediate between the monopolar and bipolar stimulation: more current flows into the tissue than in the bipolar configuration, but less so than in the monopolar configuration. The sharpening of the electric field is better than with bipolar configuration, since a significant portion of the current leaves the working (central) electrode in the direction perpendicular to the axis connecting the three electrodes ("beam forming"). This is particularly advantageous considering that the currents flowing between the contacts are limited by the electrode lead body that is, as previously discussed, non-conductive. The effectiveness of current focusing is critically dependent on the mutual distance of the stimulating electrodes relative to the position of the targeted excitable elements. Multi-electrode phased array approaches have been introduced to cochlear implants. Here more electrodes are used in stimulation, and the calculation of the individual currents are based on the desired excitation profile and are computed backwards from this profile. However, the more distant electrodes have increasingly smaller influence on the current and the effectiveness of adding more than five electrodes may be small, as observed in cochlear implants. Outcomes reached are not significantly better than with tripolar stimulation.

Electrode/tissue orientation

We consider the mutual geometric relation of the neuronal elements and the electric field next. There are favorable directions of current making stimulation more efficient.

Imagine an axon running at 90 degrees to the current path (Fig. 7.2, right panel). In this configuration, some fraction of the current will enter the cell through the neuronal membrane. If the axon is closer to the anode, the extracellular space becomes more positive and the current entering the neuron at this place will hyperpolarize the cell. However, following the current path the current will exit the cell through the RC circuit close to the entry point, thus depolarizing this other membrane patch. Consequently, the neuron has a nearby hyperpolarized and a depolarized membrane patch, partly canceling each other's effects. A similar effect will be observed with a cathode, only the entry point will depolarize the membrane and the exit point will hyperpolarize the membrane.

A more favorable condition will be if the angle of the axon and the current path will be 0 degrees, in other words, if the current runs along the axon (Fig. 7.2, left panel). Here, since the current path is parallel to the axon, once entering the axon it propagates a significant distance along the fiber's course. In this case patches of hyperpolarization and depolarization are more remote and cannot cancel each other's effect. It is known that for fibers oriented parallel to the current path, the threshold is about four times lower than in cases where the directions are perpendicular (i.e., 12 dB better, see Box 7.1). Of course, this is also influenced by the polarity of the stimulating electrode contact.

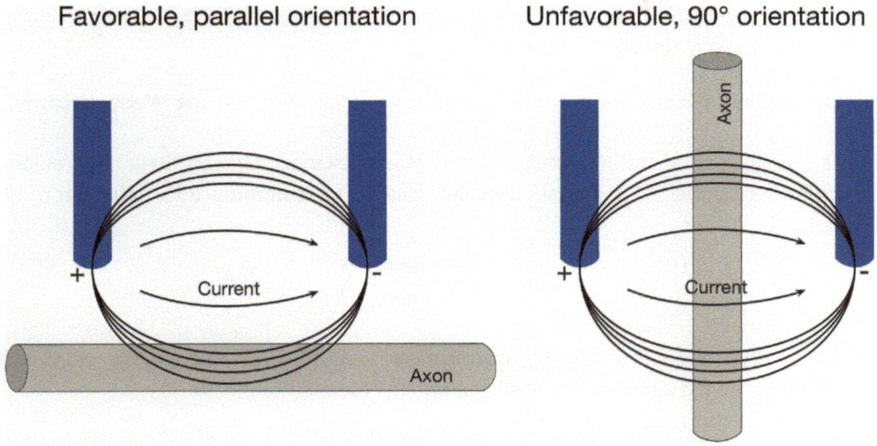

Fig. 7.2 The favorable *(left)* and unfavorable *(right)* orientation of the electrical field to the neural fiber (axon). In the unfavorable orientation, the current enters and exits the fiber in closely neighboring places so that the effects can cancel out more easily than in the favorable orientation.

Box 7.1: Factors and dBs

A frequently used concept is that of decibels (dBs). However, for most students this concept is confusing and instead of facilitating understanding, it complicates it. Therefore this Box provides a very simple explanation of where dBs come from and how they relate to factors.

A dB expresses relative relations between measures. Factors can serve the same function ($x=5*x_{ref}$, thus x is five times larger than x_{ref}, there is factor 5 between x and x_{ref}). Similarly, relations can be expressed in percent. However, such linear relations often fail to cover physiological sensory processes that are not linear, but rather exponential. Intensities are perceived logarithmically as a consequence of the Weber-Fechner law and Stevens's law. Thus, between perceived loudness and sound pressure (in Pascal) is a logarithmic equation, and this relation can be expressed in dBs.

A dB can easily be put into relation with a factor. Imagine that some value (x) is a factor f (f-times) larger than a reference value x_{ref}. Then we can write

$$f=\frac{x}{x_{ref}}$$

Now instead of using a scale of factors in the range from 1 to 1,000,000, we may want to use smaller numbers that are closer to the way how sensory organs operate. For example, since $1=10^0$ and thus $\log(1)=0$, a factor $f=1$ would correspond to a logarithmic measure of $L=0$. Similarly, instead of a factor $f=100$ we might use $L=2$, since $100=10*10=10^2$ and $\log(100)=2$. Finally, instead of a factor $f=1000$ we might write $L=3$, since $1000=10*10*10=10^3$. Logarithms compress the value axis more in the high values than in the low values. This is also how we perceive stimulus intensity: we are very sensitive to increments if stimulus intensities are small, but we are less sensitive to increments if the intensities are large. That is biologically meaningful. Thus using dB scales not only we can use smaller numbers that are easier to put into tables and understand, we might also be

Continued

Box 7.1: Factors and dBs—cont'd

closer to the way how we humans perceive physical quantities—as the Weber-Fechner law suggests.

This is the basic idea of the Bell scale, named after Alexander Graham Bell. Bell Telephone Laboratories introduced the dimensionless Bell scale in telecommunication, characterized by the equation

$$L = \log\left(\frac{Intensity}{Intensity_{ref}}\right)$$

However, often the factors can be much smaller than 10. The value was therefore further multiplied by 10, giving a measure of tenths of one bel (deci-bel, dB):

$$L = 10 \cdot \log\left(\frac{Intensity}{Intensity_{ref}}\right)$$

The final modification of this equation was the use of signal amplitude instead of intensity. Since intensity relates to squared amplitudes, the final equation is

$$L = 10 \cdot \log\left(\frac{x^2}{x_{ref}^2}\right)$$

This can be simplified by putting the square in front of the logarithm, since the logarithm of a squared value equals the double of the logarithm:

$$L = 20 \cdot \log\left(\frac{x}{x_{ref}}\right)$$

Such an equation has been very useful in many applications. While with electrical stimulation the perception of stimulus current does neither equal current in μA nor dB, dB is often used to express the current relative to some meaningful value (e.g., threshold). By that one can easily normalize the value (in this case it is a simple difference between the reference and the given value, both in dBs).

When using dB we no longer speak of factors, but of levels (sound pressure level, current level, etc.). Relation of factors to levels is given in the table below (a factor to remember is that doubling corresponds to 6dB!):

Factor	dB
0.3	~ -10
1.5	$\sim$3.5
2	$\sim$6
3	$\sim$10
10	20
100	40

Box 7.1: Factors and dBs—cont'd

As one can see, negative dBs correspond to factors <1. Multiplying factors equals adding dB, thus if the amplitude is increased by a factor of two and subsequently once again by a factor of two, this results in factor of $2*2=4$, but in dB it is $6+6=12$ dB. Division of factors corresponds to subtractions of dB.
dB is of importance in the context of neural prostheses, particularly auditory prostheses, given that also here the relation of the response to current is often logarithmic.

Consequently, the mutual orientation of current path and neurons are of importance, provided the neurons have an elongated morphology. As mentioned, the cathode is more likely to excite the neurons than the anode is, although the anode can also do this, as we will see later in the chapter. However, things are a bit more complicated, as the next section will show. Eventually, the hyperpolarizing and depolarizing effects are not symmetric in their overall impact. Whereas the hyperpolarization has only a local effect, the depolarization may trigger an action potential. Action potentials will affect target neurons and cause downstream (distant) effects that hyperpolarization does not have.

Activation function

So far we have discussed what is the more favorable direction of the electrical field if we want to stimulate fiber tracts. This allows a conclusion on how to orient the electrical field. However, we still lack the information about where within the fiber the excitation will be greatest.

To be able to assess where exactly neurons will be excited, we introduce the concept of the **activation function**. The largest excitation occurs where the largest current gradient (change) along the neuronal structures is found. Imagine an electrical field in the tissue that is generated by an electrode near an excitable axon (Fig. 7.3). Measuring the potential distribution with an imaginary microelectrode along the axon allows for computing potential differences in the electric field (the first spatial derivative of the potential, a value proportional to the current under the assumption of homogeneous resistance). In any volume the sum of entering and exiting currents has to be zero (Kirchoff's law). If there is a change in this resulting current, it means that part of the current leaves the given direction. Computing the current gradient along the neurons (axons), that is, the first spatial derivative of the current and the second spatial derivative of the potential, allows for detecting places where the charges move towards the axon and thus may enter (or leave) the neuron. This is the place of the highest likelihood of excitation. The activating function is thus defined as a second spatial derivative of the potential. The activation function is proportional to the inward and outward currents along a neuron and to its deviation from the resting potential.

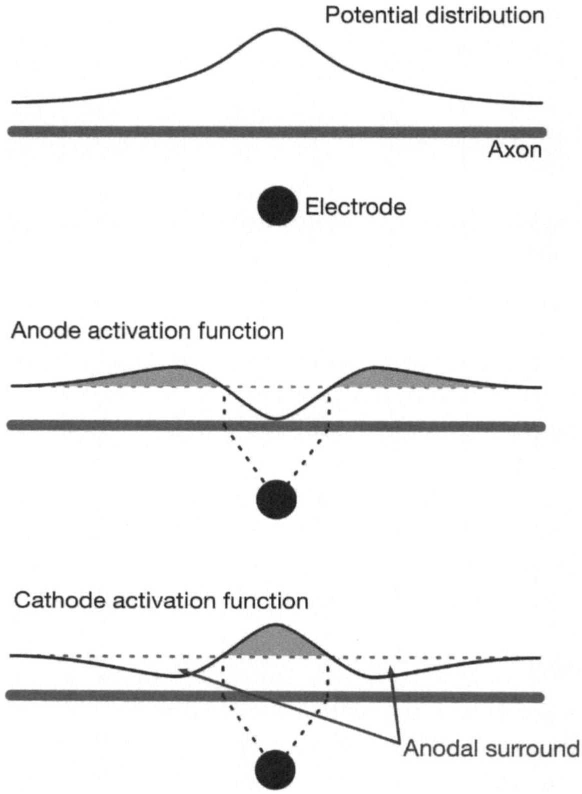

Fig. 7.3 Stimulation of an unmyelinated nerve fiber. *Top*: A monopolar stimulation electrode generates an external electrical field that causes, when measured along the axon *(green)*, a potential distribution shown above as solid line. *Middle*: Activation function for an anode computed from the potential distribution, *dotted line* represents resting condition. The *grey area* denotes depolarization, and *white (unfilled) area* denotes hyperpolarization. At a given current, the central hyperpolarization is larger than the side peaks of depolarization. Since the action potentials do not have to cross the hyperpolarized region, the hyperpolarization does not prevent excitation, but for effective stimulation larger currents are required since the stimulation takes place more distant from the electrode. *Below*: The cathode's activation function, with a lateral anodal (hyperpolarizing) surround. Normally, the central effects are stronger than the side peak effects, but with increasing stimulation current the hyperpolarization may interfere with the generation or the propagation of an action potential.

In principle, the activation function for monopolar stimulation with an axon passing by shows a central peak, which can be hyperpolarizing or depolarizing, and two side peaks that are smaller and are of opposite polarity (Fig. 7.3). As a rule, to ensure overall electrical neutrality, the sum of the inward- and outward-oriented currents should be equal. For the anode, the central peak is hyperpolarizing, and the side (lateral) peaks are smaller and depolarizing. With the cathode, the central peak is depolarizing and the side peaks are smaller and hyperpolarizing. This means that the cathode

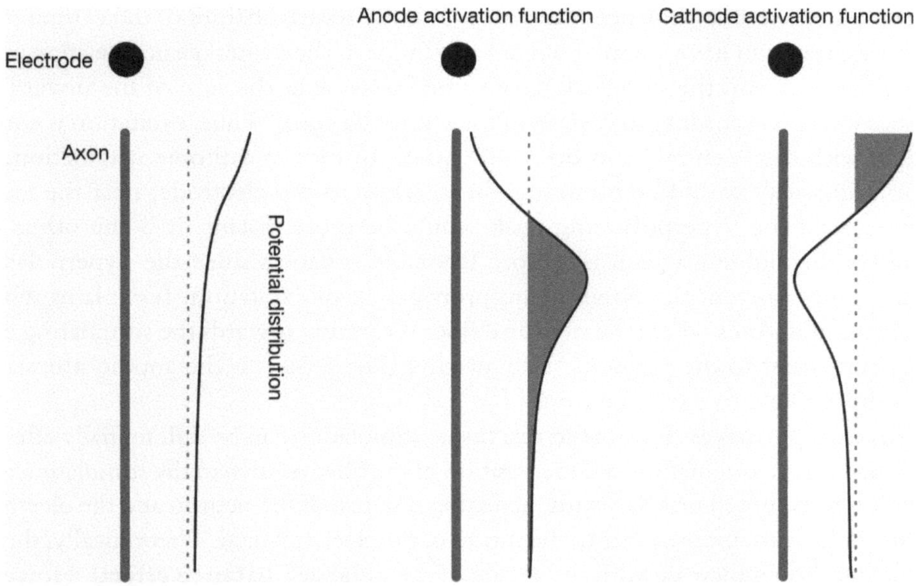

Fig. 7.4 Activation functions for a fiber *(green)* running towards the stimulating electrode. In this case there is only one falling flank in the potential distribution, and thus only one side peak in the activation function. Since the charge under both polarities must be equal, the area of the central peak and the side peaks are similar. Due to the depolarizing portion of activation function *(grey area)* being further downstream the fiber and thus closer to its target in anodic stimulation, anodic stimulation is more efficient than cathodic stimulation in this arrangement. Which polarity is more efficient thus depends on the orientation of the fiber towards the electrode.

has a greater probability of exciting neurons in this spatial configuration, since it is the larger central peak that leads to excitation (the effect on threshold is that cathodic stimulation in such configuration has a 15%–30% lower threshold than anodic stimulation). The activation function thus predicts excitation close to the active electrode for cathodic stimulation, whereas it predicts lateral excitation on both sides of the electrode for anodic stimulation (Fig. 7.3). The reverse phenomenon with cathodic stimulation, the hyperpolarizing **anodal surround**, may prevent excitation in cathodic stimulation by blocking the conduction of action potentials generated in the excited region of the fiber.

Although the activation function is not always an accurate predictor of excitation (in part because the surrounding of the axon may not be homogenous and the current can change direction without entering a neuron), it is a good and simple approximation if computed along the course of axons (fiber tracts). This of course assumes a certain spatial relationship between the electrode and the fiber. Here, a point source and a fiber running besides of it are assumed. If the fiber, on the other hand, would have a different course, for example, would run against the electrode, the activating function would be very different (Fig. 7.4). There would be only one "central" peak and one side peak present. Since the side peak needs to encompass the return charges of the central peak, in this case it would have a similar overall amplitude as the central peak (the areas under the central peak and the side peak have to be the same as the sum of the inward and outward current according to Kirchhoff's law must be zero). Thus, excitation is equally possible with the "central" and the "side" peak. In case of cathodic stimulation, the depolarizing peak would be more peripheral (close to the electrode, near the end of the fiber) and the hyperpolarizing peak would be more distant. It is the other way around in the anode - which is a more favorable situation since the hyperpolarized region cannot prevent the downstream propagation of excitation. It explains why in spatial configurations where the neuronal fiber is running towards the stimulating electrode, in contrast to the previous configuration (Fig. 7.3), it is the anodic stimulation that is more likely to excite neurons.

This example makes clear that in real tissue, stimulation can be differentially effective depending on the orientation and the position of the fiber relative to the stimulating electrode. It is to be noted first that with increasing distance of the neuron and the electrode, the thresholds must increase due to the spread of the electrical field. Theoretically, threshold current should increase with the square of the distance (**distance effect**). However, the real situation is more complex. Similar to conduction velocity mentioned in previous chapters, *stimulation is more effective for fibers with larger diameter.* For this, an inverse square relationship exists: for each doubling of axon diameter, the electrical stimulation threshold drops by 12 dB (to one fourth). In cathodic stimulation, fibers running in very close proximity of the cathode may be even inhibited by anodal surround and by inactivation of sodium channels due to strong depolarization (depolarization block). Fibers located further away may be sufficiently far to yield the anodal surround ineffective. That can sometimes lead to the paradox that closer fibers are less easily stimulated than more distant fibers, and thinner fibers are more stimulated than thicker fibers. Computation for thin fibers reveals that this effect can extend over a millimeter from the electrode (Fig. 7.5). Again, also in this simulation many assumptions have been used, so that stimulation effects in central nervous system is complex.

For longer duration pulses (>1 ms, rarely used in clinical applications), where resistance of the cell membrane plays a more important role than capacitance, the activation function is less accurate and its modifications have been proposed (e.g., the *mirror estimate*). Furthermore, most tissue includes neuronal somata and fibers running in different directions relative to the electrode, so that predictions about neuronal excitation are more difficult. The concept of activation function is thus a simplification of the existing rules and more complex models exist.

For well-controlled stimulation, a regular arrangement of the fibers that are the targets for the stimulation is of substantial advantage. The majority of cortical axons and dendrites are oriented perpendicularly to cortical surface. Early studies indeed documented that

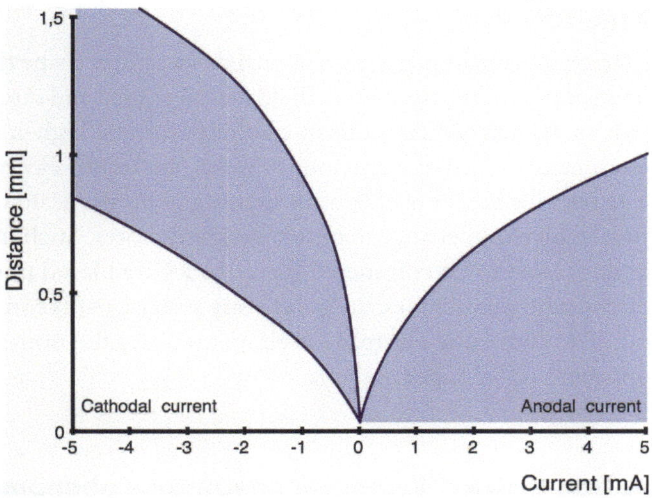

Fig. 7.5 Current-distance relations for stimulation thresholds calculated for a fiber with ~10-μm diameter. The stimulated regions are shaded blue. For cathodal currents, stimulation occurs at some distance from the electrode, whereas for anodal stimulation this is not the case. For fibers that have a larger diameter, the shaded regions move further away from the electrode. *(Figure modified from Rattay et al. (1987).)*

stimulation at the cortical surface is more effective in anodic configuration, given by the fact that the fibers (dendrites) of cortical neurons run towards the stimulating electrode and do not pass along, not as in Fig. 7.3 but more in the way as shown in Fig. 7.4. As discussed, anodal stimulation might preferentially activate fibers running towards the electrode, whereas bypassing fibers or other orientations may lead anodal stimulation to become suppressive. It may explain why cortical surface stimulation yields stronger effects with anodal stimulation. Spatial orientation may explain also some data indicating differences of polarity sensitivity in the same structure for different species.

One possibility to differentiate the stimulation site is to determine the strength-duration curve for the response to electric stimulation (by measuring action potentials or compound action potentials). This allows for the determination of the time constants for the excitable membranes. These depend on the size of the membrane and its resistance (affected by myelination; see **Chapter 4**). The resulting chronaxies are longest for stimulation of somata (in the cortex in the order of few ms), shorter for dendrites and non-myelinated axons and shortest for myelinated axons (200–400 μs). However, when performing stimulation within the neuronal tissue, often chronaxies are measured that are in between of these values and thus demonstrate mixed stimulation at all these sites.

Impedance of the tissue

Another limiting factor is tissue impedance. Impedance variations shape the electric field. Close to high-impedance barriers, the electric field is compressed and directed away from it, forming **boundary effects.** As the current cannot pass these high-impedance structures, it flows preferentially in other directions to reach the return electrode. Boundary phenomena may be responsible for problems in exciting neurons located close to surface of the brain or close to high-impedance membranes or structures. Such inhomogeneities represent an important issue to be considered if electrodes are placed in electrically heterogeneous structures with membranes, cells and bony structures (like in the inner ear in cochlear implants). The prosthetic electrode itself, particularly the non-conducting carrier, may also contribute to such phenomena.

Previous activation history: Temporal adaptation phenomena

Excitability depends on previous history of stimulation. The simplest of these phenomena relates to the **refractory period**. As long as the fast sodium channels are in the inactive phase, further stimulation cannot generate action potentials. These periods are the same as the one described in the physiological section (**Chapter 4**). The duration of the refractory period is in the order of 1–3 ms. The consequence is a masking of following stimuli during high stimulus repetition rates. The refractory period has an *absolute component* where no action potentials can be elicited, and a *relative component* when only a part of the sodium channels have overcome inactivation, a smaller-amplitude action potential may be elicited. This is typically observed near the end of the refractory period.

Even when stimulation does not reach action potential generation threshold, such inactivation can still appear in some channels of the membrane and can lead to reduced excitability. This process is called electrical **accommodation**: long duration stimulation, even below threshold, increases the stimulation threshold. With repeated above-threshold stimulation at high repetition rates, the evoked spiking activity also reduces over time. This phenomenon is called **spike-rate adaptation**. This refers to a reduced firing rate with ongoing electrical stimulation and has been observed under many different stimulation conditions. In ongoing high-frequency stimulation in the order of one or several thousand pulses per second, as is frequently used for peripheral nerve stimulation, such adaptation is likely to occur. Consequently, with ongoing constant stimulation rates the nerve fibers become less responsive. This may be different in different types of neurons, but some adaptation is likely to occur in all of them, of course with different time constants. In the auditory nerve, for example, it takes place within time-windows of 5–100 ms. The mechanism relates to potassium channels in the neuronal membrane that gradually open during prolonged depolarization of a neuron and reduce its excitability (for details see the recommended literature in **Chapter 4**).

Hyperpolarization can cause an overshooting depolarization after the hyperpolarization has been terminated. Following a strong recruitment of inhibitory synaptic processes hyperpolarizing the neuronal membrane, neurons show a phenomenon called postinhibitory rebound (**Chapter 4**). This is due to faster activation-gate kinetics of the sodium channel compared to its inactivation gate (a phenomenon with opposite direction, but same mechanism as accommodation). Thus, following hyperpolarization, activation is back to normal, yet the inactivation is still blocked, leading to net sodium conductance higher than normal, favoring depolarization and generation of action potentials. This means that if a hyperpolarization of neurons is abruptly terminated (e.g., with pulsatile electric stimulation that is suddenly stopped), the neurons may generate action potentials. Preferentially, this occurs with anodic stimulation that is more likely to hyperpolarize neurons; therefore, the phenomenon has been called **anodic break**. It may, however, appear also with cathodic stimulation, since in parts of the neurons surrounding the working electrode it may lead to hyperpolarization, too (e.g., due to the anodic surround phenomenon mentioned above). Using a slowly decaying electrical stimulus (e.g., using exponential or ramped offset) can prevent the anodic break.

Additionally, a **depolarization block** is observed with prolonged or supra-threshold excitation. If the neuron is depolarized so that the membrane potential is near 0 mV, the sodium channels enter the refractory state (sodium channels are inactivated) and action potentials cannot be generated anymore. An additional input to these neurons will not allow for the generation of action potentials. High-intensity, long-term excitation is therefore similarly undesirable as hyperpolarization if the aim is to stimulate neurons.

Signal forms

Considering the temporal morphology of the electrical stimulus, safety aspects suggest the need for charge-balancing (**Chapter 6**). Biphasic stimulation (with a positive and a negative part) using sinusoidal, pulsatile, but also sawtooth and other shapes are possible. Commercially, only pulsatile and sinusoidal stimulation have been used so far. Pulsatile stimulation has been used most frequently. Simultaneous stimulation through more than one electrode at a time can lead to varying current flow between electrodes and thus unwanted and unpredictable interactions at the level of electrical fields, reducing the effectiveness of the stimulation. To avoid this, stimulation in such cases is as a rule **interleaved** between electrodes so that the electrical fields of two neighboring electrodes cannot interact. Thus whenever one electrode stimulates, the other electrodes in the vicinity are inactive. Pulsatile stimulation has the advantage of better defining the moment of onset and offset of the stimulus in time and, at the same time, allows high stimulation rates using interleaved stimulation protocols. Additionally, when considering the phenomena in the time domain, one can observe that individual neuron variability (e.g., measured by stimulation threshold) increases with decreasing pulse duration. Therefore, selecting short pulses will grade responses in the activated neuronal population, and thus provides better options for coding, for example, stimulus intensity. This type of stimulation dominates commercial applications.

Optimum **pulse duration** is another important factor for brain prostheses. Charge delivery needs to be in relation to the leaky integrator properties of the neuronal membrane, as expressed by the strength duration curves discussed in **Chapter 4**. Theoretically, doubling the active phase duration of the pulse should reduce the threshold by factor of two; however, this is pragmatically not the case, as mentioned in **Chapter 6**. With increasing pulse duration the current required to reach the excitation threshold decreases, but rather than the expected 6 dB (reduced by half) it is in the range of ~4 dB (reduced by one third) per doubling the phase duration.

It is interesting to consider the overall *charge* rather than the current that is required to reach threshold. Short pulses require less charge to reach thresholds, but also require high voltage to deliver this charge quickly. The charge threshold (in nC/phase) is lowest with short pulses and increase up to duration of 800–1000 μs (see **Chapter 11**). This means that with long pulse durations, while thresholds are reached at lower currents (over longer time), some of the delivered charge already leaves the neuron before the action potential is generated. The optimum value for low energy charge delivery at still relatively low voltages is considered experimentally between 100 and 200 μs/phase. However, due to the need for high stimulation rate many applications use even shorter pulses, down to 30 μs/phase. Higher thresholds mean correspondingly high voltages at the electrodes during operation, which can create safety concerns since high voltage can cause chemical reactions on the electrode.

With pulsatile stimulation, due to the need for charge balancing, **symmetrical biphasic pulses** are being used most frequently (Fig. 7.6). Effects caused by one phase are combined with effects of the other phase, which can be opposite. Remember, anodic stimulation has different effects than cathodic stimulation (Fig. 7.3)! The second phase thus not only compensates faradaic reactions but also excites or inhibits neurons. Since it has opposite polarity, it can partially interact with the excitation building up due to the first phase. In some unfortunate cases, one phase can excite while the other phase can inhibit the same neurons. This explains why thresholds for monophasic pulses are generally lower than thresholds for biphasic pulses. Nonetheless, monophasic pulses violate the charge balance condition and thus are rarely used chronically due to safety issues.

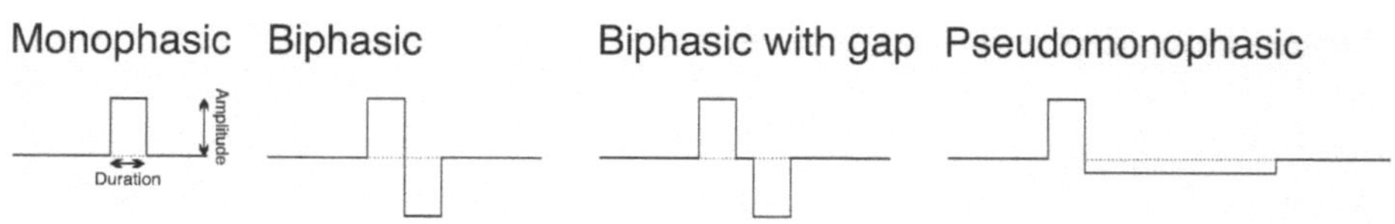

Fig. 7.6 Current amplitude vs. time relation of different pulse shapes used for electrical stimulation. All pulse shapes have to fulfill the charge-balance condition.

Since the return electrode provides a current pulse with inverted polarity, the use of bipolar configurations will initiate opposite effects on the return electrode that starts with the opposite phase. Thus whenever there is the cathodic phase on the working electrode there is the anodic phase in the return electrode. Both the working and the return electrode thus excite or inhibit neurons, with reverse effects in time and space. The high diversity of ionic channels and the phenomena described previously can make the polarity effect asymmetric. The stimulation effects may then differ between cathodic leading and anodic leading biphasic pulses, even though both involve a cathodic and anodic phase. The temporal sequence matters! This complicates the interpretation of the effects of biphasic pulses, particularly when applied in bipolar or tripolar configurations.

One possible workaround is the use of asymmetric **pseudomonophasic pulses** (Fig. 7.6): one phase is brief and has a high amplitude (i.e. high current), the other phase is long and has a correspondingly smaller amplitude (i.e. small current) so that overall the pulse remains charge-balanced. If the amplitude of the second phase should be small enough not to reach the excitation threshold, one could effectively achieve monophasic stimulation effects with charge-balanced and thus safe stimulation. However, the threshold difference for the two phases is not large, since it is the charge that determines the excitation. Since the short and the long phase of the pseudomonophasic pulse have the same charge, they should have the same stimulation thresholds. But, as shown in Fig. 6.1 and mentioned previously, the true thresholds deviate from this rule due to the leaky nature of the neuronal membrane. In other words, long pulses are slightly less effective in exciting neurons than short pulses. Thus relative to the dynamic range (see below), one can still gain a few dB difference in thresholds between the short and the long phase of a pseudomonophasic stimulus. Pseudomonophasic pulses are often used in research since the results have a more straightforward interpretation of polarity effects than bipolar pulses. They are only rarely used in a modified form clinically (e.g., for some cochlear implants and for deep brain stimulation).

A way of improving the thresholds with symmetrical biphasic pulses is to introduce a short **delay ("interphase gap") between the two phases** of the biphasic pulse. Such a configuration gives the first phase more time to "operate" before the other phase comes, resulting in slightly lower stimulation thresholds. This approach has been used in some commercial applications of neuroprostheses. Finally, other pulse shapes have also been tested, including trapezoid pulses with either slowly increasing onset or offset, sawtooth shapes, and many more. While small differences in physiological characteristics of the responses to these pulses have been noted, the critical parameter for the response was charge delivered by the stimulus. In clinical applications, mostly biphasic charge-balanced pulses with or without interphase gap have been used.

In some neuroprosthetic devices, sinusoidal stimulation has been used. This has similar properties to biphasic pulses; however, the synchronization to the electric stimulus is weaker due to the smoother signal shape. No safety issues have been observed down to stimulation frequencies <100 Hz (periods of >10 ms). However, sinusoidal stimulation has the disadvantage that interleaved stimulation is not possible and that at low frequencies the periods are long; thus, channel interactions in multi-channel stimulation becomes an issue. Theoretically, when neuronal elements are very close to the electrode and currents can be low, channel interaction is less and sinusoidal stimulation might be a suitable option for some applications as well.

Suprathreshold responses: Current level functions

Electrical pulsatile stimulation using brief biphasic charge-balanced pulses as a rule synchronizes nearby neurons very strongly and generates only a few (often one or two) spikes in response to one current pulse. However, not each period of the stimulus may be responded to, and the number of responded periods increases with increasing current. These pulses have a very stereotyped temporal relationship to the electric stimulus. **Phase locking** refers to the coupling of the action potentials to the phase of the electric stimulus that evoked them. If stimulating peripheral nerves, a population phase locking can also be observed with responses recorded using electrodes placed on the skin surface that measure activity from many axons together.

The **dynamic range** of the responses (Fig. 7.7), that is, the range of currents over which responses show a monotonically growing response strength with increasing stimulation intensity (in which the response can be taken as an unequivocal measure of stimulus intensity) in individual electrically stimulated neurons is quite narrow, and due to the high phase locking the firing rate saturates within ~3 dB for pulsatile and ~6 dB for sinusoidal stimulation (Fig. 7.7A). This dynamic range increases in downstream neuronal structures, particularly if there is a large population of directly stimulated neurons, since downstream neurons integrate activity from many directly stimulated neurons. If the directly stimulated neurons have different thresholds (which is typical), their dynamic range sums up and can reach 20 dB. This small dynamic range is the consequence of electric stimulation that bypasses the normal transduction process with chemical intensity coding at a sensor cell-neuron synapse and directly intervenes at the voltage-sensitive sodium channels of the neuron. For example, if in the same auditory organ (the ear) responses are obtained through a functional sensory organ, the phase locking is weaker and the dynamic range of responses is much larger (40–80 dB, see Fig. 7.7A and C). This is given by the chemical character of the synapse between the receptor (sensor) cell and the first neuron generating action potentials. The chemical synapse can have spontaneous transmitter release, generating spontaneous activity as well as noise during evoked responses. Furthermore, the kinetics of the ligand-gated channels can transform the intensity of the chemical signal into a graded electrical signal with high resolution. The relationship between transmitter concentration and depolarization is consequently shallow, providing detailed coding of stimulus intensity. Electric stimulation bypasses this

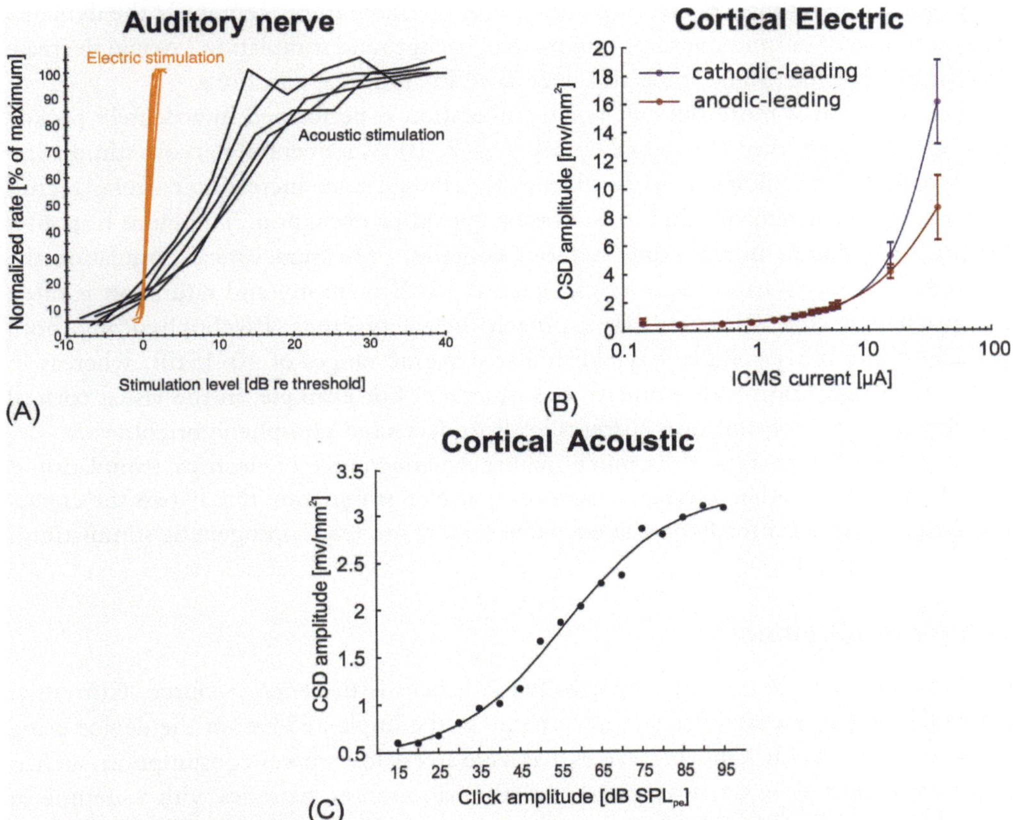

Fig. 7.7 Rate-level functions for responses to biphasic charge-balanced pulses compared to physiological responses to a corresponding sensory stimulus. (A) Direct comparison of rate-level functions in the auditory nerve, where responses to electric stimulation show fast saturation. Abscissa in dB SPL for acoustic and dB μA for electric stimulation. (B) Intracortical microstimulation (ICMS) in the auditory cortex of a guinea pig leads to an increase in evoked current source density (CSD) signals in the auditory cortex that continue to increase up to the maximum safe current. Cathodic-leading and anodic-leading biphasic charge balanced pulses at 200 μs/phase were used. The dynamic range observed covers 12 dB. (C) Same responses for acoustic click stimulation. For acoustic stimulation, the dynamic range is 40–60 dB. *(A: Data from Javel and Viemeister (2000), reprinted from Kral and Tillein (2021). B, C: Data from Voigt et al. (2019).)*

mechanism and electrically activates the axon directly. All this leads to the loss of dynamic range in electric stimulation, as shown in Fig. 7.7.

To increase the dynamic range, subthreshold stochastic background stimulation has been previously suggested with the goal to bring the membrane potential closer to the firing threshold. In addition, this intervention would increase the stochasticity of the electric stimulus, since a previously subthreshold stimulus would sometimes (depending on the previous background activity) bring the neuron above threshold. This approach, called stochastic resonance, however, did not bring much improvement of the dynamic range and due to current consumption by the "background stimulation" would decrease the battery lifetime. So far it has not been used in clinical applications.

The situation is more difficult when stimulation is performed in a densely packed neuronal structure like the cerebral cortex (Fig. 7.7B). With central nervous stimulation the dynamic range often cannot be objectively assessed since increasing currents recruit ever more distant neurons due to increasing spread of excitation. Therefore responses continue to increase in amplitude without saturation. For intracortical stimulation the dynamic range of synaptic activity can exceed 12 dB or more, and saturation is often not reached at currents levels that approach the safety limits. Psychophysically, both central and peripheral implants yield similar dynamic ranges of 10–15 dB, whereas in some applications non-monotonicity was observed. For example, in the visual cortical prostheses increase stimulation currents leads to decreased phosphene brightness.

At present it appears as if the much smaller dynamic range of electrical stimulation is also observed with other alternative ways of neuronal stimulation that bypass the chemical synapse and act directly on the excitable membrane (e.g., optogenetic stimulation).

Energy requirements

One essential issue in present-day prosthetic devices is the energy source. Currently, external batteries are used that provide energy to the implanted part of the device using electromagnetic fields. Only in devices that have a very low power consumption, such as pacemakers with slow processing and low stimulation rates, batteries with a lifetime of several years are feasible. These can be implanted with the device and replaced surgically after several years. To avoid the need for an external battery source, and in the attempt to achieve fully implantable devices, several suggestions have been made to exploit energy from within the body. Can passive energy harvesters provide enough energy for stimulation of neurons? In other words, how much energy do we need to elicit one action potential using a current source?

To estimate the energy requirements, we use the example from the most successful prosthetic device, the cochlear implant. To stimulate the auditory nerve requires ca. 30 μA and 30 μs phase duration biphasic pulses (i.e., 60 μs in total), with electrode impedance of ca. 5 kΩ. From impedance and current one can calculate the voltage on the electrode using Ohm's law. The energy consumption (requirement) per such threshold single pulse is given by

$$E_{electric} = U \cdot I_e \cdot t \approx 2.7 \cdot 10^{-10} [J]$$

where U is the voltage, I_e is the current, and t is the time. The resulting minimum energy required to evoke one action potential is thus ~0.27 nJ for electrodes with impedance in kOhm range (this determines the driving voltage for the given current). However, perceptions that allow more than detection, including discrimination of complex patterns, require as a rule more than one action potential, and 100% efficacy of any device is improbable. An energy of 0.27 nJ is therefore the lowest estimate of the energy to be provided by the devices to generate any perception. While central auditory implants require less current to reach the neuronal thresholds, the electrodes are smaller and have therefore much higher impedances (and require higher voltages for stimulation), partly counterbalancing the lower thresholds.

At present purely passive energy harvesters cannot collect enough energy (from sound, body temperature, muscle activity, etc.) to operate without an external energy source. Prosthetic devices thus require external or rechargeable batteries (or another energy source) for operation. Many suggestions in the literature did not consider these simple energy considerations and later proved not enough to drive neurons.

Brief summary

- Electric fields can be focused using bipolar or tripolar configurations.
- Activations functions help predict the areas of tissue that receive strongest excitation.
- The geometry of the stimulation electric field generates surround regions with weaker and opposite effects.
- The mutual relationship of the electrical field and the major direction of the neuronal elements in the proximity of the electrode determines the effectiveness of the stimulation.
- Currents with directions parallel to the direction of axons are typically more likely to reach excitation thresholds than those with perpendicular orientations.
- Different temporal adaptation phenomena can modify responses of neural tissue to electric stimulation.
- Biphasic bipolar configurations have complex effects in the tissue that require consideration.
- Electric stimulation has a very narrow dynamic range compared to natural types of neuronal activity.

Key literature and further reading

Anderson, D.N., Duffley, G., Vorwerk, J., Dorval, A.C., Butson, C.R., 2018. Anodic stimulation misunderstood: preferential activation of fiber orientations with anodic waveforms in deep brain stimulation. J. Neural Eng. 16, 016026.

Bari, B.A., Ollerenshaw, D.R., Millard, D.C., Wang, Q., Stanley, G.B., 2013. Behavioral and electrophysiological effects of cortical microstimulation parameters. PLoS One 8, e82170.

BeMent, S.L., Ranck, J.B., 1969. A quantitative study of electrical stimulation of central myelinated fibers. Exp. Neurol. 24, 147–170.

Boulet, J., White, M., Bruce, I.C., 2016. Temporal considerations for stimulating spiral ganglion neurons with cochlear implants. J. Assoc. Res. Otolaryngol. 17, 1–17.
Grill, W.M., 2015. Model-based analysis and design of waveforms for efficient neural stimulation. Prog. Brain Res. 222, 147–162.
Grill, W.M., Mortimer, J.T., 1996. The effect of stimulus pulse duration on selectivity of neural stimulation. IEEE Trans. Biomed. Eng. 43, 161–166.
Hern, J.E., Phillips, C.G., Porter, R., 1962. Electrical thresholds of unimpaled corticospinal cells in the cat. Q. J. Exp. Physiol. Cogn. Med. Sci. 47, 134–140.
Javel, E., Viemeister, N.F., 2000. Stochastic properties of cat auditory nerve responses to electric and acoustic stimuli and application to intensity discrimination. J. Acoust. Soc. Am. 107, 908–921.
Joucla, S., Yvert, B., 2009. The "mirror" estimate: an intuitive predictor of membrane polarization during extracellular stimulation. Biophys. J. 96, 3495–3508.
Kral, A., Tillein, J., 2021. Cochlear implants. In: Fritzsch, B. (Ed.), Senses: A Comprehensive Reference (2nd ed.). Vol 2 (Audition). Elsevier Academic Press, p. 923–944.
Litvak, L., Delgutte, B., Eddington, D., 2001. Auditory nerve fiber responses to electric stimulation: modulated and unmodulated pulse trains. J. Acoust. Soc. Am. 110, 368–379.
McIntyre, C.C., Grill, W.M., 2002. Extracellular stimulation of central neurons: influence of stimulus waveform and frequency on neuronal output. J. Neurophysiol. 88, 1592–1604.
McNeal, D.R., 1976. Analysis of a model for excitation of myelinated nerve. IEEE Trans. Biomed. Eng. 23, 329–337.
Merrill, D.R., 2010. The electrochemistry of charge injection at the electrode/tissue interface. In: Zhou, D., Greenbaum, E. (Eds.), Implantable Prostheses 2: Techniques and Engineering Approaches. Springer Verlag, pp. 86–135.
Nowak, L.G., Bullier, J., 1998a. Axons, but not cell bodies, are activated by electrical stimulation in cortical gray matter. I. Evidence from chronaxie measurements. Exp. Brain Res. 118, 477–488.
Nowak, L.G., Bullier, J., 1998b. Axons, but not cell bodies, are activated by electrical stimulation in cortical gray matter. II. Evidence from selective inactivation of cell bodies and axon initial segments. Exp. Brain Res. 118, 489–500.
Oberlaender, M., de Kock, C.P.J., Bruno, R.M., Ramirez, A., Meyer, H.S., Dercksen, V.J., Helmstaedter, M., Sakmann, B., 2012. Cell type-specific three-dimensional structure of thalamocortical circuits in a column of rat vibrissal cortex. Cereb. Cortex 22, 2375–2391.
Parkins, C.W., Colombo, J., 1987. Auditory-nerve single-neuron thresholds to electrical stimulation from scala tympani electrodes. Hear. Res. 31, 267–285.
Ranck, J.B., 1975. Which elements are excited in electrical stimulation in mammalian central nervous system: a review. Brain Res. 98, 417–440.
Rattay, F., 1987. Ways to approximate current-distance relations for electrically stimulated fibers. J. Theor. Biol. 125, 339–349.
Shannon, R.V., Otto, S.R., 1990. Psychophysical measures from electrical stimulation of the human cochlear nucleus. Hear. Res. 47, 159–168.
Shepherd, R.K., Hatsushika, S., Clark, G.M., 1993. Electrical stimulation of the auditory nerve: the effect of electrode position on neural excitation. Hear. Res. 66, 108–120.
Voigt, M.B., Hubka, P., Kral, A., 2017. Intracortical microstimultion differentially activates cortical layers based on stimulation depth. Brain Stimul. 10, 684–694.
Voigt, M.B., Kral, A., 2019. Cathodic-leading pulses are more effective than anodic-leading pulses in intracortical microstimulation of the auditory cortex. J. Neural Eng. 16, 036002.

CHAPTER 8

Tissue reaction to neuroprostheses

An implant in the body causes reactions by the body. Even though the implant consists of inert materials like silicone and platinum, it is recognized as a foreign material and evokes immune reactions. These need to be considered and monitored in clinical use. This chapter focuses on the mechanisms of these reactions and the way they can be monitored.

Surrounding tissue adaptations: The implant as a foreign body

Implanting any material into the body inherently causes reactions that are caused by either the physical presence of the electrode (passive reactions) or due to the stimulation current (active reactions). Two phases of passive reactions to the implant can be differentiated.

- Acute reactions, caused mainly by the trauma of implantation and surgery. The surgery related to the implantation is the largest insult that also causes the most massive adaptations that are usually observed within the first weeks following implantation. It is dominated by the healing process of the implantation trauma.
- Chronic reactions that are observed in the course of the following months. They typically consist of the reaction to the implant and the exposed materials. These reactions are primarily dependent on the form of and the materials used in the device, and are aggravated by mechanical stability of the implant in the tissue. The reader is reminded here that biocompatibility and reactivity of the material, as discussed in **Chapter 6**, are key aspects of chronic reactions to the implant.

Tissue reactions to the implant are involved in both acute and chronic reactions. They are caused by the immune system, which as a rule recognizes the implant as a foreign material (it lacks the human leukocyte antigen—HLA—tag of the "own" cells of the body), and induces what medicine calls a **foreign body reaction** (Fig. 8.1). This is an immune reaction in which the tissue-resident immune cells secrete biologically active substances that cause more directed molecular responses through antibodies and cellular immune responses (even in absence of infection, thus causing a sterile inflammation response). Tissue-resident histiocytes such as microglia in the brain (tissue-resident immune cells with phagocytic activity) can react to the mechanical irritation by the implant. In the brain, another group of cells called astrocytes react to the foreign body. The extent of foreign body reaction may vary depending on the immune activity of the tissue where the prosthesis is implanted. As a rule it is a local response: an immune reaction that leads to

Prostheses for the Brain
https://doi.org/10.1016/B978-0-12-818892-7.00007-9

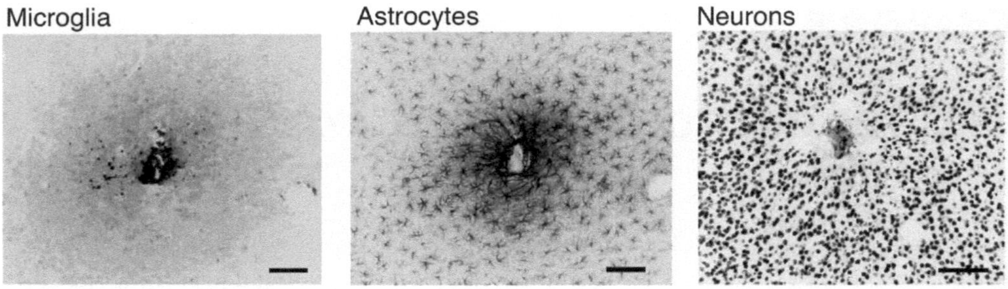

Fig. 8.1 Tissue reaction to an electrode that was in the brain for 4weeks; reactions by microglia, astrocytes, and neurons are shown. Microglia and astrocytes cause a foreign body reaction that displaces the neurons away from the electrode. Bar: 100 μm. *(Reproduced with permission from Biran et al. (2005).)*

formation of granulation tissue that encapsulates the foreign body into a fibrous capsule (or, in the case of the brain, glial capsule), and by that separates it from the rest of the body. This is a meaningful reaction that ensures the material does not release any substances into the body or does not disseminate within the organ due to chemical and biological activity. This reaction can be facilitated by infections (i.e., when bacterial or viral components infect surrounding tissue). Accompanying this reaction, and a possible consequence of it, is a displacement of neurons from the proximity of the foreign body either as a consequence of injury and cell death or as a consequence of the growing volume of glial reaction.

Foreign body reactions are facilitated in cases where there is mechanical instability of the implant within the body (e.g., when the implant moves relative to the tissue and mechanically irritates adjacent cells that can secrete biologically active substances further boosting immune reactions). The brain is embedded in cerebrospinal fluid that can be displaced by the brain during accelerations or decelerations of the body. It protects the brain from damage by mechanical contact with the skull (there is of course a limit for this). In the cerebrospinal fluid the brain is moving relative to the skull. Another source of brain movement comes from breathing that causes changes in intrathoracic pressure. This is translated via the veins onto the brain. Finally, heartbeat can also cause movements of the brain due to the pressure waves in large arteries. Consequently, an implant electrode, particularly when stiffer than the brain tissue and connected through stiff lead wires with a pedestal, connector, or processor fixed in the skull, will interact with the movement of the brain. The resulting force of the implant acting on the neuronal tissue will exacerbate the glial reaction to the implant.

Such foreign body reactions will cover the implant with glial tissue and will potentially isolate and displace excitable elements (neurons) from the implant, or in the worst case even destroy them in the proximity of the implant. These reactions take weeks to months and may be accelerated in cases of injury or infection. The consequence is an increase in stimulation thresholds, an increase in effective current spread, and an increase of electrical impedances of the electrodes (see below). In the case of recording implants, this may lead to loss of recorded neurons and poorer signal-to-noise ratio. A possible work-around are more flexible implants that better adapt to the movement of the brain.

The tissue reaction is very specific to the neuroprosthesis, its target structure, and the local specifics of the environment. Therefore the reactions of the tissue to the individual implants will be discussed in more detail the *Applications* section of this textbook (Chapters 11–16).

Electrode impedance and its clinical value

Resistance refers to the inverse electrical conductivity of a medium during DC stimulation. In AC stimulation, conductivity depends on frequency of the current. In physics this is captured by the frequency-dependent resistance called impedance (**Chapter 5**).

The simplest case for checking the integrity of a device is therefore testing the **impedance of the electrodes**, since both a short circuit of the lead wires as well as break of a lead wire can be detected as a decreased or an increased impedance. Also foreign body reaction affects the impedance. Electrical impedance is defined as the frequency-dependent ratio of voltage to current. Current and voltage may differ in amplitudes and in their phase shift against each other and both properties of the impedance can be mathematically expressed by a complex number. However, for present purposes it is sufficient to use the absolute value of the complex impedance and understand it as a frequency-dependent resistance. In contrast to electrochemical testing on the bench, measurements with reference to the standard hydrogen electrode are not an option in clinical use. Here the reference electrode is either another electrode on the implant or the housing of the implant. Since measurements are often performed at low currents, the reader is also reminded that impedance depends on current density and thus may depend on the absolute current applied. Finally, the measurement includes two bilayers: that of the working and that of the return electrode, so that the circuit in Fig. 8.2 needs to be considered in these cases. However, in case of the reference on the housing electrode, which is much larger than the stimulating contacts, the impedance of the reference is substantially smaller than that of the stimulation contacts and thus its influence can be practically neglected.

The result of such impedance measurement in a subject is a frequency-dependent resistance function (as introduced in Fig. 5.5 and elaborated in **Chapter 10**). In an idealized case the function is similar to Fig. 8.3. Three different regions of the impedance can be defined.

1. One dominated by the leakage (R_{e1} and R_{e2}) and series (R_{s1} and R_{s2}) resistances, here called the "faradaic region." This is the region that is present only if faradaic reactions

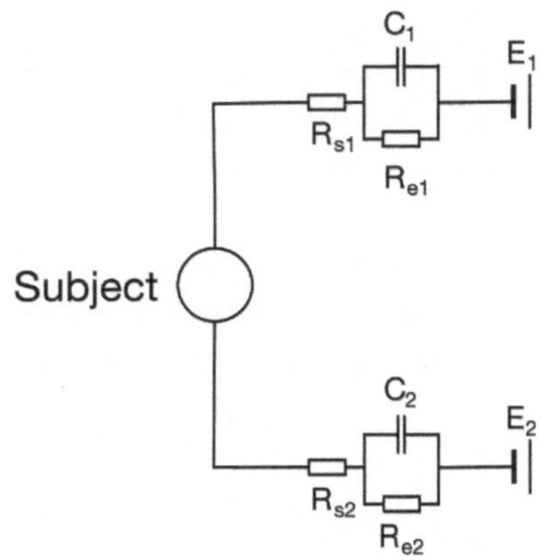

Fig. 8.2 Simplified circuit of the measurement of electrode impedance on a subject. The working and the return electrodes both have an electrode potential (E_1 and E_2), two RC circuits with the capacitance (C) and the leakage resistance (R_e), and two series resistances (R_s). The tissue that the current has to pass on the way from working to return electrode may additionally add electrical components. These are marked here as the circle denoted "Subject." The sum of all these effects is measured with impedance when applied in a clinical setting.

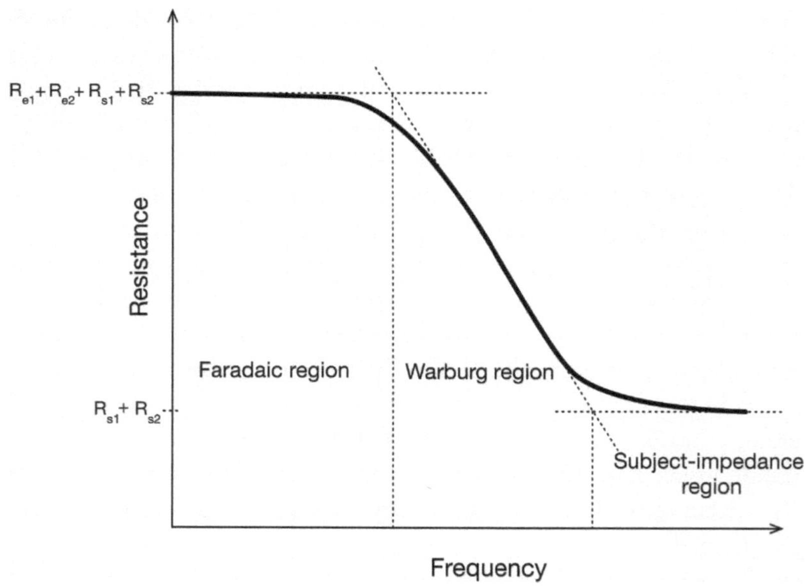

Fig. 8.3 Idealized resistance dependence on frequency. As discussed in **Chapter 5**, the limits of the impedance function is defined by series and leakage resistances, if measured on the subject than both working and return electrode need to be considered. The first region is dominated by faradaic components (it exists only if there is a finite leakage resistance, and thus a faradaic component). The region mainly defined by the capacitance of the bilayer is called the Warburg region. The highest frequency region is unaffected by the capacitance and thus mainly defined by the resistance of the tissue between the electrodes (the series resistances).

are possible and thus current may flow through the leakage resistance. Whether this region is observed in the curve depends also on the voltage on the electrode and the value of a possible dielectric breakdown, as described in **Chapter 6**.

2. At higher frequencies the impedance curve is defined by the capacitances (C_1 and C_2) of the bilayer and the series resistances (R_{s1} and R_{s2}). This region is called the "Warburg region," named after Emil Warburg (1846–1931) who was the first to describe the capacitive properties of the electrode in electrolyte and to suggest the first equivalent electric circuit.
3. Finally, at highest frequencies only the series resistances determine the impedance. The high frequency impedance is dominated by the series resistances (R_{s1} and R_{s2}) since the capacitor of the double-layer is a short circuit (and thus the leakage resistor, R_e, does not play a role, only the series resistor remains; see also **Chapters 5 and 6**) This is consequently the region where only the body of the subject, that is, the electrical conductivity of the tissue between the electrodes, determines the impedance.

Such an idealized impedance curve is pragmatically never obtained, for many reasons. One of them is that in clinical applications, the low-frequency region of this curve (the faradaic region) cannot be measured since the stimulator does not provide the appropriate low-frequency stimulus. Furthermore, the reference electrode for impedance measurement is often the housing of the implant. Titanium, frequently used for the housing, is covered with a layer of titanium oxide, making it a purely capacitive electrode with negligible faradaic currents. Also by design of the processors, the amplification and processing steps usually include high-pass filters. A possible experimental result would be similar to the function shown in Fig. 8.4. A constant sinusoidal current of 5 μA is applied and the resulting voltage is measured at the same electrodes. The four electrodes of the implant were located in the cochlea and were measured relative to a reference located under the skin in the neck. As a rule, resistance of an electrode in tissue decreases with increasing frequency as predicted by the Warburg region of the idealized function. This means that when we keep the current constant, the voltage drops with frequency as a consequence of decreasing resistance (implication of Ohm's law, $U=R*I$).

Another technical implication from Fig. 8.4 is that since all electrodes show a similar impedance profile, the electrodes are intact. Wire breakage of individual electrodes (revealed by an increase in impedance) or short circuit between two electrodes (revealed by a drop in impedance) can be excluded based on these measurements.

Since the applied current is constant and the voltage drops with increasing frequency, the resistance drops correspondingly as well. However, this is not the whole story. When the signals are considered in time, a change in amplitude with frequency is noted as is an increasing delay (phase shift) of the voltage relative to the current (see insets in Fig. 8.4). This is a consequence of the bilayer capacitance, which requires some time to charge and

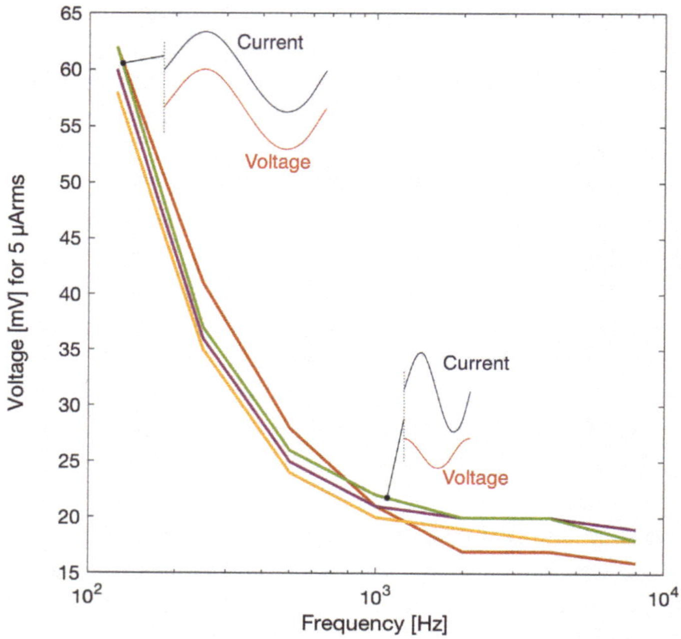

Fig. 8.4 Voltage measurements in an experimental neuroprosthesis, here in a feline model of cochlear implantation, showing the typical drop of voltage with increasing frequency at all four electrode contacts tested. The constant current source delivered $5\,\mu A_{rms}$. In this case, the reference is a remote subcutaneous electrode, and thus the voltage includes the effect of both the stimulating and return electrodes. In addition, the DC component of voltage due to the electrode potential is not included. The voltage drop with increasing frequency results in corresponding drop of resistance with frequency (Fig. 6.3). Insets show the relation of voltage and current for two frequencies. The current has the same amplitude, but the voltage does not. Furthermore, the voltage and current show phase shifts at the higher frequencies. The resulting individual resistances of these electrodes are between ~4 to 12 kΩ. *(Data taken from Kral et al. (2013).)*

discharge the bilayer; the consequence of this phenomenon is a frequency-dependent phase shift.[1] In the example in Fig. 8.3, voltage and current at high and low frequencies (at the faradaic and the subject-impedance regions) would be in phase. However, in the Warburg region in between, voltage and current would be out of phase and the amplitude ratio varied with frequency.

Since electrical sinusoids were used in Figs. 8.3 and 8.4 and many clinical processors cannot generate sinusoidal signals, another useful way of evaluating impedance is analyzing the current and voltage curve during pulsatile stimulation, as shown in Fig. 8.5. Pulsatile stimulation includes several frequency components that underlie frequency

[1] Therefore, the capacitance has, in addition to an amplitude dependence on frequency, a phase dependence on frequency. This is can be displayed by a Bode plot.

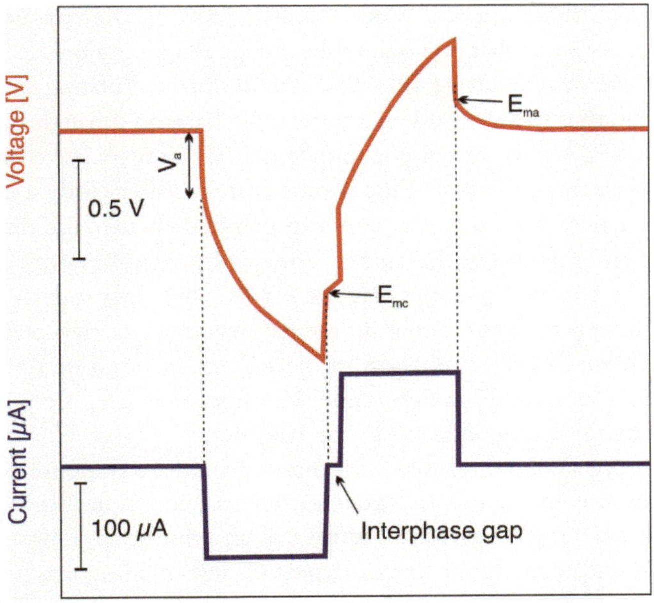

Fig. 8.5 Voltage *(red)* and current *(blue)* time functions of the current source during stimulation with a biphasic pulse (with a brief interface gap). V_a is the initial rise (in this case drop) in voltage called access voltage, which is given by the ohmic resistance of the tissue-electrode interface (series resistance, or R_{s1} and R_{ss} in the circuit shown in Fig. 8.3). The subsequently decreasing voltage during the plateau of the current pulse is caused by the parallel RC part of the interface, i.e., R_{e1}, R_{e2} and the capacitance. E_{mc} is the maximal cathodal potential excursion (at the time when the current source stopped generating current) and E_{ma} is the maximal anodal potential excursion.

dependent current/voltage ratios and phase shifts like those shown in the inset of Fig. 8.4. Unlike sinusoidal signals that contain only one frequency, pulses capture the phase and amplitude effects at many frequencies. Therefore, while for sinusoidal stimulation the shape of the stimulus was identical in voltage and current (the shapes were scaled and shifted version of each other, but the functions for current and voltage had the same morphology in the insets of Fig. 8.4), for pulsatile stimulation the voltage curve in time domain is very different from the current curve. Remember that here a current source is used and thus only current is controlled.

With a current source, by definition the current (blue) curve in Fig. 8.5 follows the desired time function. The voltage (red curve) is consequently shaped by the filtering characteristics of the RC circuit. The voltage function starts with a steep decline due to the cathodic phase of the current; the voltage drop is called **access voltage** (V_a) and is caused by series resistances that respond without delay to the current. Afterwards there is a slowing decline of the voltage caused by the parallel RC circuits. The change (decrease) in voltage becomes smaller with increasing charge on the capacitors and stops when the current pulse terminates. When the current stops, the voltage first falls to the maximal cathodal potential that is given by the charge remaining on the bilayer (currents to the electrodes are switched to zero by the current source, isolating the electrode from the current source; thus the electrode has to start discharging through the tissue). When the anodic phase of the current pulse is initiated, a fast increase in voltage appears, followed by an increase up to the end of the anodic current. Afterwards, a drop to the maximal anodal potential is observed, and a slow exponential return to 0 V that is given by the passive currents, circumventing the current source. Under laboratory conditions with exact measurement, the voltage curve may show a DC shift (may start or end at non-zero voltage due to the electrode potential difference between the two electrodes used for measurement). Given this time function of the voltage in response to the current (red curve in Fig. 8.5), it is possible to determine the impedance (i.e., frequency-dependent resistance) at all frequencies contained in the stimulus.

Stimulating using a current source with pulses provides a response containing many frequencies. Thus, measuring the voltage time response function measures the complex impedance quite well, too (in technical terms it is an impulse response). Moreover, the combined voltage and current time functions provide information on whether the current source is still in the working range with the given electrode–tissue interface. If the device cannot produce enough voltage to drive the necessary current, both the current time function and the voltage time function will show characteristic changes: the voltage function will reach a ceiling voltage and the current function will deviate from the defined value and will not provide the required clean biphasic pulse (Fig. 8.6). These signals thus can detect that the impedance is too high for this current source. The current source is then out of

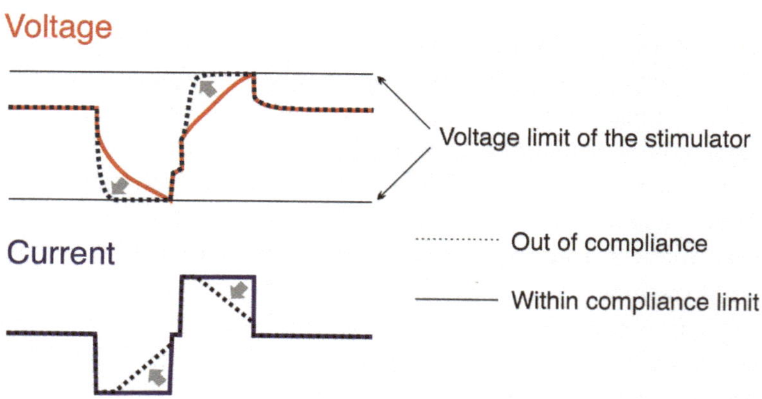

Fig. 8.6 Compliance limits of current source. When the current source cannot provide enough voltage to generate the required current, typical changes in the time functions appear: the voltage saturates at the maximum voltage of the source, and the current deviates from the set value. *Dashed lines* show the functions out of compliance limit of the stimulator, and *gray arrows* point to the "out of compliance" effects. Current sources must be operated only within the specified compliance limits.

compliance limits (compliance in this case referring to the maximum voltage the device is capable producing). The condition is shown with the dashed line in Fig. 8.6 where the charge delivery is not controlled anymore. This might concern both the cathodic and anodic phase of the pulse, but sometimes only one of them. Depending on the architecture of the stimulator, charge imbalance may occur if only one phase is out of compliance. This is a serious safety issue and therefore channels out of compliance should be detected and switched off as soon as possible. A technical workaround to provide enough charge despite high impedance may involve increasing phase duration of the pulse applied at this electrode. By that, lower voltage is required for the same charge delivery.

Commercial systems provide resistance information, but only for a single frequency or as an absolute value of the impedance for the given pulse and do not provide the voltage function. Although a few tested frequencies would suffice to determine the parameters of the circuit shown in Fig. 8.3, impedance testing in clinical devices is simplified to a single value resistance used as a part of the routine check-ups of the integrity of implants. Short circuits in the lead wire will cause a decrease in impedance, whereas wire breakage causes an increase in impedance.

Foreign body reactions to the implant can also be detected by an increasing impedance of the electrode(s) over time, which is particularly prominent within the first few week to months following implantation. The processes involved in this slow increase in impedance over time are many:

1. Fibrous or glial tissue adhering to the implant commonly has a greater resistance compared to fluids or surrounding tissue. Cell adhesion to the implants can be detected using impedance measurements, particularly since it may cause a specific change of the resistance in a specific frequency range. While this has not been so far in clinical use so far due to the restrictions in the processors of clinical implants, it provides a possible way to monitor the processes on the surface of the electrode contact. Stimulation with current can reduce the coverage of the surface of electrodes if these are embedded in fluids, so that after stimulation less cells cover the electrode contact than before stimulation. These effects can be studied by investigation of frequency-dependent resistance using impedance spectroscopy.
2. Changes in the composition of the electrolyte also affect impedance. Chemical changes affecting the concentration of ions in the electrolyte also directly affect impedance. Different types of ions and charged molecules contribute to the specific conductivity of electrolytes differently in a broad range depending on their respective mobility. More mobile (charged) molecules contribute more to conductance (see **Chapter 10**). Acidity can directly (pH is a direct measure of H^+ concentration that is of low absolute concentration under physiological conditions) and indirectly (by affecting the dissociation of other substances) change conductivity of the tissue and thus impedance. Whether conductivity is increased or decreased with increased acidity depends on the specific pH-dependent reactions in the given tissue.

3. Impedance changes can also result from changes in the extracellular matrix. Inflammation near the implant can affect the amount of ions and their mobility in the solution, and thus affect impedances. These processes can also directly affect the bilayer and the electrode reactions that take place.
4. Electrical current, particularly DC, may induce the migration of immune cells towards the implant (a phenomenon called **electrotaxis**) and can cause a sterile inflammation due to electrical stimulation itself. Immune reactions are likely to affect the bilayer and consequently are the reason why in cases of inflammation (even under non-infected condition) the impedances of the electrodes can increase. While DCs are avoided in clinical devices by providing charge-balanced stimulation, with technical failures small direct currents may appear, corrode the electrode and attract immune cells. Corticosteroids attenuate immune activity. Therefore, under sterile (non-infected conditions) the administration of corticosteroids that enter the tissue around the implant may decrease abnormally high impedance in some cases back to a normal range.

In experimental electrophysiology, microelectrode impedances are commonly measured with pulsatile stimulation at 1000 Hz. This technique is used in many commercial implants and the reported impedance is typically the result of the relation of peak current and peak voltage obtained in such conditions.

Transimpedance measurements

Another diagnostic method is measuring the voltage distribution within the tissue by applying current through one electrode and measuring the voltage through another electrode(s). This provides information on the spread of the stimulating electric field, and the tissue the implant is located in, and is therefore of potential clinical use. Obviously, now two electrodes (the stimulating and the measuring) and their electrical properties are directly involved in the measurement, in addition to a remote reference electrode, and thus the voltage measured is affected by even more parameters than in the simple impedance measurements with a common reference electrode. In case of N electrodes N^2-N symmetric combinations of electrode pairs exist. If the measured potentials at the electrodes are devided by the injected current, this recording setting in neuroprosthetics is often referred to as a **transimpedance measurement** and the resulting symmetric matrix of values (abscissa stimulation electrode, ordinate measurement electrode) is called **transimpedance matrix**. Since resistance increases with distance (the specific tissue resistance is multiplied by the tissue volume between the stimulating and recording electrodes), the highest voltages are observed symmetrically around the diagonal of the matrix and decrease with increasing distance from the stimulating electrode (the closest electrodes showing the largest voltages). The transimpedance matrix provides information on the distance of the electrodes relative to each other and the conductivity of the structures in between. In cochlear implants, for example, these measurements may inform which contact is located outside of the cochlea, or detect fold-over of the electrode tip during implantation. If electrodes distant to the given stimulating electrode on the electrode carrier are showing abnormally high voltages, than it is very likely that the implant has formed a fold-over and the distant electrodes were brought into proximity of the stimulating electrode.

Cyclic voltammetry

A laboratory method that has been used to characterize the electrode and the electrochemistry of the electrode surface is cyclic voltammetry. Here, a voltage source is used and the voltage is first slowly increased linearly in time (approximately 100 mV/sec), and after reaching a maximum voltage linearly decreased again. This is repeated (therefore "cyclic") so that the voltage time plot looks like a sawtooth. During these voltage changes the current that flows through the electrode is measured and plotted as voltage-current relation. Due to electrochemical reactions at the electrode surface, the current does not follow voltage changes as predicted by Ohm's law. Furthermore, the current for increasing and decreasing voltage differs as the electrode coverage with molecules depends on the preceding state, leading to a hysteresis. The deviations of voltage-current relationships measured during up and downregulation of the voltage and the voltages where chemical surface reactions affect the current are used to identify specific reactions and to understand the electrochemistry of the electrode surface.

Pragmatically, this procedure is not used in clinical applications, since it requires a voltage that conventional prosthetic devices cannot deliver (sawtooth shape), the voltages required are rather high and faradaic reactions are intentionally initiated, violating safety principles. It is, however, a widely used research tool when investigating new materials and electrode designs.

Infection of the implants

A foreign body reaction with subsequent encapsulation of the implant forms a body niche that in a way is more isolated from the immune system than other parts of the body. Bacteria may enter the body during the surgical implantation procedure and can adhere to the body of the implant. Due to the placement of the implants in natural and artificial cavities, often crossing different tissues and entering the brain or sensory organs, the access of the immune system to the implant is less than normal and the implant provides a route to structures where infections are not normally common and so are difficult to defend. On the foreign body of the implant, the microbes may form a **biofilm**, a structure that involves a high density of bacteria that tightly adheres to the material and are encased in a matrix of extracellular polymers (Fig. 8.7). The biofilm may be formed by bacteria like *Staphylococcus aureus* and is a serious complication.

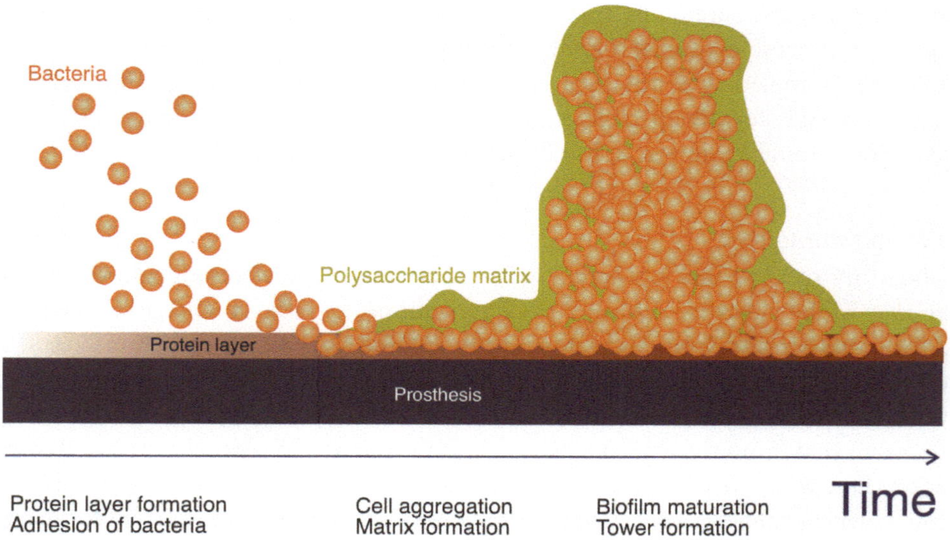

Fig. 8.7 Formation of a biofilm on the surface of a prosthesis. The first step of biofilm formation is the fast adherence of extracellular proteins on the surface of the prosthesis. If bacteria are present in close proximity, they adhere to the proteins as well as to the material of the prosthesis by colloidal absorption. Bacteria start forming a layer by adherence to each other, and produce a polysaccharide matrix that covers them. Biofilm maturation is further related to formation of bacterial "towers" with living and dead bacteria. The matrix in the towers may disrupt and release the bacteria into the systemic circulation, causing a generalized infection. *(Adapted after Le et al. (2014) (Creative Commons Attribution License).)*

Biofilm formation proceeds in steps. First, the implant, when placed in a tissue, will be very quickly covered by a film of extracellular proteins (collagen, fibrinogen, or fibronectin). This is a normal process involved in the foreign body reaction that takes place in absence of an infection. The bacteria, if present, initially behave like colloidal microparticles and adhere non-specifically to the implant body or to the protein layer covering it in a process of colloidal adhesion. However, with time the bacterial filamentous cell appendages start functioning as adhesive structures that interact with the proteins of the protein film. Bacteria can adhere to the prosthesis by colloidal adhesion, with help from the proteins in bacterial membranes called adhesins on their surface, and by interaction with the protein layer formed on the surface of the prosthesis. Bacteria are often smaller than immune cells and therefore can hide in small cavities or structures on the surface of the prosthesis.

The next step is the adherence of the bacteria to each other by adhesins. The bacteria subsequently produce a layer of polysaccharides that covers them (polysaccharide matrix). This further protects the developing biofilm and allows additional bacteria to migrate into it. The maturation stage of the biofilm is characterized by division of the bacteria, their multiplication, and often formation of microbial groups (called towers) on the surface of the implant. Since the matrix in towers may be disrupted, the microbes in such towers can be released into systemic circulation and cause a generalized spread of infection.

Whether an infected biofilm will be formed depends on how fast the implant is integrated into the host tissue compared to the speed in which bacteria adhere to it (the "race to the surface"). After a biofilm has formed, it becomes very difficult to eliminate it by antibiotics, since the concentration that reaches the biofilm is substantially less than the concentration in other tissues, and thus some of the bacteria in the film (the "persister cells") survive, often develop a resistance to the antibiotics, and finally divide and form a new antibiotic-resistant biofilm. Biofilm formation is always a serious complication. The key to preventing it is care of sterile conditions during implantation. Some implants have nanostructures on the surface that prevent adhesion of bacteria (exploiting the "lotus effect") and thus further reduce the risk of biofilm formation.

While there is little information on biofilm development with regard to impedance changes, it is obvious that infections with biofilm formation would affect both series resistance as well as capacitance of the electrode and should be reflected by an increase in electrode impedance. Nonetheless, it is not the leading clinical diagnostic tool, since local inflammation will cause reactions of the tissue that will cause clinical symptoms beyond impedance increase.

Infections of neuroprostheses are very serious complications due to the intimate contact of the prosthesis with the brain. The brain is separated from systemic circulation through the blood-brain barrier. Therefore all interventions that cross the dura mater (**Chapter 4**), the outer barrier between cerebrospinal fluid and the rest of the body, are linked to great danger of infections entering the brain and causing encephalitis (inflammation of the brain) or meningitis (inflammation of the meninges), both of which are life-threatening complications. Furthermore, the body of the implant is often anchored in bone, and bone infections are often persistent and difficult to treat. Therefore any local infection around an implant with connection to the sensory organs or the brain needs to be aggressively treated. Generally, due to these complications and biofilms, an infected implant has to be removed from the body. Reimplantation is only possible after the infection has been successfully treated.

Summary

This chapter outlines a secondary important function of a neuroprosthetic device: not only does it stimulate neurons, the means used to check integrity of the electrode can also be used to determine the reaction of the tissue to the implant. A neuroprosthetic constitutes a probe in the brain; it can be used as a device to measure neuronal and, in part, metabolic activity in the target tissue. As such, a neuroprosthetic device provides an access to the brain and can be used for diagnostic purposes, too. Some scientists call such a device "theragnostic," combining therapeutic and diagnostic functions.

Brief summary

- Following implantation, acute and chronic reactions of the tissue are observed.
- Foreign body reactions encapsulate the implant in connective tissue over longer time.
- Encapsulation of the implant affects the impedance of the electrodes
- Mechanical instability and infections may augment foreign body reactions.
- Voltage of the current source shows both amplitude and phase dependence on frequency.
- Impedance informs on the integrity of the implant as well as the tissue reaction in the body.
- In infections, biofilms may be created on implants and are a serious complication.

Key literature and further reading

Arciola, C.R., Campoccia, D., Montanaro, L., 2018. Implant infections: adhesion, biofilm formation and immune evasion. Nat. Rev. Microbiol. 16, 397–409.

Biran, R., Martin, D.C., Tresco, P.A., 2005. Neuronal cell loss accompanies the brain tissue response to chronically implanted silicon microelectrode arrays. Exp. Neurol. 195, 115–126.

Choi, J., Payne, M.R., Campbell, L.J., Bester, C.W., Newbold, C., Eastwood, H., O'Leary, S.J., 2017. Electrode impedance fluctuations as a biomarker for inner ear pathology after Cochlear implantation. Otol. Neurotol. 38, 1433–1439.

Cogan, S.F., Garrett, D.J., Green, R.A., 2016. Electrochemical principles of safe current injection. In: Shepherd, R.K. (Ed.), Neurobionics. John Wiley & Sons, Inc, Hoboken, NJ, pp. 55–88.

Geddes, L.A., Baker, L.E., 1989. Principles of Applied Biomedical Instrumentation. Wiley & Sons, Inc, Hoboken, NJ.

Grill, W.M., 2005. Safety considerations for deep brain stimulation: review and analysis. Expert Rev. Med. Dev. 2, 409–420.

Kral, A., Hubka, P., Heid, S., Tillein, J., 2013. Single-sided deafness leads to unilateral aural preference within an early sensitive period. Brain 136, 180–193.

Le, K.Y., Dastgheyb, S., Ho, T.V., Otto, M., 2014. Molecular determinants of staphylococcal biofilm dispersal and structuring. Front. Cell. Infect. Microbiol. 4, 167.

Neuburger, J., Lenarz, T., Lesinski-Schiedat, A., Büchner, A., 2009. Spontaneous increases in impedance following cochlear implantation: suspected causes and management. Int. J. Audiol. 48, 233–239.

Newbold, C., Richardson, R., Huang, C.Q., Milojevic, D., Cowan, R., Shepherd, R., 2004. An in vitro model for investigating impedance changes with cell growth and electrical stimulation: implications for cochlear implants. J. Neural Eng. 1, 218–227.

Newbold, C., Richardson, R., Millard, R., Huang, C., Milojevic, D., Shepherd, R., Cowan, R., 2010. Changes in biphasic electrode impedance with protein adsorption and cell growth. J. Neural Eng. 7, 056011.

Seligman, P.M., Shepherd, R.K., 2004. Cochlear implants. In: Horch, K.W., Gurpeet, D.S. (Eds.), Neuroprosthetics: Theory and Practice. World Scientific Publishing Co., Singapore, pp. 878–904

CHAPTER 9

Brain adaptations to neuroprostheses

The brain processes sensory input and in response activates muscles to interact with the physical environment. The brain also adapts to the activity it is processing within its neuronal circuits. We learn (i.e., change our behavior) as a consequence of experience. The brain is therefore not a rigid structure; it is sculptured depending on the type of tasks it is confronted with, depending on the history and demands of the individual organism. The brain substrate for such changes is called neuronal plasticity.

Neuronal plasticity is defined as a persistent change in the functional properties of neurons or neuronal aggregates caused by neuronal activity. Because of neuronal plasticity, activity may leave a lasting trace in the brain and provide the neural mechanism of learning.

The psychology of learning, as well as the physiology of neuronal plasticity, are rich scientific fields that cannot possibly be comprehensively discussed in this context. We instead want to provide some introductory information on physiological mechanisms of neuronal plasticity and then focus on plasticity relevant for neuroprosthetic devices.

Neuronal plasticity and neuroprosthetic devices

Since any significant change of neuronal activity may induce corresponding changes in the neuronal connections of the brain, even loss of activity can cause major changes in excitability of neurons and neuronal networks. Therefore, neuroplasticity is a key player in clinical conditions related to loss of function. For example, a person suffering from loss of visual sensitivity in one spot of the retina (called scotoma) shows a rearrangement of the visual resources to those parts of the retina that are still functional and so provide input for the visual system. This is to the cost of those portions of the retina that became blind. This is a reasonable change, an adaptation that best exploits all neuronal resources for the residual visual input. However, after a successful restoration of visual function in the scotoma this plastic process will reduce the outcome of that intervention, since the restored portion of the retina is not appropriately represented and processed by the central visual system. Over time and with use of the restored function this effect may be compensated by the same neuronal plasticity. Thus, plasticity has to be considered in assessing the outcome of neuronal pathology and all therapeutic interventions.

From the perspective of prosthetic therapy, two types of consequences of neuroplasticity can be considered.

Prostheses for the Brain
https://doi.org/10.1016/B978-0-12-818892-7.00006-7

(1) Beneficial effects: Some forms of plasticity are directly induced by neuroprostheses and affect neuronal circuits within the stimulated system. The brain learns to adapt to the artificial prosthetic stimulation and to maximize the extraction of information from such input. This is beneficial for the subject and provides increased efficacy in use of the neuroprosthesis.

(2) Adverse effects (maladaptive plasticity): A reallocation of the central resources after a lesion in the sensory system, as in the case of scotoma, or of one sensory system by another sensory system during complete sensory loss, are examples of maladaptive processes. These can provide supranormal performance in the spared functions or sensory systems, but degrade the potential of sensory restoration in the affected system (by removing neuronal resources from it). In such a condition, while the sensory input may be restored, the brain regions required for processing of the restored input are occupied by another task. Therefore, from a therapeutic perspective such plastic change is maladaptive. Similarly, in some forms of pain, neural plasticity may lead to its persistence and thus a chronic condition that is difficult to handle. Such plasticity is maladaptive.

It needs to be emphasized that neural plasticity is in the majority of cases an adaptive process. It is the task for doctors to find ways of making optimal use of neuroplasticity for the subject with a disease. As we will see later in this chapter, neuroprostheses can induce maturational processes in the brain that would be otherwise missed and allow, for example, children with hearing impairment to establish complex auditory processing and an acoustic form of communication (speech understanding). That is the most prominent example of beneficial plastic effects of prosthetic therapy, allowing a brain system that otherwise would miss key developmental processes and remain dysfunctional to functionally mature.

Forms of neuronal plasticity

Aristotle and Plato realized that humans learn by forming associations. The neuroscience of associative learning dates back to the work of Ivan Petrovitsh Pavlov (1849–1936) who, interested in digestion, discovered that certain digestive reactions can be trained. When an otherwise irrelevant sensory stimulus (e.g., light or sound) is repeatedly paired with food in brief succession, the stimulus alone starts to initiate digestive processes (e.g., salivation) even when presented alone. Pavlov suggested that brain structures responding to the sensory stimuli become associated with brain regions responsible for controlling this digestive processes. His paradigm, tested on dogs, is called conditioning.

Most scientists at the beginning of the twentieth century thought that the brain is a syncytium, where the cells are not isolated but rather form a network with their inner volume communicating with each other. Camillo Golgi (1843–1926) introduced the first staining that allowed for visualizing isolated neurons (see **Chapter 1**). The first ideas that neuronal contacts called synapses represent the substrate of learning dates back to Santiago

Ramon y Cajal (1852–1934) who, by inspecting Golgi-stained neurons, realized a large variability in the morphology of individual synaptic contacts. He therefore suspected that the synapses change as a consequence of experience. His thoughts were further developed by many who followed, including Jerzy Konorski (1903–1973) and Donald O. Hebb (1904–1985). Konorski and Hebb coined the term neural plasticity and suggested that coincident activity causes a change in synaptic efficacy. Later Warren McCulloch (1898–1969) and Walter Pitts (1923–1969) demonstrated that a neuron can perform logical operations, which clarified that brains can perform computations similar to a computer (or, more accurately, a Turing machine). In combination, these suggestions clarified that a neuronal network can perform meaningful computational operations at the level of synapses and that it can adapt to the tasks it performs, and thus can learn.

Brief, strong activation of a synapse may cause a short-term depletion of neurotransmitter at the synapse (decrease in synaptic effects) or an accumulation of calcium in the postsynaptic cells (increase in synaptic effects). These changes are called adaptation (desensitization) and sensitization, respectively. They are not a true correlate of learning since their effect is only transient (sometimes referred to collectively as short-term plasticity), but as such may contribute to subsequent persistent changes in synaptic efficacy.

Plastic change in synaptic efficacy can result from repeated activation of the same synapse (*homosynaptic plasticity*) or neighboring synapses on the same neuron (*heterosynaptic plasticity*). If postsynaptic neurons are activated above a certain level or plasticity threshold, a molecular process is initiated that changes the synapse, including the presynaptic ending and postsynaptic membrane. In total these processes lead to a persistent increase in synaptic efficacy termed **long-term potentiation** (Fig. 9.1). Today it is well understood at the molecular level.

The reverse process, **long-term depression**, also contributes to neuronal plasticity. Long-term depression results from desynchronized or weak activation of the presynaptic and postsynaptic neuron, leading to a decoupling of the two neurons (weakening of the synapse). Carla Shatz, a neuroscientist from Stanford University, summarized these concepts in the words "what fires together, wires together." Both potentiation and depression can happen in many regions of the central nervous system from the spinal cord up to the cerebral cortex (see below).

There are many different forms of such neuronal plasticity. Some require an active involvement of the individual and take place if a sensory stimulus is of great biological relevance. Others take place more or less passively, even in cases when the individual ignores the stimulus. This latter type of plasticity is based on the statistics of stimulation: more frequent or often co-occurring stimuli will reorganize the brain such that it responds better to the given stimulus or stimulus combination. This is particularly prominent in juvenile age. Juvenile brains, due to the different composition of the molecular machinery of synaptic transmission, show much greater potential for synaptic change and thus for plasticity (**juvenile plasticity**). Inhibition matures later than excitation, favoring

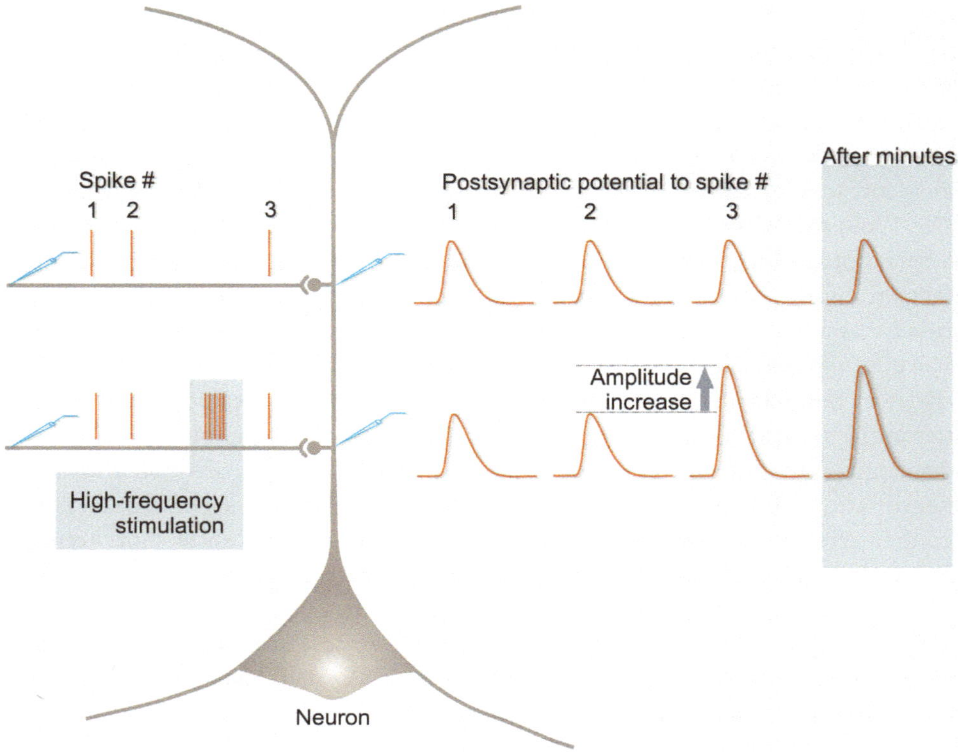

Fig. 9.1 The mechanism of long-term potentiation. Two synapses of the neuron are shown, both of them receiving the same triplet of spikes (# 1, 2, 3) from the presynaptic axons. However, on the lower synapse in the figure, the axons transiently shows a high frequency activity before spike #3, strongly stimulating the synapse. Here, the last postsynaptic potential (#3) demonstrates an amplitude increase that persists for many minutes or even hours after this event. Thus, the efficacy of the synapse has increased, and the synapse has been "long-term potentiated."

excitation over inhibition in juvenile age. This additionally increases the likelihood of reaching the plasticity threshold. Synaptic number also changes during development, with fast synaptogenesis and a prominent peak in juvenile age, followed by synaptic elimination (pruning) causing adult brains to have less synapses than juvenile brains. More synapses, and more plastic synaptic processing, make children better learners. Even passive stimulus presentation, without active engagement of the child, may lead to reorganization of the brain structures activated by the stimulus. This is particularly pronounced if such stimulation is frequently repeated. Similar conditions as a rule do not change the adult brain. Consequently, learning shows **sensitive (or critical) periods** during development, where skills not learned in early childhood require more effort later in life, and sometimes peak performance is limited compared to what can be achieved if learned during early childhood. Certain types of skill acquisition show critical periods. For example, auditory, visual, and language development are all highly dependent on early plasticity and will fail to functionally develop if there is no early experience. We discuss this later in the chapter.

Genetic makeup causes adult synapses to be different in their molecular composition and consequently less plastic. In adult age, the composition of synapses has reached the mature state and the molecular substrate for juvenile plasticity has expired. Inhibition (and thus the excitation/inhibition ratio) has matured and the plasticity threshold has increased. This is a reasonable change, since passive learning based on frequency of exposure is not a meaningful strategy for an entire lifetime. The maturing subject has presumably learned all essential skills required to survive in the given environment and "unlearning" of these skills could be detrimental. However, adults are capable of a controlled, **"gated" plasticity**. Organisms do not always learn all what they are exposed to; we have to select relevant from irrelevant information, and learn only what helps us to better cope with our environment. It is meaningful at this stage to start selecting the information that is to be stored. This is achieved by boosting plasticity using reinforcing neuromodulatory systems. These are networks of neurons producing a neurotransmitter with a lasting modulating function on the target neurons (e.g., cholinergic, serotoninergic, or noradrenergic) activated in biologically relevant conditions (e.g., fear or focused attention). Such modulatory systems either reduce activity of inhibitory neurons or directly modulate (activate) the excitatory neurons that are supposed to learn. This is called gated (adult) plasticity, since this plasticity is "gated" or "allowed" by the subject themself. Thus, our adult learning is internally controlled and not (only) driven by the environment. This helps to focus plasticity towards particularly relevant environmental aspects and prevents that plasticity from erasing or overwriting stored information.

Furthermore, neurons have the tendency to maintain a constant average activity level. To ensure this, spike initiation thresholds adapt to overall activity. Synaptic processes can rescale, and the balance between excitation and inhibition can shift in favor of excitation if mean activity is reduced and vice versa. Such processes ensure a stable level of activity over long time scales and are called **homeostatic plasticity**. In absence of a major driving input, this leads to an increase in sensitivity of the neurons to excitation. Neurons become more responsive to weak inputs that previously only modulated the activity caused by other inputs. This is relevant for neuroprosthetic devices that are used to replace lost function. Both of the underlying pathologies as well as the initiation of neuroprosthetic stimulation will involve processes of homeostatic plasticity.

A very special type of plasticity can be observed if part of the sensory epithelium in the sensory organs is damaged (called **injury-related plasticity**). Here, only parts of a given neural system (that represent the injured regions of the sensory organ, as in the case of a scotoma) receive no input. Based on synaptic and homeostatic mechanisms, this leads to loss of inhibition in the target neurons from the injured part of the sensory organ, and conseqeuntly the excitatory-inhibitory balance is shifted towards excitation, assisted also by homeostatic mechanisms. Due to such processes, the plasticity threshold is exceeded, even in absence of any "gating" in adult brains. The representation of the healthy part of the receptor organ expands into the non-active regions. Based on this mechanism, following injury in the sensory organs, the brains of adults may reorganize passively. Therapeutic interventions that then restore the sensory function need to consider how this mechanism interacts with the restored sensory input.

As the reader can appreciate, the many forms of plasticity may lead to the idea that the term plasticity is too general to capture all the underlying processes related to learning. However, out of historic and pragmatic reasons, the term is still widely used to describe the ability of the neural tissue to change according to the level of activity.

Finally, another neural process that is relevant is **excitotoxicity**, which is overstimulation of neurons that leads to their programmed cell death (apoptosis). A very strong stimulation of a synapse leads to opening of voltage-sensitive calcium channels in many neurons. A strong inflow of calcium increases the otherwise very low intracellular calcium concentration. While calcium often acts as a secondary messenger activating enzymatic reactions in the cell, an abnormally high intracellular calcium concentration may also activate several apoptotic metabolic pathways, finally activating caspases, which are enzymes that facilitate intracellular proteolysis and eventually lead to programmed cell death. A similar process is likely responsible for the observed "hidden hearing loss" where hearing thresholds (hair cells) are not affected directly, but the synapses of hair cells to auditory nerve are lost. By that, the drive to the auditory system is reduced, and while the subjects have normal hearing thresholds, they develop difficulties in understanding speech in noise. As experiments on mice and primates have shown, this condition may arise due to overstimulation of the synapses and loss of spiral ganglion cells and/or their primary afferents.

Plasticity is, however, not the same as memory. Memory is the substrate of information storage and retrieval. It requires a dedicated circuitry that stores information in a distributed way, but also circuitry to access and retrieve it actively, based on the demands of the organism. Plasticity is the substrate of memory, but memory is more. While plasticity may require only one synapse, memory requires networks of neurons and many neuronal structures that allow information storage and retrieval (including hippocampus and the neocortex). The interested reader is referred to textbooks of psychology and neuroscience for more detail.

Plasticity and brain structures

Before we dive deeper into the effects of prostheses on the brain, we need to clarify that not all brain structures have the same potential for plastic adaptations. Some structures have synapses that do not adapt on a long-term basis. Typically, such non-plastic synapses are located in the periphery of the nervous systems and secure a reliable transmission of control signals from and to other organs. For example, the synapse between the axon of motor neurons in the spinal cord and the muscles (the neuromuscular junction) has to be reliable and is thus not plastic. It is important that the nervous system can evoke a certain well-defined muscular reaction (the muscles have their own sensory organs that detect the tension in the tendons and the length of the muscle fibers and report these back to the spinal cord and the brain; thus there is still homeostatic feedback in this system). Similarly, synapses at the onset of the visual and auditory pathways are nonplastic to ensure reliable transmissin from receptor cells to the first neurons of the pathway (however, the sensor can adapt, and there are efferent, from the brain to the sensory organ, connections that can modify their function).

The most plastic synapses, on the other hand, are located in the cerebral and cerebellar cortex and in the hippocampal formation. These structures are responsible for learning and memory and therefore contain the most adaptable neurons. Adult learning mostly happens in the circuits between cortex and hippocampus, but some, for example motor learning, may involve subcortical structures and the cerebellum, too. There is a range between these two extremes, so that other brain regions may also adapt to activity to different extents. Often efferent connections from the cerebral cortex are involved in such adaptations.

The cerebral cortex is the structure where most of the learning is initiated, where first neuronal adaptations to loss of function or regain of function are observed, and where long-term memory is stored. The cerebral cortex is particularly large (relative to the rest of the brain) in humans. It is a convoluted structure with sulci and gyri that allow an approximate orientation on the surface of the brain (Fig. 9.2A). The cortex is further organized into histologically distinct Brodmann areas, to which some functions of the cortex can be approximately assigned. For example, Brodmann area 17 (BA 17) is the area where the visual information in the cortex arrives (primary visual cortex), and BA 41 is the area where auditory information arrives.

The cells found in the cortex have a large variety of forms and functions. The most prominent cells are pyramidal cells. They are excitatory neurons and have a large pyramid-shaped soma and a dense dendritic tree with usually one prominent dendrite (the apical dendrite) that reaches out towards the surface of the cortex (Fig. 5.1; Fig. 9.2B). Pyramidal cells often send their axon to another Brodmann area, or to a subcortical structure, and therefore can be considered output elements of the cortex. The remaining cells are typically intrinsic neurons that process incoming information within the column or in nearby columns; about 30% are inhibitory neurons of many different shapes.

The cortex is furthermore organized into functional vertical units (i.e., oriented perpendicularly to the cortical surface) called columns (Fig. 9.2C). They span all six layers of the cortex (from surface layer I to deepest layer VI) and have a relatively uniform circuitry throughout all Brodmann areas. Activity from the thalamus arrives most abundantly in layer IV (the granular layer); from there it proceeds to layers II and III (the supragranular layers) and from there to layers V and VI (the infragranular layers). Information to other cortical areas is sent from layers II and III to layer IV of the other area, whereas the column receives feedback information from layers V and VI of other cortical areas, mainly

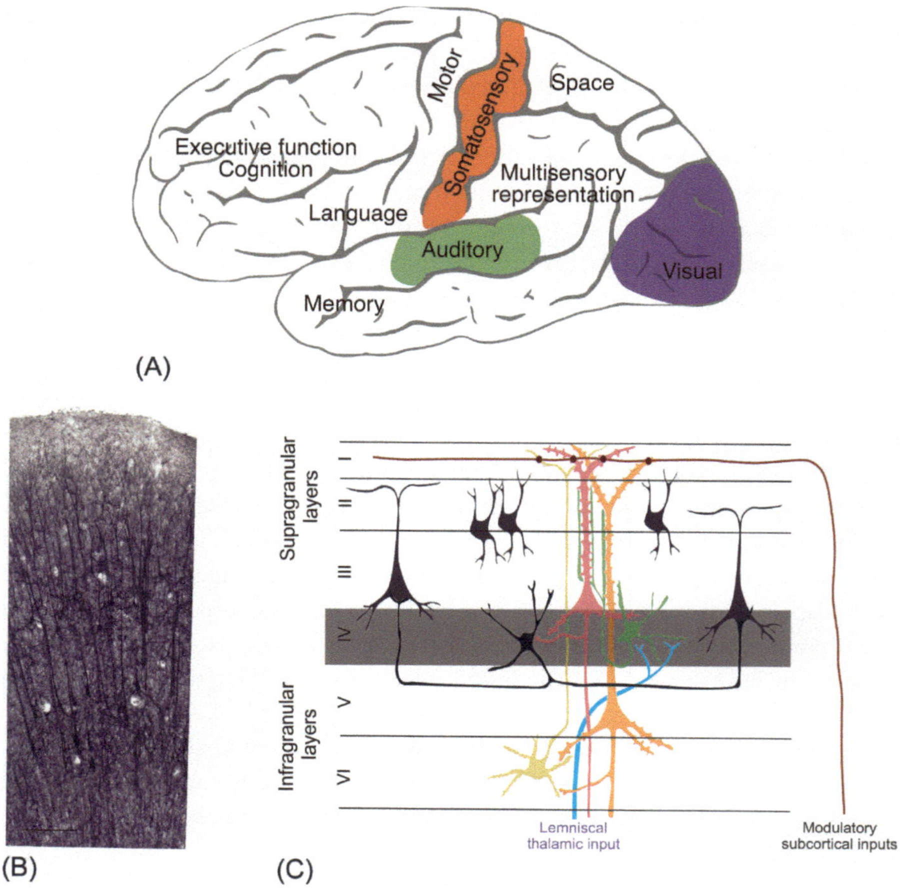

Fig. 9.2 The cerebral cortex is responsible for conscious perception and is a central place of learning in the brain. (A) Side view on the cortex with main gyri. Very simplified functional organization is indicated by the text. (B) Example of a staining of auditory cortex (SMI-32) of a cat visualizing pyramidal cells organized into columns, with long apical dendrites. (C) Functional model of the cortical column showing the diversity of different cells (pyramidal: *pink* and *orange color*; Stellate: *green*; inhibitory basket cells: *black*. Pyramidal cells of neighboring column: *gray*; cortex contains further intrinsic neurons of different morphology: *gray* layer II cells as examples). Layer IV is the granular layer, layers I–III are collectively referred to as supragranular and layers V and VI as infragranular layers.

into layers I, V, and VI. Layer I has few neurons and mainly contains axons from distant neurons and apical dendrites of neurons from the given column. Layer I has a predominantly modulating function for the cortical column, acting through synapses with the apical dendrites of neurons within the cortical column. This circuitry is generally conserved across cortical areas and is therefore called the canonical circuit. This will be of importance when discussing implants for the cortex (**Chapters 12 and 15**).

Cortical columns have lateral connections between neighboring columns that are both excitatory and inhibitory in character. Lateral inhibition observed in so-called basket cells (Fig. 9.2C) is used to preserve or even increase the spatial contrast, such as those found within the sensory system as a representation of the sensory epithelium. There are many forms of inhibition mediated by neurons that are positive to some specific proteins such as somatostatin-positive neurons, parvalbumin-positive neurons, and vasoactive intestinal peptide-positive neurons. The latter are of key importance for the formation of the gated plasticity mentioned previously, since they are in a position to inhibit other inhibitory neurons and therefore disinhibit the cortical column to increase plasticity.

Brain plasticity affects outcomes of prosthetic therapy

There are several principal changes in the nervous system related to prosthetic devices:

- The inducing pathology introduces plastic adaptations due to either loss of function (inactivity) or abnormal function. The loss of function could have happened suddenly or progressively over many months and years, with different consequences for the downstream structures in the brain. In sensory organs, loss of function is related to loss of activity. As explained previously, partial deprivation induces injury-related plasticity. Total sensory loss is a problem for neurons, since they lose the majority of their excitatory drive. Homeostatic plasticity then reorganizes synapses of these neurons, changing the spike-initiation threshold, increasing excitatory transmission, and reducing inhibitory transmission with the goal of maintaining the same overall mean activity levels. In absence of major input, this leads to an increase in the sensitivity of the network. By such adaptation, neurons become more responsive to weak inputs that previously only modulated their activity. One consequence is the overtaking of networks by new functions that can be observed following sensory loss. This can be, as in the case of multimodal areas, helpful to reorganize towards new inputs. The result may be crossmodal plasticity, which is the takeover of one system by another. This can happen, for example, in the auditory cortex of a deaf individual that becomes more responsive to visual stimuli or the visual cortex of a blind individual that responds to auditory stimuli. As mentioned, this may become a problem for later restoration of the sensory system, since the brain regions responsible for processing the lost modality now have attained a new function and may no longer effectively process the original input. Indeed, with cochlear implants (**Chapter 11**) this has become an important clinical issue, since fostering visually guided communication (e.g., in children using sign language) might interfere with acoustic communication in the brain. The question is not yet resolved, but what has become clear is that children with inborn deafness and subjects with adult onset of deafness might differ in the extent of such plastic interactions.
- Use of the device itself initiates plastic processes. Due to synaptic plasticity, the brain adapts to the new stimulation and learns to more effectively extract information from

it, and to ignore any meaningless variation (noise) in the stimulation. This can lead to more proficient use of the prosthetic device over time. Such processes are as a rule observed within the first few months of device use, but in some cases may last many years (see **Chapter 11**).

- The prosthetic device generates abnormal activity in the brain. Typically, electrical stimulation is characterized by large current spread in the neuronal tissue, high synchronization of activity (all active neurons respond within a brief time window), and a small dynamic range. This leads to widespread adaptations. If the prosthesis is acting on central portions of the brain, for example the cerebral cortex, one essential concern is that such highly synchronized activity may cause seizures, a known side effect in cortical visual prostheses (**Chapter 12**). Furthermore, such repeated stimulation may induce plastic synaptic changes (like long-term potentiation in synapses that convey the effect of stimulation) that might further favor propagation of activity and seizures. Using strong cortical stimulation, scientists used to deliberately induce epileptic activity in experimental animal models, a procedure known as "kindling." While this is the desired effect in studies of synaptic plasticity or epilepsy, it is a harmful side effect in clinical applications of central prostheses and needs to be avoided. Interestingly, so far these effects have been observed solely with cortical implants. It is very likely that the less plastic subcortical structures (like with auditory brainstem or midbrain implants discussed in **Chapter 11**, or deep brain stimulation discussed in **Chapter 13**) do not adapt to the stimulation in the same way as the cortex. However, devices that aim to interrupt or suppress abnormal activity, such as systems for deep brain stimulation, may lose a part of the effectiveness due to central adaptations to the device.

Cochlear implants are the best prosthetic example for exploiting neuroplasticity to the benefit of the subject. In fact, they have provided new insights into processes of brain plasticity themselves.

Initially, these devices were used to restore hearing in subjects who became deaf in adulthood. After cochlear implantation and the first fitting session, some of the subjects, while noting an abnormal quality of the perceived sounds, could immediately discriminate language sounds. Some of them could even pick up the phone and understand their spouse for the first time after decades of complete deafness. However, as described later in this book, usually about 12 months are necessary to reach peak performance, indicating that plastic processes make electric hearing more efficient.

Early onset of deafness is, however, a different issue. Congenital deafness, one of the three most frequent inborn diseases, interferes with the acquisition of spoken language. Deaf children as a rule do not learn to speak; they are mute not because they cannot speak, but because they did not learn spoken language. However, they can still vocalize (i.e., cry, laugh, etc.). Until a few decades ago, congenitally deaf subjects relied on sign language and lived in their own social groups. Cochlear implants provided a new therapeutic option to them. When these subjects were implanted in adulthood, the intervention ended in disappointment; while they could hear electric stimuli, they could neither identify them nor discriminate them efficiently. Some were satisfied since they could hear their doorbell or their phone, and could be alerted by danger, but the device did not help them to discriminate complex sounds, categorize them, and by that also understand speech, despite long periods of use. These results generally supported the idea that to hear and to understand speech needs to be learned in childhood. In other words, as mentioned, there is a critical period for language development.

It is known from historic studies that brain injury in juvenile age can be compensated better than brain injury in adult age. Margaret A. Kennard (1899–1975), a neurologist studying brain lesions in primates and human infants, discovered this negative correlation of the outcome expectancy and age at lesion (now called the "Kennard principle"). The brain exploits the large capacity for plastic change in juvenile age (juvenile plasticity) to adapt to lesions; parts of the brain without lesions can better take over functions of the injured parts of the brain if this takes place during early childhood. Kennard observed that such compensations show a critical period of three years, after which they are less well expressed or even absent.

This raised the question, was the failure of cochlear implants in adult prelingually deaf patients a consequence of high age at implantation as well? Some courageous clinicians like William House tried to answer this, despite extensive criticism from colleagues and non-medical critics. The outcome proved him right. Deaf-born children implanted early now belong to the best performers among implanted subjects, provided they are implanted within a critical period of two to three years (the earlier the better). The results of the most comprehensive study on these subjects are shown in Fig. 9.3. Speech comprehension drops with implantation age, and in this population of subjects, age at implantation is the strongest predictor of success. Of course the implant is not enough for this; it requires caring parents who dedicate time and energy to talk to their child and neuroplasticity to adapt to the cochlear implant.

To persuade the medical community for pediatric implantations, and particularly the wide non-medical deaf community, objective evidence was required. This was obtained from animals where neuronal processes could be directly observed. Cochlear implant stimulation on cats has provided insights into the deficits caused by congenital deafness and the positive developmental effects of electric stimulation. In the auditory cortex the correlate of the critical period was found (Fig. 9.4): a maturational arrest has been documented in deaf-born cats, with an induced maturation observed using early cochlear implantation. It has also been demonstrated that the process of synaptic development in the cerebral cortex is crucially dependent on experience, and in absence of sensory input, the auditory cortex loses too many synapses. Consequently, the computational power of the cerebral cortex is reduced. In particular, synapses that connect the different auditory areas together are lost. Therefore, the binding of auditory stimuli into a meaningful representation is compromised. This explains the neuronal mechanism behind the

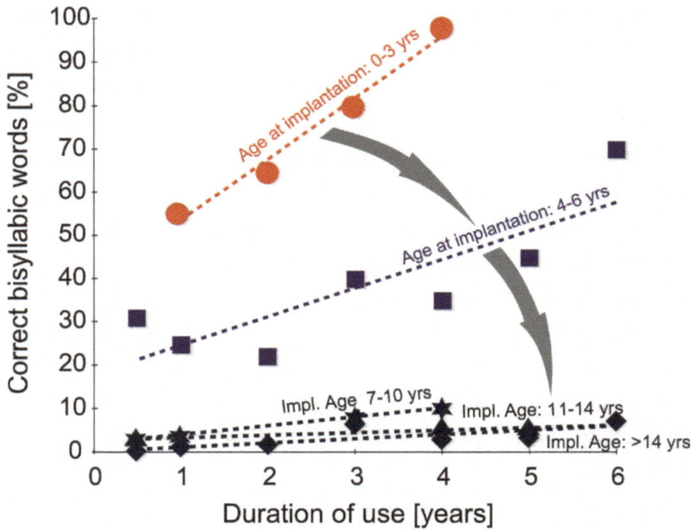

Fig. 9.3 Correct identified bisyllabic words (mama, papa) as a function of duration of cochlear implant use in congenitally deaf children. Age at implantation shown by color. Children implanted early reach near 100% in the test, whereas children implanted after age 7 years do not progress. *(Data from Manrique et al. (1999).)*

difficulties to discriminate and categorize complex sounds in late-implanted congenitally deaf subjects.

Objective electrophysiological measures obtained at the same time in implanted children were consistent with such outcomes. They documented the positive effects of cochlear implant in the human brain and allowed to delineate the end of the critical period at around three years of age. The exquisite consistency in both lines of research demonstrated that similar processes take place in the cat and human brain and that the critical periods are related to auditory processing and only downstream to language (in children). Since deaf children show a mean of 7 years delay in reading ability (sign language and written spoken language are two different languages), educational success in children with inborn deafness is in mean significantly lower than in hearing children. Cochlear implants allowed for the integration of many deaf children into mainstream schooling and improved their educational outcomes.

In many countries, newborn hearing screening has allowed the initiation of therapy within the critical period for therapy of deafness.

Another example is single-sided deafness in childhood, where the brain receives input through one ear only. The cortex reorganizes towards the remaining hearing ear, and the capacity to process input through the deaf ear is progressively reduced. As such, it loses the capacity to appropriately process the input on the deaf ear. This phenomenon does not occur in adult onset of single-sided deafness; in fact, also here there is a brief critical

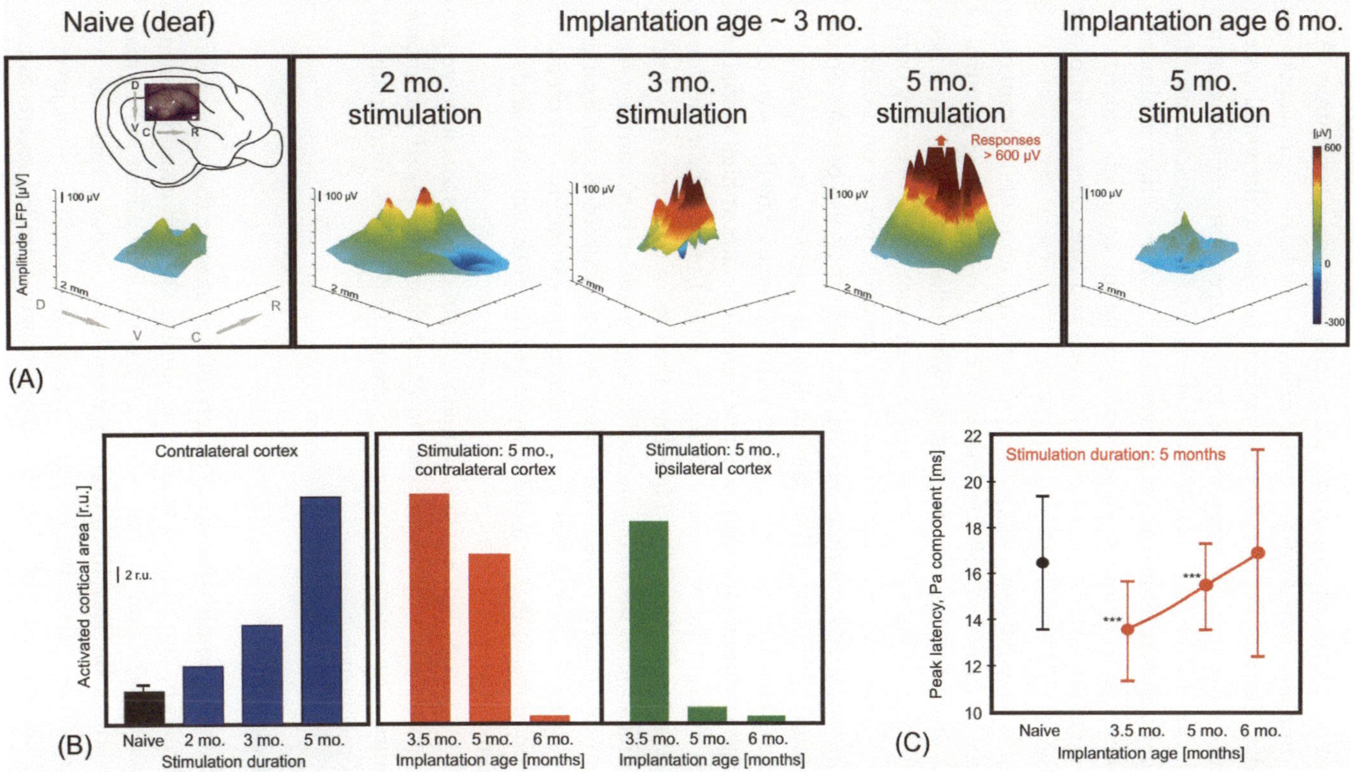

Fig. 9.4 Cochlear implant stimulation in cats induces maturational changes in the auditory cortex. (A) Even in deaf cats, acute cochlear implant stimulation induces responses in the auditory cortex. However, following early implantation and chronic electrostimulation, the active cortical area expands and the responses increase in amplitude. The same is not observed if implantation is performed in adult age (at 6 months in the cat). Anatomical direction labels: D ~ dorsal; V ~ ventral; R ~ rostral; C ~ caudal; LFP stand for local field potential, the type of response recorded. (B) Quantification of active areas. Stimulation duration over several months increases the responsive region *(left)*, whereas increasing implantation age decreases it *(middle and right)*. (C) Quantification of response latencies, demonstrating that early implantation reduces latencies of the responses, but late implantation does not, corresponding to findings in children with electroencephalography. *(Figure reproduced with permission from Kral and Sharma (2012).)*

period (lasting few years after birth). If therapy of single-sided deafness is requested, it has to take place early in life so that the implanted ear profits from the intervention. Also single-sided cochlear implantations lead to similar effects, thus bilateral implantations are recommended today. Similar effects, even more extensive, exist in the visual system: loss of visual acuity in one eye requires intervention in early age to prevent long-lasting maladaptive effects. In the visual system, single-sided absence of vision (monocular deprivation) in cats, monkeys, and children leads to an even more dramatic effect of blindness in the deprived eye. Restoration of vision (either in reopening the artificially closed eyelids or by removing cataracts surgically), when performed too late, does not improve vision in the affected eye.

Brain development is an extensively interrelated process and none of the brain functions exist in isolation. An increased risk for deficits in executive functions (control of behavior and thought processes) and attention (along with other functions) have been shown in deaf-born children. This is the consequence of the fact that the sensory organs are not redundant with respect to each other. Not only do they operate on a different physical signal (light in vision, and sound in hearing, etc.), but they also operate on different qualities of the signal. Hearing, vision, and smell are distance senses, scanning the world at larger distances. Touch and taste are senses related primarily to the own body. Hearing operates at high temporal precision, whereas vision operates at high spatial precision. Touch helps to differentiate own from foreign (is what I see and hear the consequence of my own action on the world?). Therefore, the loss of one sense may lead to more profound reorganization of the brain, including higher-order functions not traditionally considered sensory related. The connectome model of deafness, for example, suggests that hearing loss in childhood may lead to changes in attention and memory, but also in executive functions, so that deaf children tend to be more impulsive and show less capacity for sustained attention.

Critical periods are the consequence of developmental brain changes that involve also neural plasticity. Therefore, critical periods exists in many domains. Visual and motor diseases may also require early intervention once appropriate therapies, potentially via neuroprostheses, become available.

Plasticity in adult age

Neuroprostheses try to either mimic the natural pattern of activation in the brain or interrupt pathological activities by introducing interfering stimuli. In both cases, the stimulation may induce plastic adaptations in the brain that have to be understood to make effective use of the prosthetic devices. In contrast to juvenile age, these adaptations, with the exception of injury-related plasticity, are less extensive and persistent than juvenile plasticity. As such, the consequences of a loss of a neural function are less severe. Sometimes, many decades after the primary insult resulting in functional loss, neuroprosthetic devices can provide their full spectrum of benefit for the subject, implying that the corresponding neuronal circuits were not extensively suffering from the inactivity.

Adaptation in senior age

Another clinically important neuroplasticity aspect is aging. The potential for plastic changes, including adaptations to a neuroprosthetic device, decrease with old age. The use of complicated technical equipment becomes more difficult for the elderly. Aging is related with cognitive decline in many subjects, and consequently the free cognitive resources available for handling a neuroprosthetic device decrease. Surgical interventions require more careful consideration, since side effects of anesthesia and the surgical procedure increase. On the other hand, neural deficits, particularly age-related impairment of vision and hearing, isolate the impaired subject from the society and likely contribute to further cognitive decline. Restoration of sensory-motor abilities therefore contribute to healthy aging.

Given all these aspects, age is not a contraindication for neuroprosthetic therapy. This has been particularly well documented in cochlear implants. Elderly subjects significantly profit from neuroprosthetic devices; of course, performance may be less than in the average user, and may not improve as fast and extensively as in younger subjects. Hearing loss in middle age is the most important modifiable factor involved in cognitive decline at old age; therefore, restoration of hearing, including with neuroprostheses (**Chapter 11**), is key in reducing this cognitive decline. For example, first data on cochlear-implanted elderly subjects suggests that the progression of cognitive decline might be reduced following therapy of hearing. This might be a cardinal beneficial effect of restoring even limited functionality, allowing social interactions and an active, more self-determined life.

Detecting adaptations and maladaptations to the implant

Looking at the future, one outstanding area of research is the identification of changes in the brain that may be limiting the benefit of prosthetic therapy in the brain. Such changes may include significant loss of target neuronal tissue due to the underlying disease as well as plastic changes in the target and connected structures.

It is important to identify these changes. Better knowledge on the underlying disease and use of animal models of the disease provides mechanisms and allows the development of objective measures that can trace these changes based on neuronal signals recorded from the given subject. This would enable better predictions of clinical outcomes and therapeutic progress. Knowledge of neuronal plasticity will help to unlock the full potential of these devices.

In the case of central adaptations, responses to stimulation provide information on changes in brain plasticity related to the implants. This can be measured by different methods, e.g., using electroencephalography, and may provide information on how well the brain responds to stimulation, objectively tracing the progress following implantation and thus quantifying the effectiveness of the therapy. Rehabilitation approaches can subsequently be adapted based on identification of neuronal plasticity following implantation.

Brief summary

- The brain is plastic and adapts to loss of function and neuroprosthetic stimulation.
- Long-term potentiation and depression of synapses are the brain correlate of learning.
- Juvenile neuronal plasticity is greater than adult plasticity.
- The brain has critical development periods of learning, which, if missed, limit the outcome of later therapy.
- Functional sensory input promotes cognitive performance in the elderly and may beneficially influence cognitive decline with age.
- Tracing neuronal adaptations using objective (e.g., electrophysiological) measures can allow for monitoring effectiveness of neuroprostheses.

Key literature and further reading

Bavelier, D., Neville, H.J., 2002. Cross-modal plasticity: where and how? Nat. Rev. Neurosci. 3, 443–452.

Campbell, J., Sharma, A., 2016. Visual cross-modal re-organization in children with cochlear implants. PLoS One. 11, e0147793.

DeFelipe, J., López-Cruz, P.L., Benavides-Piccione, R., Bielza, C., Larrañaga, P., Anderson, S., Burkhalter, A., Cauli, B., Fairén, A., Feldmeyer, D., Fishell, G., Fitzpatrick, D., Freund, T.F., González-Burgos, G., Hestrin, S., Hill, S., Hof, P.R., Huang, J., Jones, E.G., Kawaguchi, Y., Kisvárday, Z., et al., 2013. New insights into the classification and nomenclature of cortical GABAergic interneurons. Nat. Rev. Neurosci. 14, 202–216.

Dorman, M.F., Sharma, A., Gilley, P., Martin, K., Roland, P., 2007. Central auditory development: evidence from CAEP measurements in children fit with cochlear implants. J. Commun. Disord. 40, 284–294.

Fallon, J.B., Irvine, D.R.F., Shepherd, R.K., 2009. Neural prostheses and brain plasticity. J. Neural Eng. 6, 65008.

Fallon, J.B., Shepherd, R.K., Nayagam, D.A.X., Wise, A.K., Heffer, L.F., Landry, T.G., Irvine, D.R.F., 2014. Effects of deafness and cochlear implant use on temporal response characteristics in cat primary auditory cortex. Hear. Res. 315, 1–9.

Kral, A., Eggermont, J.J., 2007. What's to lose and what's to learn: development under auditory deprivation, cochlear implants and limits of cortical plasticity. Brain Res. Rev. 56, 259–269.

Kral, A., Sharma, A., 2012. Developmental neuroplasticity after cochlear implantation. Trends Neurosci. 35, 111–122.

Kral, A., Kronenberger, W.G., Pisoni, D.B., O'Donoghue, G.M., 2016. Neurocognitive factors in sensory restoration of early deafness: a connectome model. Lancet Neurol. 15, 610–621.

Kral, A., Popper, A.N., Fay, R.R., 2013. Deafness. Springer Verlag, New York, Heidelberg, Dordrecht, London.

Kral, A., Dorman, M.F., Wilson, B.S., 2019. Neuronal development of hearing and language: cochlear implants and critical periods. Annu. Rev. Neurosci. 42, 47–65.

Kronenberger, W.G., Beer, J., Castellanos, I., Pisoni, D.B., Miyamoto, R.T., 2014. Neurocognitive risk in children with cochlear implants. JAMA Otolaryngol. Head Neck Surg. 140, 608–615.

Livingston, G., Sommerlad, A., Orgeta, V., Costafreda, S.G., Huntley, J., Ames, D., Ballard, C., Banerjee, S., Burns, A., Cohen-Mansfield, J., Cooper, C., Fox, N., Gitlin, L.N., Howard, R., Kales, H.C., Larson, E.B., Ritchie, K., Rockwood, K., Sampson, E.L., Samus, Q., Schneider, L.S., et al., 2017. Dementia prevention, intervention, and care. Lancet 390, 2673–2734.

Lomber, S.G., Meredith, M.A., Kral, A., 2010. Cross-modal plasticity in specific auditory cortices underlies visual compensations in the deaf. Nat. Neurosci. 13, 1421–1427.

Manrique, M., Cervera-Paz, F.J., Huarte, A., Perez, N., Molina, M., Garcia-Tapia, R., 1999. Cerebral auditory plasticity and cochlear implants. Int. J. Pediatr. Otorhinolaryngol. 49, S193–S197.

Merabet, L.B., Pascual-Leone, A., 2010. Neural reorganization following sensory loss: the opportunity of change. Nat. Rev. Neurosci. 11, 44–52.

Neville, H.J., Lawson, D., 1987. Attention to central and peripheral visual space in a movement detection task: an event-related potential and behavioral study. II. Congenitally deaf adults. Brain Res. 405, 268–283.

Niparko, J.K., Tobey, E.A., Thal, D.J., Eisenberg, L.S., Wang, N.-Y., Quittner, A.L., Fink, N.E., Team, C.D.I., 2010. Spoken language development in children following cochlear implantation. JAMA 303, 1498–1506.

Ponton, C.W., Eggermont, J.J., 2001. Of kittens and kids: altered cortical maturation following profound deafness and cochlear implant use. Audiol. Neurootol. 6, 363–380.

Sharma, A., Dorman, M.F., Kral, A., 2005. The influence of a sensitive period on central auditory development in children with unilateral and bilateral cochlear implants. Hear. Res. 203, 134–143.

Sharma, A., Gilley, P.M., Dorman, M.F., Baldwin, R., 2007. Deprivation-induced cortical reorganization in children with cochlear implants. Int. J. Audiol. 46, 494–499.

Snyder, R.L., Rebscher, S.J., Cao, K.L., Leake, P.A., Kelly, K., 1990. Chronic intracochlear electrical stimulation in the neonatally deafened cat. I: expansion of central representation. Hear. Res. 50, 7–33.

Snyder, R.L., Rebscher, S.J., Leake, P.A., Kelly, K., Cao, K., 1991. Chronic intracochlear electrical stimulation in the neonatally deafened cat. II. Temporal properties of neurons in the inferior colliculus. Hear. Res. 56, 246–264.

CHAPTER 10

Advanced concepts physical chemistry: Electrodes and electrolytes

Introduction

This chapter summarizes and extends previous chapters from the standpoint of physical chemistry. This chapter is more oriented toward readers with mathematical and physical backgrounds or those who want to acquire it and introduces the mathematical treatment of conduction in electrolytes. However, profound physical knowledge is not essential for the basic understanding of the mechanisms discussed in this section. It extends the "Principles" section by an in-depth analysis of the underlying processes discussed in **Chapters 5–8**.

Conductivity of electrical current in electrolytes differs from conduction in metallic conductors, such as wires, in several fundamental aspects. In a simple aqueous electrolyte solution, such as a solution of HCl in water, with two metal electrodes of different electrical potential, the resulting electric field E_0 exerts an electrostatic force on both dissolved ions H_30^+ and Cl^- in opposite directions[a]. If no mechanism exists that allows charge transfer from the solution to an electrode, ions will accumulate around the electrode and will charge the environment of the electrode with opposite polarity until all movements come to rest, creating a polarizable electrode (see **Chapter 5**). The charged boundary between the electrode and the solution, the double layer of the electrode, constitutes a perfect capacitor. This means that direct current flow (DC) will stop after the initial phase, but alternating currents (AC) can still be conducted by alternating movement of ions. If charge *can* be transferred across the boundary from the electrode, ions can be transported from the positively charged electrode (anode) to the negative electrode (cathode), leaving discharged components around the electrodes in the solution. This would decrease the electrical potential of the boundary layer. However, the ions are rapidly replaced by other ions from the solution by electrostatic forces. If we take hydrochloric acid (HCl) at low concentrations dissolved in water as the electrolyte, it will be fully dissociated in the aqueous solution. Consequently, only chloride ions Cl^- and hydronium ions H_3O^+ ($H_2O + H^+$) will exist in the solution. If we now apply a voltage to the two inert (that do not participate in chemical reactions) electrodes, both ions will

[a] Single protons in aqueous solutions do not exist alone, but only in the form of hydronium ions $H_2O + H^+ = H_3O^+$.

Prostheses for the Brain
https://doi.org/10.1016/B978-0-12-818892-7.00014-6

be attracted by the electric field in opposite directions to the electrodes (Fig. 10.1) and from a certain voltage on both ions will be discharged by chemical reactions at the electrodes. Summing up the chemical reactions at both electrodes, we can write:

Electrode 1	$2\ Cl^-$			$\Leftrightarrow$	Cl_2	+	$2e^-$
Electrode 2	$2\ H_3O^+$	+	$2e^-$	$\Leftrightarrow$	H_2	+	$2\ H_2O$
	$2\ HCl$			$\Leftrightarrow$	H_2	+	Cl_2

This process is called electrolysis when driven by an external voltage, charging electrode 1 positively (the anode) and electrode 2 negatively (the cathode). However, without an externally applied voltage the reaction may work also in the opposite direction as a fuel cell, converting chemical components directly into electric energy (voltage and current). This simple example illustrates some fundamental differences between electric conduction in metals and electrolytes.

(1) Whereas conduction in metal leaves the conductor unchanged, conduction of static current in electrolytes changes the concentration of the compounds.

(2) Electric current in electrolytes is combined with the physical movement of ions that are distinguishable even if they have the same charge. This is in contrast to electric current in wires where individual electrons are indistinguishable. For example, a current of K^+ ions can be differentiated from a current of Na^+ ions even if they are similar in size. Hence, multiple distinguishable currents from different components can coexist summing up to a total current.

(3) Transfer of charge to an electrode requires a chemical reaction, leaving the involved components in different states.

Faraday constant

Physicists and chemists use different units to count particles. Whereas chemists use mol ($1\,\text{mol} = 6.02 \cdot 10^{23} = N_A$; Avogadro constant) to count atoms and molecules, physicists use single particles, for example, the elementary charge of a single particle is $e^0 = 1.602 \cdot 10^{-19}\text{C}$ ($1\text{C} = 1\ \text{As} = 6.24 \cdot 10^{18}\ e^{\pm}$), to count charges. These are equivalent approaches; in physical chemistry, both ways are used and the conversion is possible through the Faraday constant[b]:

$$F = 96495 \frac{\text{As}}{\text{mol}} \tag{10.1}$$

However, using both in parallel is appropriate to treat different systems. For example, cell membranes generally have a thickness of approximately 4 nm and a specific capacitance of

[b] "The chemical power of a current of electricity is in direct proportion to the absolute quantity of electricity which passes"; quote from Faraday M (1834): VI. Experimental researches in electricity. Seventh Series. Philosophical Transactions of the Royal Society of London;124:77–122.

approximately 1 μF/cm^2. Hence, charging 1 cm^2 of this membrane to 0.1 V requires 10^{-7} As. In chemical terms this would require 10^{-7} As/96495 As/mol ≈ 1 fmol difference in ion concentration, being much too low to be detected chemically. However, small amounts of salts in neuronal cells can establish a cell potential long after active processes have stopped to keep a steady state by replenishing concentrations of ions in neuronal cells. Hence, chemically small amounts of ion differences in such cells provide a powerful battery and buffer for neuronal (electric) activity.

Specific conductivity

The resistance of a homogeneous material is inversely proportional to the cross-sectional area A and proportional to the length l of the conductor. Hence, with the specific resistivity ρ and the specific conductivity $\kappa = 1/\rho$ the resistance of a (conducting) material can be written as:

$$R = \rho \frac{l}{A} = \frac{1}{\kappa} \frac{l}{A} \tag{10.2}$$

In many cases it is more convenient to use the reciprocal of R: the conductance $G = 1/R$, having the unit Siemens [$S = \Omega^{-1}$]. The unit mho (Ohms inversely written for Ω^{-1}) is also commonly used for Siemens in some publications. Hence, the units of the specific conductivity are κ [Sm^{-1}], although for convenience [S/cm] is generally used. To determine the conductivity of solutions various types of conductivity (measurement) cells are used that usually have platinum electrodes in a capacitor like the configuration shown in Fig. 10.1.

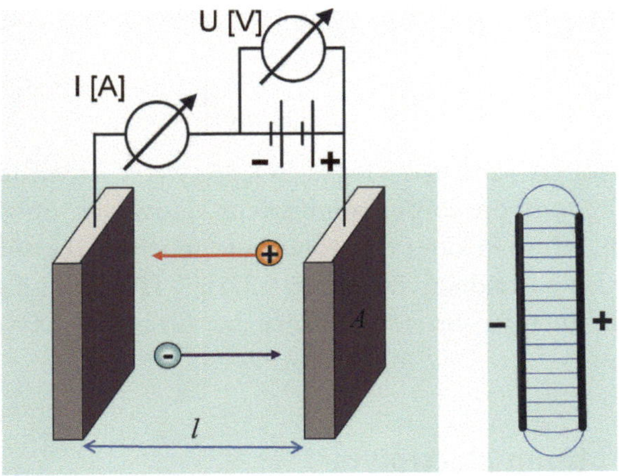

Fig. 10.1 *Left*: Principle of a conductivity cell. Between two electrodes of area A at a distance l an electric field is applied. *Right*: In conductivity cells where the condition $l << \sqrt{A}$ is not fulfilled, the electric field cannot be assumed homogeneous. In this case, the calibration to determine the cell constant is usually performed using a standard solution at known conductivity and temperature. In contrast to the illustration, AC currents are mostly used to reduce polarization effects and electrolysis.

As it is unreliable to determine the conductivity from the geometric dimensions of the cell due to boundary effects (Fig. 10.1, right), cells are usually calibrated with a solution of known conductivity (and temperature) to determine the cell constant A/l. Although electrolytically deposited platinum black on the electrodes reduces the electrode impedance (see **Chapter 6**), polarization may lead to significant errors in measured resistances. For this reason and in contrast to Fig. 10.1 usually AC currents of a few kHz are used to determine the conductivity of solution. Lower frequencies are subject to inaccuracies from electrode polarization, and higher frequencies may lead to errors due to inductivities of connection and cables (C_s in Fig. 5.2). Another way to compensate for polarization errors arising from the resistance of the solution-electrode interface is 4-pole cells where one pair of electrodes is used as the current pathway and another independent pair is used to measure the voltage along the current path. With high impedances of the input, the voltage-sensing pair of electrodes, which carries no significant current, is less affected by the polarization. Frequencies of $2\pi f = 1000\,\text{Hz}$ ($f = 159.1\,\text{Hz}$) and $2\pi f = 10{,}000\,\text{Hz}$ ($f = 1591.5\,\text{Hz}$) are common to simplify calculations (**Chapter 8**).

In solutions the specific conductivity also depends on the amount of ions available. Hence, using the specific conductivity κ [S/cm] and the bulk concentration of electrolyte we can define the molar conductivity as:

$$\Lambda_m = \frac{\kappa}{c}\left[\frac{\text{cm}^2}{\Omega\ \text{mol}}\right] \tag{10.3}$$

Note: (1) As κ is commonly given in [S/cm] concentrations, c in [mol/cm^3] are used here instead of SI units; (2) One mol of 1–1 salt[c] may dissociate into 2 mol of ions maximally. Furthermore the equivalent conductivity can be defined taking the number of charges (n_e) that are created by the dissociation of an electrolyte into account:

$$\Lambda_{eq} = \frac{\kappa}{n_e c}\left[\frac{\text{cm}^2}{\Omega\ \text{mol}}\right] \tag{10.4}$$

For example, n_e is 1 for HCl and n_e is 2 for H_2SO_4. As water is itself an electrolyte, H_3O^+ and HO^- ions will contribute to the conductivity. However, only a small fraction of water is dissociated and water does not contribute much to the specific conductivity, as very pure water has a conductivity of $\kappa = 4.3\ 10^{-6}\,\Omega^{-1}\,\text{m}^{-1}$. Exposing pure water to ambient air will increase its conductivity by dissolved CO_2 to approximately $\kappa = 70.0\ 10^{-6}\,\Omega^{-1}\,\text{m}^{-1}$.

Conductivity of strong electrolytes

As ions interact by Coulomb forces that depend on the average distance between them, conductivities (10.3), (10.4) depend on the concentration of the electrolyte; the greater

[c] A 1-1 salt describes a salt that dissociates into two monovalent ions, e.g., sodium chloride (NaCl).

the concentration, the greater the interaction, and only for $\lim c \to 0$ do interactions disappear. For strong electrolytes the concentration dependence was investigated experimentally and led to the phenomenological **Kohlrausch's law**:

$$\Lambda_m = \Lambda_m^\infty - k_c\sqrt{c} \tag{10.5}$$

where $\Lambda_m^\infty = \lim_{c\to 0}\Lambda_m$ is the limiting molar conductivity and k_c is a constant. Λ_m^∞ cannot be measured directly because the conductivity disappears at low concentrations, so it is determined by extrapolation of concentration series. Fig. 10.2 shows some examples of the molar conductivity of strong electrolytes. In contrast to the conductivity of an electrolyte solution that usually increases with concentration, the molar conductivity (i.e., the conductivity per mol) decreases with the concentration. With increasing concentrations the average distance between ions becomes smaller and electrostatic interactions between ions become stronger, leading to a reduction of the conductivity per ion (or mol). Further, as the illustration shows, Kohlrausch's law only applies to **strong electrolytes** such as HCL in contrast to **weak electrolytes** such as acetic acid (C_3COOH) (see the following section). Kohlrausch demonstrated that in the absence of interaction, for $\lim c \to 0$, ions contribute independently to the conductivity. For a strong electrolyte that dissociates into n_+ cations and n_- anions the limiting molar conductivity can be calculated as the sum of limiting conductivities of the components:

$$\Lambda_m^\infty = n_+\lambda_\infty^+ + n_-\lambda_\infty^- \tag{10.6}$$

According to Kohlrausch, this is the law of independent migration of ions. It can be used to calculate the limiting conductivity of weak electrolytes where the linear interpolation (Fig. 10.2) fails. For example, the limiting molar conductivity of CH_3COOH can be calculated as:

$$\begin{aligned}\Lambda_m^\infty(CH_3COOH) &= \lambda_\infty^+(H_3O^+) + \lambda_\infty^-(CH_3COO^-)\\ \Lambda_m^\infty(CH_3COOH) &= \lambda_\infty^+(H_3O^+) + \lambda_\infty^-(CH_3COO^-) + \lambda_\infty^+(Na^+) - \lambda_\infty^+(Na^+) + \lambda_\infty^-(Cl^-) - \lambda_\infty^-(Cl^-)\end{aligned} \tag{10.7}$$

$$\Lambda_m^\infty(CH_3COOH) = \Lambda_m^\infty(HCl) + \Lambda_m^\infty(CH_3COONa) - \Lambda_m^\infty(NaCl) \tag{10.8}$$

As CH_3COONa, HCl, and NaCl are strong electrolytes, the linear interpolation provides accurate results. Thus the limiting molar conductivity can be calculated from Eq. (10.8).

Strong and weak electrolytes

In contrast to strong electrolytes that are completely dissociated with all molecules as ions available in the solution, weak electrolytes are only partially dissociated into ions in the solution. Hence, the chemical equilibrium for the reaction of an acid HA $HA + H_2O \underset{k_r}{\overset{k_f}{\rightleftharpoons}} A^- + H_3O^+$ with the rates of reaction k_f and k_r can be described with the law of mass action as:

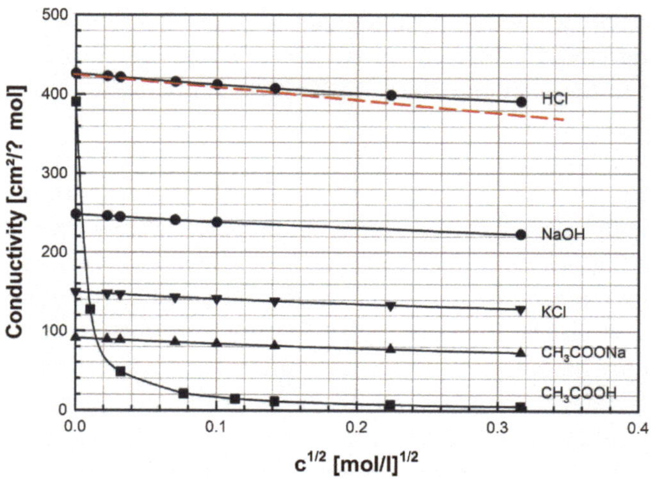

Fig. 10.2 The specific molar conductivity as a function of $\sqrt{c}$ for some strong electrolytes. The *dashed line* shows the linear approximation for HCl $\lim c \to 0$. As an example, the weak electrolyte CH_3COOH is also shown having a different characteristic function of molar concentration. *(Data from CRC Handbook of Chemistry and Physics (1995).)*

$$K_c = \frac{[A^-][H_3O^+]}{HA} \tag{10.9}$$

where K_c is the dissociation constant. However, as K_c will depend on the total concentration, this can be taken into account by the assumption that not all concentrations contribute fully but only "effective" concentrations a_i. This is done by multiplying the concentrations c_i of ions i with activity coefficients f_i that depend on the ionic strength of the solution I to obtain the "active" concentrations a_i:

$$a_i = f_i(I)c_i \tag{10.10}$$

Generally, for finite concentrations, the activity coefficient f_i is less than 1, taking into account that only a fraction of ions contributes to the effective concentration a_i. Only for infinite dilution can the factors $\lim_{c\to 0} f_i = 1$ and the interaction between ions be disregarded. Let's assume in the following that the weak acid is only partially dissociated and the activity coefficients can be ignored ($f_i = 1$). In this case, the concentrations in Eq. (10.9) can be replaced by using the fraction α of dissociated salt molecules:

$$[H_3O^+] = [A^-] = \alpha c \text{ and } [HA] = (1-\alpha)c \tag{10.11}$$

leading to:

$$K_c = \frac{\alpha^2 c}{1-\alpha} \tag{10.12}$$

with the solution for a:

$$a = \frac{K_c}{2c}\left(\sqrt{1 + \frac{4c}{K_c}} - 1\right) \tag{10.13}$$

At low concentrations the hypothetical conductivity with all molecules dissociated can be approximated by the limiting conductivity Λ_∞. Hence, the conductivity is determined by the fraction of dissociated molecules and limiting conductivity:

$$a = \frac{\Lambda_m}{\Lambda_\infty} \tag{10.14}$$

From Eqs. (10.13), (10.14) follows **Ostwald's dilution law** for weak electrolytes:

$$\frac{1}{\Lambda_m} = \frac{1}{\Lambda_m^\infty} + \frac{\Lambda_m c}{K_c(\Lambda_m^\infty)^2} \tag{10.15}$$

The hyperbolic function for weak electrolytes (10.15) describes the characteristic of CH_3COOH well for low concentrations in contrast to Kohlrausch's linear relationship for strong electrolytes. In summary, strong electrolytes dissociate completely and the concentration dependence is governed by Coulomb interactions between charges that increase with concentration and disappear at low concentrations. In contrast, in weak electrolytes, only a fraction of molecules dissociate and the concentration dependence is governed by the law of mass action.

Ion mobilities and solvation of ions

In a homogeneous electric field, for example, in the middle of a capacitor like the configuration shown in Fig. 10.1, the electric field is given by:

$$\vec{E} = -\frac{\partial\varphi}{\partial x} = -\frac{\Delta\varphi}{l} \tag{10.16}$$

An external electric field $\vec{E}$ will exert a force $\vec{F}$ on an ion with z charges that is given by:

$$\vec{F} = ze^0\vec{E} \tag{10.17}$$

This force results in an acceleration of the ion that moves with a time-dependent velocity $\vec{v}$. On the other hand, the ion experiences an increasing frictional force in the opposite direction with increasing velocity. Assuming that the Stokes formula for a sphere of radius r applies in a microscopic system, the viscous drag in a fluid with the viscosity η according to the Stokes' relation is:

$$\vec{\mathrm{F}} = -6\pi\eta r\vec{v} = -f\vec{v} \tag{10.18}$$

with the frictional coefficient *f*. Solving:

$$ma = m\frac{\partial \vec{v}}{\partial t} = ze^0 \vec{E} - 6\pi\eta r \vec{v} \tag{10.19}$$

leads to the solution:

$$v(t) = \frac{ze^0 E}{6\pi\eta r}\left(1 + e^{-\frac{ze^0 E}{6\pi\eta r}t}\right) \tag{10.20}$$

Hence, after a short time of acceleration given by the exponent in Eq. (10.20), forces are balanced and the ion moves with a constant **drift speed** v_s:

$$v_s = \frac{ze^0}{6\pi\eta r}E = uE \tag{10.21}$$

The coefficient u is the **ion mobility** that determines the transport rate of ions responsible for the conductivity of an electrolyte solution.

Hittorf first observed that different ions have different mobilities and hence contribute differently to the total conductivity. Although Stokes law applies to macroscopic spheres such as cells, caution has to be taken when applying classical hydrodynamics to microscopic objects the size of molecules and atoms. The radius r of ions is an experimentally determined effective hydrodynamic radius that includes the hydration shell (general solvation shell) of water dipoles attracted by electrostatic forces. However, here the problem of a microscopic system remains, as the relative dielectric constant of water ($\varepsilon = 78.5$, 298 K) can be only macroscopically defined and forces can only be estimated. The hydration shell can be characterized by the hydration number N_{eq}, which is the number of water molecules creating the shell. Relative hydration numbers can be found experimentally by the determination of water molecules transported together with the respective ion (cotransport) in electrolysis leading to a dilution. Estimated hydration numbers are 5.4 for K^+, 8.4 for Na^+, and 10–12 for Mg^{++}. Generally, radii of bivalent ions such as Ca^{++} tend to have lower conductivities due to bigger hydration shells. As can be seen from Table 10.1, H_3O^+ and OH^- have exceptionally high conductivity. Due to a strong

Table 10.1 Comparison of molar conductivities $\Lambda_\infty^{\pm}$ of infinitely diluted ions, their mobility u, and diffusion coefficients at 298°K.

Ion	$\Lambda_\infty^{\pm}$ [(S/cm²)/(equiv./cm³]	*u* [(cm/s)/(V/cm)]	*D* [10^{-5} cm²/s]
H^+	349.8	36.25	9.31
Na^+	50.1	5.19	1.33
K^+	73.5	7.62	2.07
Ca^{++}	59.5	6.17	0.79
Cl^-	76.4	7.92	2.03
CH_3COO^-	40.9	4.24	1.09
NO_3^{--}	71.5	7.41	1.90

dipole moment, H_2O molecules have a very small average distance to each other. Protons may "tunnel" from one H_3O^+ to the adjacent H_2O converting it into a H_3O^+ without physical movement (and friction) of the first ion. This effect contributes to an additional conductivity without transport of the hydration shell. For OH^- a similar mechanism contributes to the conductivity. In general, the steady-state movement of different ions, underlying Stokes' friction, sums up to the total current through a solution.

Conductivity and mobility of ions

To determine the relationship between conductivity and mobility we assume a strong electrolyte of concentration c. In the steady state the current I and the current density i (flux) passing the area of size A are:

$$I = \frac{\partial Q}{\partial t} = \frac{\Delta Q}{\Delta t} \text{ and } i = \frac{1}{A}\frac{\Delta Q}{\Delta t} \tag{10.22}$$

For independently moving ions the flux will be separable into charges carried by the ions with index i:

$$i = \frac{1}{A\Delta t}\sum_i \Delta Q_i = \sum_i i_i \tag{10.23}$$

If the ion has n_i charges the charge carried by ion i through the area A in an elapsed time Δt is:

$$\Delta Q_i = n_i cF \cdot A \cdot u_i E \Delta t \tag{10.24}$$

$$i_i = n_i u_i cFE = n_i u_i cF\frac{\Delta\varphi}{l} \text{ and } i = \sum_i n_i u_i cF\frac{\Delta\varphi}{l} \tag{10.25}$$

Using Ohm's law and Eq. (10.23): $I = \frac{U}{R} = \frac{\Delta\varphi}{R}\left[\frac{V}{A}\right]$ results in the following relationships:

$$I = \frac{\kappa A \Delta\varphi}{l} \Leftrightarrow i = \frac{\kappa\Delta\varphi}{l} \tag{10.26}$$

From the comparison of Eqs. (10.25), (10.26) follows for the ion specific (i) currents:

$$\kappa_i = n_i u_i cF \text{ and } \kappa = \sum_i n_i u_i cF \tag{10.27}$$

The relationship (10.27) links the mobilities u_i to the share of the conductivity κ_i carried by this type of ion i. The total current through the solution I and the conductivity κ is given by the sum of ion currents and the conductivities κ_i carried by each type of ion, respectively. In summary, the current through a solution can be split into separable currents carried by each type of ion.

Hittorf transport numbers

We have seen in the previous that ionic currents can be split into individual contributions to the total current. Hittorf transport numbers of anions t^- and cations t^+ are defined as the fraction of the total current through the solution that is carried by the respective ion. For a total current I carried by the currents I^+ and I^- of ions in a 1–1 electrolyte solution at a given concentration:

$$t^{\pm} = \frac{|I^{\pm}|}{I^{+} + |I^{-}|} = \frac{|Q^{\pm}|}{Q^{+} + |Q^{-}|} \tag{10.28}$$

where $t^+ + t^- = 1$. By definition, transport numbers depend on the type of counter ion and on their concentrations in the solution and consequently on the properties of the entire mixture. Hence, for multiple components in the solution, the transport number of the ion with indices i is:

$$t_i^{\pm} = \frac{|I_i^{\pm}|}{\sum_i |I_i^{\pm}|} \tag{10.29}$$

The fact that anions and cations in a solution may have different velocities in an electric field and the consequences of this requires an explanation. Let's assume a 1–1 electrolyte in a solution with the cations having triple the velocity as the anions (Fig. 10.3). Before a DC current is applied we have electroneutrality $\left(\sum n_+^i c_-^i + n_+^i c_+^i = 0\right)$ and a homogeneous distribution of ions locally and globally in the solution (Fig. 10.3). We define three different compartments in the solution: two close to each electrode and one centrally between them. When applying a DC current, four quantities of anions and cations are discharged at both electrodes according to the transport numbers $t_+ = 3/4$, $t_- = 1/4$ per unit time. In the same time, three cations are moved from one compartment to the next (and more in between) and one anion in the opposite direction. This simple example illustrates that although different ions contribute differently to the total current, electroneutrality is preserved locally and globally at all times. However, the example also demonstrates that the salt concentrations around the electrodes are decreased by a 1:3 ratio.

Conductometric titration

Up to now we have focused on pairs of ions in solutions and have seen that increased concentrations of ions lead to higher conductivities of the solution. In mixtures this situation needs not to be true as reactions may take place that reduce the total number of available ions. One simple example is the titration of a strong acid (HCl) with a strong base (KOH) while observing the conductivity of the solution (conductometric titration).

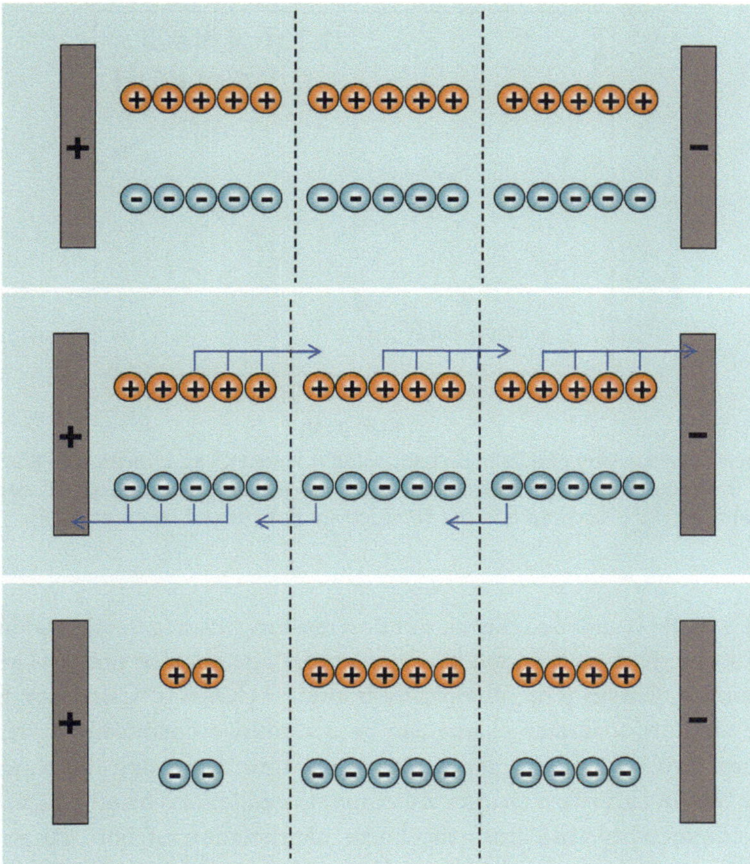

Fig. 10.3 Movement of ions of different mobility ($u^-:u^+=1:3$) in a DC electric field. *Upper panel*: Salt concentrations are homogeneously distributed. *Middle panel*: While four unit charges are removed by the cathode and anode, three cations and one anion are displaced across the imaginary boundaries, resulting in a net flow of four charges. *Lower panel*: Whereas the concentration in the middle compartment is not changed, the salt concentrations in the compartments close to the electrodes are decreased. At all times and in all compartments electo-neutrality is preserved.

$$H_3O^+ + Cl^- + K^+ + OH^- \rightarrow K^+ + Cl^- + 2H_2O$$

Let's assume 1 L of a solution of $c=0.1$ moL/L HCl, when a KOH solution of much higher concentration is added (Fig. 10.4). In this case the addition of volume by the KOH solution is negligible and we can assume a constant concentration of HCl. For low amounts of KOH the solution contains mainly HCl and the conductivity reaches a minimum when the solution contains only KCl (the contribution of H_2O to the conductivity of the solution is low compared to that of the salt). In our example, more than

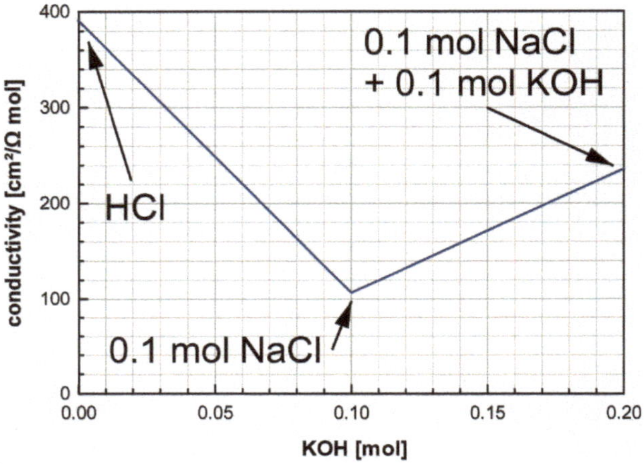

Fig. 10.4 Specific conductivity of a solution containing 0.1 mol HCl as a function of KOH added. The *x*-axis shows the amount of KOH added. Up to 0.1 mol HCl is converted to KCl decreasing the conductivity until all HCl is used up and the conductivity is increased by excess KOH.

0.1 mol excess KOH is added to the salt solution resulting in an increasing additional conductivity. This method can be used also in case that one charged group is immobilized such as in surface charges (e.g., chemically bound —COOH). Using conductometric titration the amount of surface charge can be determined chemically by reducing the amount of free H_3O^+ and replacing it by cations, thus decreasing the conductivity of the solution. When all surface charges are compensated, excess base will lead to a linear increase of conductivity, and from the linear interpolation of both ranges, the total amount of surface charge can be determined. As the concentration of H_3O^+ is equivalent to the pH value this illustrates once more that conductivity of a mixture is a function of all the chemical components.

The tissue-electrode interface: Electrochemical processes

Electrodes in prosthetic devices have to fulfill multiple requirements. Mainly, they have to be biocompatible and chronically stable. The first condition requires that no (toxic) substances be released, and the second, in addition to mechanical stability, requires that the electrode is neither altered nor consumed by the stimulation process, including corrosion. This in turn leaves as an option for such devices only electrodes that do not participate in the charge transfer process or with chemical reactions that are reversible. Hence, noble metal electrodes are the most obvious option. Such electrodes made of inert metals, such as platinum, gold, or iridium, constitute what is called a polarizable electrode (see **Chapters 5** and **6**).

When a polarizable electrode is brought into contact with the solution, ions in the solution are attracted or repelled depending on their charge. At the interface of this **double layer** (or bilayer), the bulk concentrations of ions in the solution are altered near the surface and excess charges compensate the electric potential. Several models of this double layer can be applied to determine its thickness, depending mainly on the concentration of ions in the solution or more specifically on the ionic strength (see Eq. (10.34)).

At high concentrations the simple model of a **Helmholtz layer** applies, predicting a linear electrical potential gradient in the solution. It applies when the Debye length is small compared to the size of hydrated ions in the solution and no additional charges between the ions and the surface can be assumed. When the ions have constituted a double layer with their charge centers at a distance to the surface, the intermediate space contains no charges, and from Maxwell's first law, $\nabla \vec{D} = \sigma$ follows for a non-charged surface in one dimension:

$$\frac{\partial^2 \varphi}{\partial x^2} = 0 \Rightarrow \frac{\partial \varphi}{\partial x} = \text{const.} \tag{10.30}$$

From this relationship a linear potential gradient in the intermediate double layer follows, as shown in Fig. 5.2. This is a "rigid" double layer model in contrast to the "diffuse" double layer at low ion concentrations.

Although simple, the validity of the Helmholtz model depends on the concentration and composition of ions in the solution and can be applied to many physiological systems as these usually have an ionic strength in the range of a few hundred mmol/L. In Fig. 5.2, such a contact of an inert electrode with electric potential Φ_S to a solution with electric potential Φ_L is illustrated. Due to the electrical force by the potential difference at the interface, ions of opposite charge are attracted to or repelled from the (non-permeable) boundary until they are hindered by their size. As water molecules have a strong dipole moment, isolated ions do not exist in an electrolyte solution, but rather have a solvation shell consisting of water dipoles surrounding the ion that increases the size of this complex. The effective size of such ions will not only depend on the size of the ion, number of charges, and the solvation shell but also on their orientation in the case of charged large organic molecules (e.g., —COO^-) in the tissue.

At low ion concentrations the interaction between electric and thermal forces generates a spatially more extended (thicker) layer with a non-linear potential and concentration gradient, as shown in Fig. 5.2. This **"diffuse" layer** can be described with the Gouy-Chapman model. At low concentrations and ionic strength of the solution or the extracellular medium, a diffuse double layer that extends beyond the radius of the involved ions in the Helmholtz layer has to be taken into account. Assuming for example an extended planar surface, a 1–1 electrolyte and a negatively charged electrode, positive ions are attracted and negative ions are repelled creating the Gouy-Chapman layer (Fig. 5.2). With the dimensionless electrical potential:

$$\Phi = \frac{\varphi F}{RT} \tag{10.31}$$

where φ is the electrical potential, F is the Faraday constant of 96485 [As/mol], R is the gas constant, and T is the absolute temperature (in Kelvin) follows an exponential electrical potential extending into the electrolyte (upper panel):

$$\Phi(x) = \Phi_0 e^{-\left(\frac{x}{L_D}\right)} \text{ with the Debye} - \text{length } L_D = \frac{1}{F}\sqrt{\frac{\varepsilon_l \varepsilon_0 RT}{2c}} \tag{10.32}$$

For ambient temperature of 25°C, the dimensional potential leads to a unity of the dimensionless potential of approximately 25.6 mV. In general, for other than 1–1 electrolytes and mixtures the Debye length depends on the ionic strength I of a solution that is defined by the sum of all ions in the solution. In general the Debye length is:

$$L_D = \frac{1}{F}\sqrt{\frac{\varepsilon_l \varepsilon_0 RT}{2I}} \tag{10.33}$$

with the ionic strength:

$$I = \sum_i c_i z_i^2 / 2 \tag{10.34}$$

From the Gouy-Chapman theory the dimensionless concentrations $C_{\pm} = \frac{c_{\pm}}{c_0}$ of positive and negative ions for a bulk concentration $c_0 = c(x \to \infty)$ is calculated as:

$$C_{\pm eq} = \frac{\left(1 \mp te^{-\xi}\right)^2}{\left(1 \pm te^{-\xi}\right)^2}; \quad t = \tanh \frac{\Phi_{surface}}{4} \tag{10.35}$$

The lower panel of Fig. 10.5 shows an example of a negatively charged surface in a 1–1 electrolyte where negative ions in the double layer are depleted and positive ions are accumulated. Although the Gouy-Chapman model is an approximation for $|\Phi_0| \ll \frac{RT}{F} \approx 25.6$ mV, the closed solution for higher potential can be used where the assumption does not hold. Examples of the Debye length for some concentrations of a 1–1 electrolyte are shown in Fig. 10.5.

Despite its simplicity, the Helmholtz double layer applies to most biological systems, as common ion concentrations in tissue are in a range that leads to a Debye length (see Eq. 10.33) that is below the radius of the ions with their solvation shell (Table 10.2).

As the range of validity for both models overlaps this is taken into account in the Gouy-Chapman-Stern model that combines the "rigid" Helmholtz layer in the vicinity of the boundary with the "diffuse" Gouy-Chapman layer.

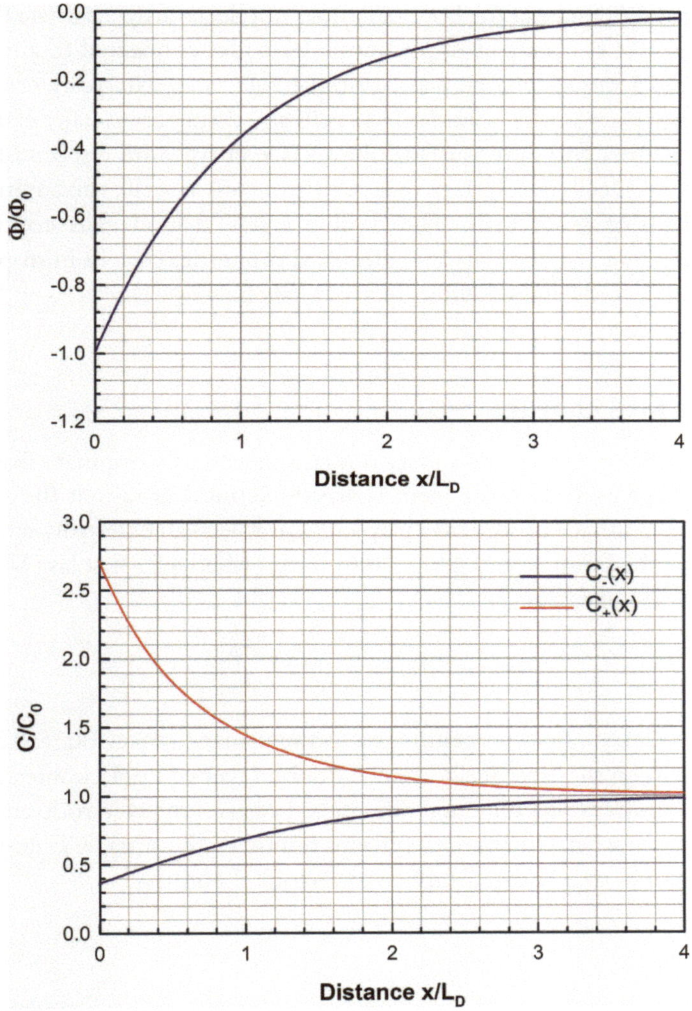

Fig. 10.5 *Upper panel*: Electrical potential distribution in the diffuse double layer near the interface of an electrode at $x=O$ with an electric potential $\Phi_0<0$ according to the Gouy-Chapman model. *Lower panel*: Concentration gradient of positive C_+ and negative ions C_- of an 1:1 electrolye solution near the electrode surface having a negative potential Φ_0 relative to the potential $\Phi_L=0$ $(x\rightarrow\infty)$ of the solution. L_D is the Debye length and c_0 the bulk concentration of the 1:1 electrolyte.

Table 10.2 Debye length L_D of a 1–1 electrolyte for different bulk concentrations *c*.

c (mol/L)	10^{-3}	10^{-2}	10^{-1}	1
L_D (nm)	9.6	3.0	0.96	0.30

The potential difference at the boundary does not necessarily originate from an external voltage source (e.g., in a pair of platinum electrodes connected to a battery). In the electrostatic case, a surface charge plays a similar role as an externally created electrical potential difference across the boundary. As cells and tissues are usually carrying charged proteins at their inner and outer surface, the surface charges are responsible for electrostatic forces between cells in solutions (e.g., erythrocytes) as well as an additional conductivity along the surface of cells. The double layers around cells contribute to the frequency-dependent conductivity and electrical properties of cells in suspensions (such as blood) as well as cells embedded in matrixes (such as tissue).

Chemical surface charges

The potential difference at the boundary does not necessarily originate from an external voltage source, but may also arise from charged chemical groups at the surface. In the electrostatic case, a surface charge may play a similar role as an externally created potential difference across the boundary (see Fig. 10.6). From Maxwell's first law $\nabla \vec{D} = \sigma$ follows in the one-dimensional case:

$$\sigma = \varepsilon_l \varepsilon_0 E_x \Rightarrow \sigma = \varepsilon_l \varepsilon_0 \left[\frac{\partial \varphi}{\partial x} \right]_{x=0} \tag{10.36}$$

where E_x is the electric field perpendicular to the planar surface. Eq. (10.36) shows the equivalence between the electrically created double layer of a polarizable electrode and a surface charge. An electrical potential difference between the electrode and the solution can be created by dissociated chemical groups bound to the surface, leading to the concept of a ζ-potential of a charged surface in colloid chemistry.

Electric models

We have seen that the processes at a solid-electrolyte boundary can be complex and depend on the material of the solid body, the composition and concentrations of the electrolytes, the electrical potential difference (voltage) across the interface, and the chemical composition of the surface. When considering polarizable boundaries, the impedance representing this interface generally will be nonlinear, depending on frequency and the potential difference across the interface. Additionally, in electrical systems we have to distinguish between two types of applications: recording and stimulating electrodes. Whereas currents in recording applications are small and voltages rarely exceed 100 mV, extra-corporal (current) stimulation across the skin sometimes requires voltages of up to a few hundred volts and currents of 10–100 mA.

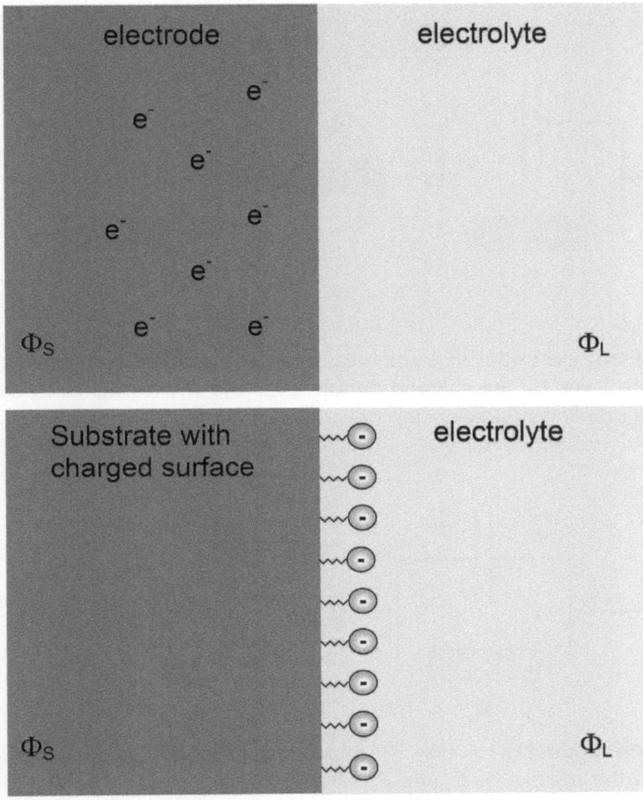

Fig. 10.6 *Upper panel*: Polarizable electrode interface with electric potential Φ_S from a voltage source to a solution with electric potential Φ_L. *Lower panel*: chemical groups carrying a charge (e.g., COO^-) creating an equivalent potential difference (ζ-potential).

However, a simplistic model for the impedance of the solid-electrolyte boundary consisting of resistors and a capacitor serves as an approximation in many cases and illustrates the principal properties (**Chapters 5 and 6**). Any circuit conducting a current requires a return electrode (Fig. 10.7). One concept is an "indifferent electrode" that is much bigger in size with $C_1 \ll C_2$ and leakage resistances $R_{e2} \ll R_{e1}$ and that can be omitted in the circuit due to its low impedance. This return electrode can be the housing of a pacemaker or implant or a separate electrode. The other concept includes two electrodes of similar size usually in proximity that allow a more constricted space to be stimulated. Both cases are equivalent to the circuit shown in Fig. 10.7. Modeling the interface as capacitors and resistors that are independent from the applied voltage and frequency has the advantage that the electrical properties can be calculated.

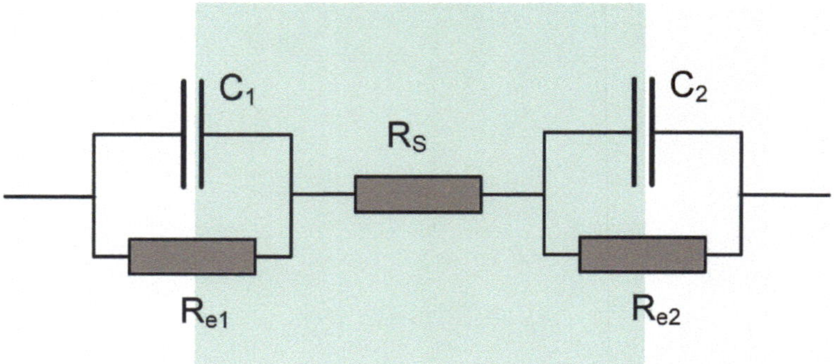

Fig. 10.7 Circuit of two electrodes in a solution. Solution is marked by the blue background. The capacitances $C_{1,2}$ are given by the charged double layer and the resistance R_S by the conductivity of the solution. The non-linear Faraday current is represented by the resistors $R_{e1,2}$.

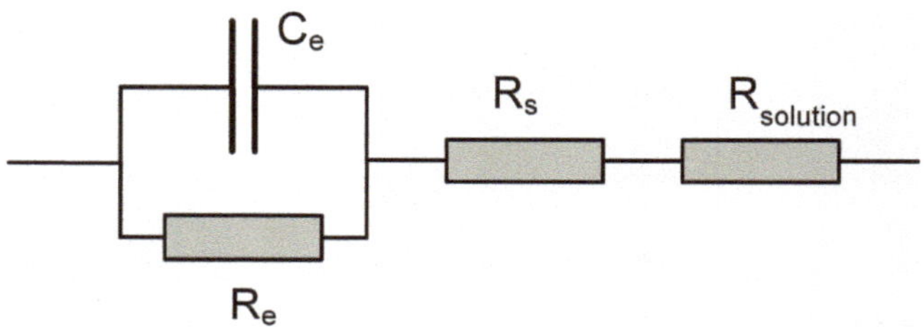

Fig. 10.8 Circuit of electrodes in a solution. The impedance of the double layer interface is given by the capacitance C_e, and the resistances R_e and R_s, whereas $R_{solution}$ is given by the conductance of the solution. C_e, R_s, and $R_{solution}$ are assumed linear here and the resistor R_e represents the pathway of the non-linear Faraday current.

However, the series resistance has in fact two different parts, one that can be attributed to the electrode and another one that is a property of the electrolyte solution, and therefore can be better approximated by the circuit shown in Fig. 10.8. Although R_s and $R_{solution}$ cannot be distinguished in a fixed electrode configuration, they can be separated (e.g., by varying the distance between the electrodes).

Mathematical treatment of the interface impedance

If no chemical reaction to transfer electrons to ions exists at the interface, the current stops when the difference in charge counterbalances the potential difference. In this aspect, the double layer resembles a charged capacitor and the polarizable electrode can be modeled as capacitor. In this case no chemical reaction takes place and the resistances for the

Faraday component in Fig. 10.7 are R_{e1}, $R_{e2}=\infty$, conducting no current, and can be omitted. Independent of whether or not one boundary or the entire circuit is modeled, this system can be described by a serial circuit consisting of a resistor R and a capacitor C. With the angular frequency $\omega=2\pi f$ and the impedance of the capacitance $Z=1/i\omega C$ in complex numbers (where $i=\sqrt{-1}$) the frequency dependent impedance of the circuit can be calculated. Using the characteristic frequency $\omega_0=\frac{1}{RC}\left[\frac{A}{V}\frac{V}{As}\right]$ the impedance of the serial circuit is:

$$Z=R+\frac{1}{i\omega C}=R-\frac{i}{\omega C} \tag{10.37}$$

$$|Z|^2=\left(R-\frac{i}{\omega C}\right)\cdot\left(R+\frac{i}{\omega C}\right) \tag{10.38}$$

$$\frac{|Z|^2}{|Z_0|^2}=\frac{1+f_0^2}{f_0^2} \text{ with } f_0=\frac{\omega}{\omega_0} \text{ and } Z_0=R \tag{10.39}$$

This circuit constitutes a high-pass filter with a low frequency limit $\omega\rightarrow 0\Rightarrow|Z|\rightarrow\infty$ where $|Z|$ is the absolute value of the impedance of Z, as shown in Fig. 10.9. The practical consequence is that when a DC voltage is applied, after some time the current flow

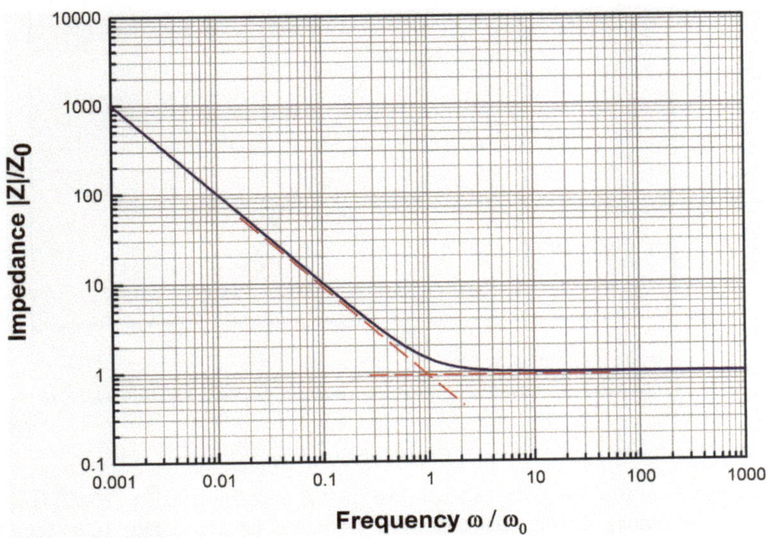

Fig. 10.9 Impedance of a simplified circuit of a double layer of characteristic frequency ω_0 without Faraday current.

stops. Hence, only transient or AC currents are conducted, resulting in a time-dependent charging and discharging of the double layer capacitance. If additional chemical reactions exist that allow a charge transfer from the electrode to the solution, the Faraday component in Fig. 10.8 has to be taken into account by assuming that $R_e \neq \infty$. With the dimensionless characteristic frequency $f_1 = \omega C_P R_F$ follows:

$$Z = R_P + \frac{1}{\left(i\omega C_P + \frac{1}{R_F}\right)} \tag{10.40}$$

$$Z = R_P + R_F \frac{1}{f_1^2 + 1} - iR_F \frac{f_1}{f_1^2 + 1} \text{ with } f_1 = \omega C_P R_F \tag{10.41}$$

$$|Z|^2 = \left(R_P + \frac{R_F}{f_1^2 + 1}\right)^2 + \left(R_F \frac{f_2}{f_1^2 + 1}\right)^2 \tag{10.42}$$

From Eq. (10.42) follows the low frequency impedance limit $\lim_{\omega \to 0} Z \to R_P + R_F$ and the high frequency limit of $\lim_{\omega \to \infty} Z \to R_P$, as illustrated in Fig. 10.10.

Although the simple model in Fig. 10.7 is commonly used in models and applications and is undoubtedly helpful to understand the coarse characteristics of a stimulation

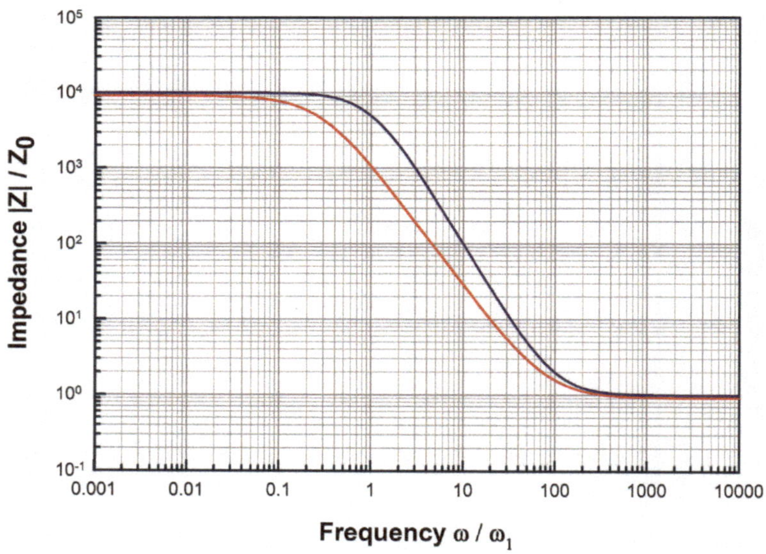

Fig. 10.10 The impedance of the circuit shown in Fig. 10.8 according to Eq. (10.42) is shown in *blue* according to the frequency characteristic derived from the circuit in Fig. 10.8 (Eq. (10.42)) with frequency-independent elements. As this is an approximation, the real double-layer impedance will look more like the characteristic shown in *red* according to Eqs. (10.44), (10.45)

system, it lacks many features of the much more complex electrical properties of the double layer. The capacity C and the resistance R_e in Fig. 10.7 will be proportional to the surface area A of the electrode, respectively $\sim 1/A$ as long as the assumption of a planar surface is valid. This will be the case if the double layer is small compared to the dimensions of the electrode and edge effects leading to inhomogeneous field distributions (e.g., in needle electrodes) are negligible.

Increasing the surface will result in a growth of the capacitance and conductance. Technically this can be done by increasing the active surface area without increasing the size of the electrode (e.g., by the application of platinum black (also known as "moor") on the electrode surface). Electrodeposition of platinum black is a standard procedure in electrochemistry to increase electrode capacitance and conductance, but it is not an option for chronic applications as it is brittle and toxic and common recipes for chloroplatinic acid contain a trace of lead acetate (Lummer solution). By depositing platinum on a platinum surface the active surface and the specific capacity and conductivity can be increased. Whereas increasing the surface geometrically (e.g., by laser cut grooves) has a moderate effect, fractal surfaces like nanostructured, porous, or platinum "grass" show promising results in terms of decreased electrode impedance as well as stability and biocompatibility. In addition, new materials such as structured metal compounds and carbon nanotubes will play a role in the future in this fast evolving field that is fueled not only by bio-applications but also new developments in battery technology.

Earlier in Fig. 10.8 we separated the impedance in an electrolyte resistance R_{s1} and a resistance R_{s2} that can be attributed to the boundary layer. However, this system is underdetermined and the determination and separation of R_{s1} and R_{s2} requires additional steps. As R_{s1} (and C_e) will be constant in the same electrolyte and R_{s2} will be proportional to the distance between the electrodes, the cell length can be varied to separate the electrode impedance from R_{s2}. However, at higher frequencies (>10 kHz) stray capacitances and inductivities of the measuring cell circuit may contribute and have to be determined beforehand and eliminated from results.

As already mentioned, the circuit shown in Fig. 10.8 is an approximation, as the double layer impedance is non-linear and the measured impedance will look more like the example shown in red in Fig. 10.10. This is a consequence of the frequency dependence of C_e and R_{s1} that are imperfectly approximated by frequency-independent electronic elements. The first attempt to describe the electronic double layer originates from Emil Warburg. In this approach, the double layer impedance Z_P is modeled by a series combination of a resistance R_{s1} and a capacitance C_e that both depend on the square root of frequency f. In this case, the phase angle δ:

$$\delta = \tanh^{-1}\left(\omega R_P C_P\right) \tag{10.43}$$

is 45 degrees and independent of frequency. Later this model was refined by Fricke who found that the polarization resistance R_{s1} and capacitance C_e can better be described as a power function of frequency:

$$\begin{aligned} C_P &\sim f^{-m} \\ R_P &\sim f^{1-m} \end{aligned} \tag{10.44}$$

with the relationship between the frequency independent power factor m and the phase angle δ:

$$\delta = m\pi/2 \tag{10.45}$$

Experimentally, Fricke's law was confirmed in a frequency range between 20 Hz and 20 kHz with power factors between 0.3 and 0.5. Platinum electrodes in simple electrolytes are probably the most carefully investigated polarizable electrode system.

Equally important, significant non-linearities arise from Faraday currents, as Faraday currents have a diode-like voltage-current characteristic (i.e., the current remains low until a threshold is exceeded). The threshold is determined by the available electrode reactions and the current level depends on the concentrations of reaction components available at the electrode. Consequently, the Faraday resistance strongly depends on voltage. An example of a simple reaction is the Clark electrode in the following section that illustrates the non-linear voltage dependence of the Faraday current.

Although charged components can be assumed to be in a steady state, local concentrations of non-charged chemical components at the interface depend on the much slower diffusion. Hence, steady-state concentrations may require significant time to establish and local concentrations at the interface may differ significantly from bulk concentrations. Consequently, diffusion barriers like adhering tissue layers or convection (e.g., stirring of the solution) at the interface may have a significant effect on Faraday currents and R_e.

Non-polarizing electrodes

Any electrical stimulation of tissue requires a circuit having at least two electrodes to establish a closed electrical loop. These two conducting electrodes in electrolyte solution(s) constitute an **electrochemical cell**. Both electrodes may be in the same solution or in separate **electrode compartments** that contain solutions of different composition and concentration. These compartments may be have the same or different temperatures and/or pressures and can be connected electrically, for example, by a salt bridge[d] or a diaphragm. A spontaneous (exothermic) reaction that produces an electrical

[d] A salt bridge usually is a tube filled with a strong electrolyte that closes the electrical circuit between separate compartments by enabling ions to migrate between the two solutions without introducing a diffusion potential (see "Diffusion potential" section).

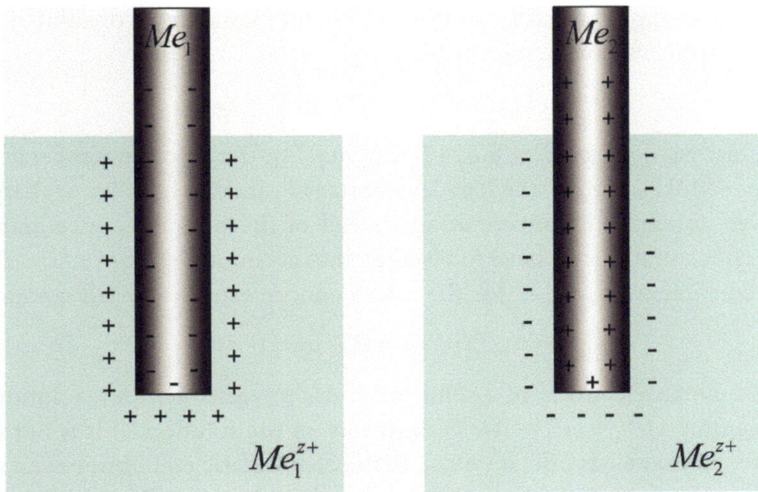

Fig. 10.11 Potential difference of metal electrodes in solutions of their ions. The *left side* shows the situation when the chemical potential of the ions of a metal Me_1 in the solid (S) and liquid (L) phase are $\mu_{Me_1^{z+}}(S) > \mu_{Me_1^{z+}}(L)$. The *right side* shows another metal Me_2 with $\mu_{Me_2^{z+}}(S) > \mu_{Me_2^{z+}}(L)$.

voltage between the electrodes is called a **galvanic cell**. When the chemical reaction is driven by an external voltage between the electrodes, it is called an **electrolytic cell**.

In general, if two phases of the electrode and the solution are brought into contact a chemical reactions can take place until the equilibrium given by the equivalence of the chemical potentials μ_i of all components (with index i) $\mu_i^{phase1} = \mu_i^{phase2}$. However, the situation in case of a metal electrode in a solution of its ions is different. If the metal has a reaction $Me \rightleftharpoons Me^{z+} + ze^-$, the ions will follow their chemical potential gradient charging the surrounding solution (Fig. 10.11, left) until the electrostatic forces counterbalance the chemical forces. For a chemical potential gradient across the boundary in the opposite direction, the reaction will also invert its direction resulting in a potential of opposite polarity (Fig. 10.11, right).

In the case of charged particles, the equilibrium across the boundary will not be given by the equivalence of the chemical potentials but rather by the electrochemical potential that takes the electrostatic interaction into account, as can be seen in the following paragraph.

Nernst equation

From the Gibb's fundamental equation:

$$dU = TdS - pdV + \Sigma \mu_i dn_i + \Phi dq \tag{10.46}$$

It follows that the thermodynamic equilibrium at constant temperature (T) and pressure (p) at the interface between two phases is given by the equivalence of the electrochemical potentials of all compounds that can flow across the boundary. For diluted electrolyte solutions the electrochemical potential is:

$$\eta_{\pm} = \mu_{\pm}^{\infty}(p, T) + RT\,\ln c_{\pm} + e_{\pm}\varphi \tag{10.47}$$

With the molar gas constant $R = 8.314$ [J K^{-1} mol^{-1}], the absolute temperature T [°K], the charge per Mol $e_{\pm} = z_{\pm} F$, the Faraday constant F, and the number of charges per ion $z_{\pm}$. However, for a finite concentration instead of the nominal concentration $c_{\pm}$ the "effective" concentrations $a_{\pm}$ have to be taken into account (see Eq. 10.10). This is done by activity coefficients $a_{\pm} = f_i\, c_{\pm}$ for the active concentrations of each component:

$$\eta_{\pm} = \mu_{\pm}^{\infty}(p, T) + RT\,\ln a_{\pm} + e_{\pm}\varphi \tag{10.48}$$

First, we assume an electrode of a solid metal *Me* in contact with a solution having a chemical reaction $Me^{z+} + ne^{-} \rightleftharpoons Me$ with its ions in the solution. If it is not electrically connected to another electrode, it will be in the electrostatic equilibrium and all currents j_i will be zero. The potential difference between the solid (*S*) and the liquid phase (*L*) of this electrode (*Me*) is the **Galvani potential** $\Delta\varphi$ that can be calculated from the electrochemical potential difference of its components i in the equilibrium $\Delta\eta_i = 0$:

$$0 = \eta_{Me^{z+}} - \eta_{Me} = \mu_{Me^{2+}}^{\infty} + RT\,\ln a_{Me^{2+}} + e_{-}\varphi_L - \left(\mu_{Me}^{\infty} + RT\,\ln a_{Me} + e_{-}\varphi_S\right) \tag{10.49}$$

From (10.49), it follows directly that the Galvani potential is:

$$\Delta\varphi = \varphi_{Me} - \varphi_L = \frac{\mu_{Me^{z+}}^{\infty} - \mu_{Me}^{\infty}}{zF} + \frac{RT}{zF}\ln\frac{a_{Me^{z+}}}{a_{Me}} \tag{10.50}$$

The activity a_{Me} of the solid metal can be assumed constant and by substituting $\varphi_0 = \left(\mu_{Me^{z+}}^{\infty} - \mu_{Me}^{\infty}\right)/zF + const.$ follows the **Nernst equation** for a metal electrode in a solution. It describes the concentration dependence of the electric equilibrium potential:

$$\Delta\varphi = \varphi_0 + \frac{RT}{zF}\ln a_{Me^{z+}} \tag{10.51}$$

where φ_0 is the standard Galvani potential at $a_{Me^{z+}} = 1$. At a room temperature of 25°C with the molar gas constant $R = 8.314$ [J °K^{-1} mol^{-1}] the dependency of the equilibrium Galvani potential on the concentration is approximately 59 mV per decade:

$$\Delta\varphi = \varphi_0 + \frac{RT}{zF}\frac{1}{\log e}\log a_{Me^{z+}} = \varphi_0 + \frac{59mV}{z}\log a_{Me^{z+}} \tag{10.52}$$

The potential difference between a single electrode and the solution cannot be measured in isolation as measuring the electrical potential of the solution would require a second contact to the solution by an electrode that also would establish a potential difference in a similar way.

In addition, an inert polarizable electrode such as a Pt electrode generates an equilibrium Galvani potential in an electrolyte solution that contains a substance *Sub* providing a redox reaction $Sub_{Ox} + ne^- \rightleftharpoons Sub_{Red}$ that can be described in the same way. The oxidized and reduced substance is called a **redox couple** Sub_{Ox}/Sub_{Red}, for example Fe^{3+}/Fe^{2+} (see section on. *Redox* reaction below). In contrast to an electrode involved in a chemical reaction, the inert electrode can only exchange electrons. When brought into contact with the solution the electrochemical potential of the electrons will equilibrate, creating an electrolytic double layer. However, as free electrons in an aqueous solution can't exist due to their short lifetime of less than 1 ms, the charge will be linked to the ion of the redox couple that determines the electric potential (see Box 10.1).

Moreover, the equilibrium condition of the electrochemical potentials η_i applies to many other systems where different phases are in contact and permit (selective) ion currents. Other important examples are cell membranes that are permeable for some components but not for all, although biological cells are not in a thermodynamic equilibrium but in a steady state.[e]

Box 10.1: Electron transfer

Using the activities of the electron in the solution $a_{e^-}(L)$ and in the metal $a_{e^-}(S)$, the electrochemical potentials at equilibrium for the boundary can be given as:

$$\begin{aligned} 0 &= \eta_{e^-}(L) - \eta_{e^-}(S) \\ &= \mu_{e^-}^{\infty}(L) + RT \ln a_{e^-}(L) + e_- \varphi_L - \left(\mu_{e^-}^{\infty}(S) + RT \ln a_{e^-}(S) + e_- \varphi_S\right) \end{aligned} \tag{10.83}$$

For the electrons in the metal, $a_{e^-}(S)$ can be assumed constant. With the charge of an electron $z=1 \Rightarrow e^- = F$ follows for the electrical potential difference across the boundary as:

$$\Delta\varphi = \varphi_S - \varphi_L = \frac{\mu_{e^-}^{\infty}(S) - \mu_{e^-}^{\infty}(L)}{F} - \frac{RT}{F} \ln a_{e^-}(L) \tag{10.84}$$

The activity of the electrons in the solution follows from the chemical equilibrium according to the of the law of mass action as:

$$\frac{a_{Ox}(a_{e^-}(L))^n}{a_{Red}} = K_a \Leftrightarrow a_{e^-}(L) = \left(K_a \frac{a_{Ox}}{a_{Red}}\right)^{\frac{1}{n}} \tag{10.85}$$

And from Eqs. (10.84), (10.85) follows the Nernst equitation for the equilibrium Galvani potential of a redox electrode as:

$$\Delta\varphi = \Delta\varphi_0 + \frac{RT}{nF} \ln\left(\frac{a_{Ox}}{a_{Red}}\right) \tag{10.86}$$

[e] In a thermodynamic equilibrium all currents of all components i are zero ($j_i = 0$), whereas a steady state is given by $\sum j_i = 0$ when the sum of all components between all compartments is zero.

Redox reaction

A redox (reduction-oxidation) reaction describes a reaction where an electron is transferred from one component to another. Oxidation is the loss of electron(s) and reduction is the gain of electron(s). The reducing agent (or reductant), which loses an electron during oxidation, is the donor. The oxidizing agent (or oxidant), gaining an electron, is the acceptor. Examples are the redox couple from the previous chapter $Fe^{2+} \rightleftharpoons e^- + Fe^{3+}$ or $Cu^{2+}(L) + Zn(S) \rightarrow Cu(S) + Zn^{2+}(L)$ where $Cu^{2+}(L)$, $Zn^{2+}(L)$ denote the ions in the liquid phase and Zn(S), Cu(S) the solids (metals).

Redox reactions can be split into two **half-reactions** where the loss and gain of electron(s) in the transferal from one component to the other is separated into two redox couples. One common example is the oxidation of Cu(S) and the reduction of $Zn^{2+}(L)$:

Oxidation of Cu(S)	$Cu^{2+}(L)$	+	$2e^-$	$\rightarrow$	Cu(S)		
Reduction of $Zn^{2+}(L)$	Zn(S)	$\rightarrow$	$Zn^{2+}(L)$	+	$2e^-$		
Sum	$Cu^{2+}(L)$	+	Zn(S)	$\rightarrow$	Cu(S)	+	$Zn^{2+}(L)$

Each redox couple of the half-reaction $Ox + \nu e^- \rightleftharpoons Red$ is usually denoted as Ox/Red. As discussed earlier, the potential difference between a single electrode and the solution cannot be measured isolated. Measuring the electrical potential of the solution requires a second electrode introducing another potential difference. In contrast, potential differences between electrodes are directly accessible, as they can be measured between the metal electrodes.

Standard electrode potentials

Fig. 10.11 depicts two situations for different metal electrodes Me_1 and Me_2 in different compartments and solutions. When the two compartments are electrically connected, the electrical potential of the two compartments will equilibrate (if no additional potential differences are introduced by the connection, e.g., diffusion potentials). If the two compartments are electrically connected by a salt bridge, for example, a tube filled with KCl, the concentrations and conditions (p, T) will not change for some time. This configuration of an electrochemical cell with a spontaneous chemical reaction, when not driven by an external voltage, is called a galvanic cell and provides a voltage between the conducting electrodes. In 1780, L. Galvani discovered that a combination of two metals with an electrolyte produces electricity. Although, the Galvani potentials between each electrode and the solution cannot be measured directly, the electric potential difference (voltage) measured between the metal electrodes is the difference between the two Galvani potentials of each electrode in its solution.

The voltage depends on the temperature, pressure, and concentrations of the respective solutions. When no current between the electrodes is possible, the voltage that is generated is specific for the reactions at both electrodes. Although no single Galvani potential is measurable and only the voltage between combinations of half-cells is accessible, isolated chemical reactions can be characterized by choosing a reference electrode with appropriate standard conditions. A common reference is the standard hydrogen electrode (SHE, **Chapter 5**) that consists of an inert Pt electrode that is placed in a stream of hydrogen gas. The platinized solid Pt electrode is placed in a solution of a strong acid with an effective H_3O^+ concentration (activity) of $1\,mol/dm^3$ (liter) at 1013.25 hPa standard partial pressure of H_2 and 298.15 K. The reaction:

$$2H_3O^+ + 2e^- \rightleftharpoons 2H_2O + H_2$$

at the Pt electrode serves as a reference. The SHE redox half-cell is used to establish a scale of oxidation-reduction potentials by defining the hydrogen standard potential E^0 to be zero[f] and to measure other half-cells with different reactions that are electrically connected by a bridge against it. Table 10.3 extends Table 6.1 and shows some examples of reactions relevant for implanted electrodes and devices.

Ag/AgCl electrode

From the previous we have seen that polarizing electrodes provide different pathways for current: capacitive and resistive. The resistive Faraday current is nonlinear and depends on the voltage as illustrated in the example of the Clark electrode (see "Clark electrode"

Table 10.3 Standard electrode potentials (CRC Handbook of Chemistry and Physics (1995)) measured against a standard hydrogen electrode (SHE).

Reaction			E^0 [V]
$Al^{3+} + 3e^-$	$\rightleftharpoons$	Al	−1.662
$Ti^{2+} + 2e^-$	$\rightleftharpoons$	Ti	−1.630
$TiO_2 + 4H^+ + 2e^-$	$\rightleftharpoons$	$Ti^{2+} + 2H_2O$	−0.502
$Fe^{2+} + 2e^-$	$\rightleftharpoons$	Fe	−0.447
$2H^+ + 2e^-$	$\rightleftharpoons$	H_2	0.0000
$AgCl + e^-$	$\rightleftharpoons$	$Ag + Cl^-$	0.22233
$O_2 + 2H_3O + 2e^-$	$\rightleftharpoons$	$2H_2O_2$	0.695
$Pd^{2+} + 2e^-$	$\rightleftharpoons$	Pd	0.934
$Ir^{3+} + 3e^-$	$\rightleftharpoons$	Ir	1.156
$Pt^{2+} + 2e^-$	$\rightleftharpoons$	Pt	1.180
$Cl_2(G) + 2e^-$	$\rightleftharpoons$	$2Cl^-$	1.358
$Au^+ + e^-$	$\rightleftharpoons$	Au	1.692

S, solids; *L*, liquids; *G*, gases.

[f] Although the absolute standard hydrogen electrode potential is not directly accessible to measurements, it can be estimated from thermodynamic data to be approximately 4.44 V at 25°C.

section). The example of the Clark electrode also demonstrates that the electrode resistance will depend on the available chemical reactions, the composition of the solution and the concentrations of the involved components (O_2 in case of the Clark electrode). In solutions of unknown composition, a better way is to provide a defined reversible reaction by the electrode. In electrophysiology, the most common electrode is the silver-silver chloride electrode (**Chapter 5**), which is less poisonous and easier to handle than the calomel (mercurous chloride) electrode that is commonly used in physical chemistry. The Ag/AgCl is a silver chloride electrode in a saturated solution of dissolved AgCl. In precision experiments solid AgCl as a deposit is used to ensure a saturated solution, but it can be pragmatically assumed that the solution is saturated if the Ag/AgCl electrode is in the solution for some time as the solubility of AgCl in water (1.33 10^{-5} mol^{-1} kg^{-1}) is low. Silver-silver chloride electrodes are used in a variety of forms such as pellets, sticks, and chlorinated silver wires. All provide the reversible reaction $AgCl + e^- \rightleftharpoons Ag + Cl^-$ that allows a charge from the metal conductor to cross the boundary as a chloride ion in the solution and vice versa (Fig. 10.12).

At constant temperature and pressure the system can be assumed in the thermodynamic equilibrium given by:

$$\eta^1_{Cl^-} = \eta^2_{Cl^-} \tag{10.53}$$

As $\mu^{\infty}_{Cl^-}(p, T)$ is independent from the concentration and the pressure and temperature can be assumed equal at the electrode and the surrounding solution, the electric potential of the electrode (Fig. 10.12) will be proportional to the electrochemical potential of chloride:

$$e_- \varphi_1 = RT \ln c^2_{Cl^-} + e_- \varphi_2 + \text{const.} \tag{10.54}$$

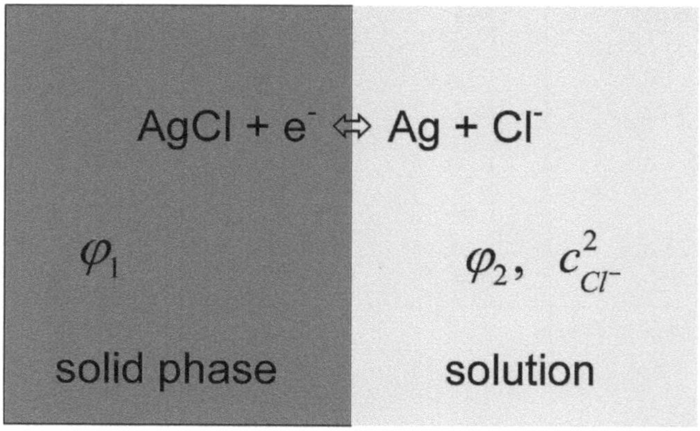

Fig. 10.12 Schematic of the boundary of an Ag/AgCl electrode to a solution. The solution is assumed to be a saturated AgCl solution having the same temperature and pressure as the electrode.

An Ag/AgCl electrode in a saturated solution of AgCl provides the reversible reaction $AgCl + e^- \rightleftharpoons Ag + Cl^-$ for charge transfer across the boundary and measures the electrochemical potential of chloride. Consequently, a pair of Ag/AgCl electrodes measures the difference in electrochemical potential as voltage between the electrode contacts:

$$\Delta E = \frac{1}{e_-} \Delta \eta_{Cl-} \tag{10.55}$$

To illustrate what is measured with a pair of Ag/AgCl electrodes, we use the following examples. First, we take a solution with a concentration gradient of KCl as shown in Fig. 10.13. Although this system is not in the thermodynamic equilibrium and concentrations will equilibrate over time, it is stable long enough to perform measurements, as diffusion in macroscopic systems is a slow process. In the absence of diffusion potentials (see "Diffusion potential" section) and currents the local electrical potentials φ' and φ'' of the solution at both electrodes sites will be the same. With the local concentrations of KCl c_1 and c_2 the voltage ΔE measured with the electrodes follows as the difference in electrochemical potential of chloride:

$$\Delta E = \varphi_1 - \varphi_2 = \frac{RT}{e_-} \ln \frac{c_1}{c_2} = \frac{RT}{e_-} \frac{1}{\log e} \log \frac{c_1}{c_2} \tag{10.56}$$

This leads to an indicated approximately 59 mV/decade concentration ratio at 25°C.

Reference electrode

In implantable stimulation devices, it is sometimes essential to measure the electrical potential. This is done with an Ag/AgCl electrode in a special configuration called a

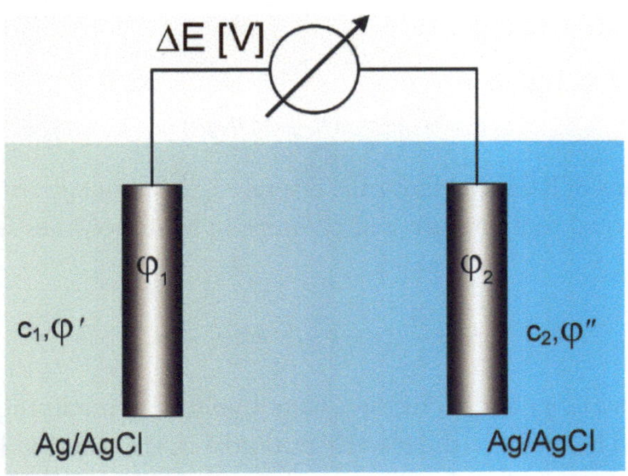

Fig. 10.13 Solution of KCl having an inhomogeneous concentration distribution. Identical Ag/AgCl electrodes are in the solution at different sites with local concentration c_1 and c_2 and local electrical potential φ' and φ''.

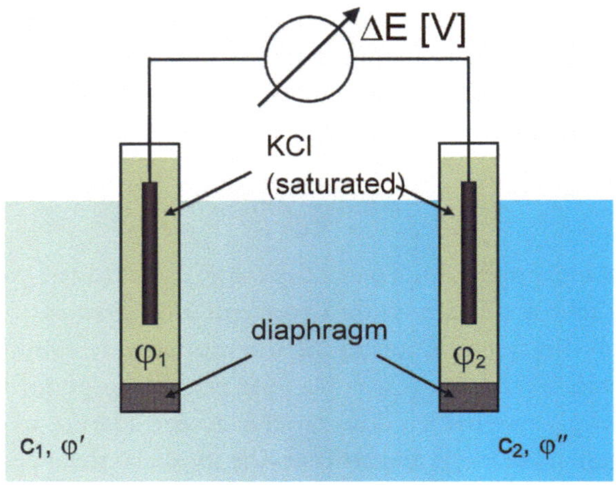

Fig. 10.14 Schematic of a pair of reference electrodes. Two Ag/AgCl electrodes measuring the difference in electrochemical potential of chloride are in separated compartments with identical concentrations of saturated KCl solution. Both electrode compartments with the electric potentials φ_1, φ_2 are connected to the solution having the local electric potentials φ', φ'' at the diaphragms.

reference electrode (Fig. 10.14). Here an Ag/AgCl electrode measuring the electrochemical potential of chloride in a solution of known concentration is used. Usually a saturated KCl solution is used to keep diffusion potential small (see "Diffusion potential" section), but other solutions, for example, physiological concentrations of NaCl are also possible to provide better biocompatibility. In the example in Fig. 10.14, two independent identical Ag/AgCl electrodes are used to measure the electrochemical potential of chloride in volumes filled with a saturated KCl solution. Hence, the potential difference measured with the voltmeter between the pair of electrodes in closed electrode volumes is:

$$\Delta E = \frac{1}{e^-}\left(\eta^1_{Cl^-} - \eta^2_{Cl^-}\right) \tag{10.57}$$

As the concentrations of KCl are identically saturated, the concentration of Cl^- are equal. Assuming further equal temperature and pressure in both volumes from Eq. (10.47), it follows that:

$$\Delta E = \frac{1}{e^-}\left(\eta_1 - \eta_2\right) = \left(\varphi_1 - \varphi_2\right) \tag{10.58}$$

The electrical potentials φ_1 and φ_2 in the isolated volumes containing the saturated KCl solution can be used to measure the electric potential in the solution by electrically connecting the inner solution of each reference electrode with the outside. This is done by adding a diaphragm as a connection to the outside solution that is penetrable for fluid but reduces the flow by convection and diffusion to a minimum. Although this is a system that will settle into equilibrium over time (equal and constant concentrations inside and outside), it provides constant concentrations for sufficient time for most measurement purposes. Although reference electrodes are a perfect tool to acutely measure electric potentials in solutions and tissue, they leak and will deplete the necessary inside concentration over time and thus they are inappropriate for long-term stable implants. Moreover, beside depletion of the salt solution, even small DC currents will use up the reservoir of AgCl of the electrode and silver ions will diffuse to the environment through the diaphragm.

Let us consider the reference electrode circuit in Fig. 10.14. The voltage difference measured between the electrodes is:

$$\Delta E = \varphi_1 - \varphi' + \varphi' - \varphi'' + \varphi'' - \varphi_2 \tag{10.59}$$

In the case that the diffusion potentials $\varphi_1 - \varphi'$ and $\varphi'' - \varphi_2$ across the diaphragm are zero or negligible (see "Diffusion potential" section) the reference electrodes measure the difference in the local electric potentials $\varphi' - \varphi''$ of the solution. This is not subject to differences in local concentrations c_1, c_2 as long as local concentrations have no impact on the diffusion potentials. The example in Fig. 10.14 is a common setup that is used to measure the potential gradient created in tissue by a current between internal (e.g., cells) or external sources and is appropriate for AC and DC potentials.

Diffusion potential

Diffusion potentials have their origin in the fact that the mobility of ions also has an impact on thermal movements. The friction of particles in a solution equally applies for Brownian motion (Einstein-Stokes relationship). Generally, in the case of diffusion at the interface between two different concentrations c_1, c_2 the more mobile ion will more quickly follow the concentration gradient (Fig. 10.15). In contrast to non-charged molecules like sugar, the faster moving ion will create an excess charge and an electric potential that generates an electrostatic force on the faster ion in the opposite direction of the movement. Hence, electrostatic forces will cause the initial movement to slow down and the electric field will accelerate the slower ion of opposite charge. In the steady-state both ions will move together with the same velocity, preserving electroneutrality except for a small excess charge at the boundary that creates the diffusion potential (difference). The steady state will remain until all concentrations are equalized in the thermodynamic equilibrium state when all concentration differences are used up.

As an example we take a system at constant temperature and pressure of two concentrations of a completely dissociated binary electrolyte that are brought in contact to each other (Fig. 10.15). We can assume that the flux $J_{\pm}$ of the ions with $z_{\pm}$ charges is proportional to the gradient of the electrochemical potential:

$$\eta_i = \mu_i(T, p) + z_i F \varphi \tag{10.60}$$

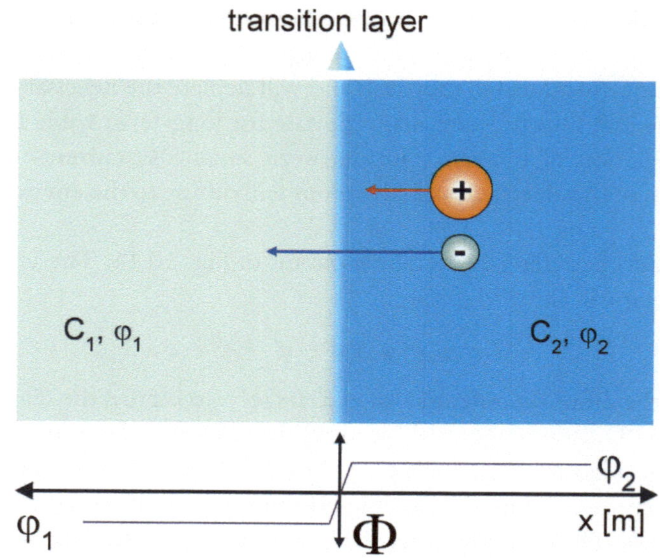

Fig. 10.15 Generation of a diffusion potential between two compartments of different concentrations. Ions with higher mobility and lower friction follow the concentration difference faster by diffusion creating a potential difference between the partitions. *Note*: The electric potential φ in the transition layer is an illustration, as the gradient needs not to be linear.

Leading in one dimension with the phenomenological factors $L\pm$ to:

$$J_{\pm} = -L_{\pm}\frac{d\eta_{\pm}}{dx} \tag{10.61}$$

In our case the total current I across the partitions is zero:

$$I = I_{+} + I_{-} = 0 \Rightarrow z_{+}J_{+} + z_{-}J_{-} = 0 \tag{10.62}$$

and from Eqs. (10.60), (10.61) it follows:

$$-F\frac{d\varphi}{dx} = \frac{z_{+}L_{+}{}^{d\mu_{+}}\Big/_{dx} + z_{-}L_{-}{}^{d\mu_{-}}\Big/_{dx}}{z_{+}^{2}L_{+} + z_{-}^{2}L_{-}} \tag{10.63}$$

For constant temperature and pressure the chemical potential is independent from x $d\mu_{\pm}/dx = 0$. By definition the transport numbers are (see Hittorf transport numbers):

$$t_{\pm} = \frac{I_{\pm}}{I} = \frac{z_{\pm}L_{\pm}}{z_{+}^{2}L_{+} + z_{-}^{2}L_{-}} \tag{10.64}$$

and it follows with $I_{\pm} = z_{\pm}FJ_{\pm}$ from Eqs. (10.63), (10.64):

$$-F\frac{d\varphi}{dx} = \frac{t_{+}}{z_{+}}\frac{d\mu_{+}}{dx} + \frac{t_{-}}{z_{-}}\frac{d\mu_{-}}{dx} \tag{10.65}$$

$$\mu_{\pm} = \mu_{\pm}^{0}(p, T) + RT\ln m_{\pm}\gamma_{\pm} \tag{10.66}$$

The integration along the x-axis from the bulk concentration c_1 (molarity m_1) to the bulk concentration c_2 (molarity m_2) leads to:

$$-\Delta\varphi_{diffusion} = \varphi_2 - \varphi_1 = \frac{1}{F}\int_{m_1}^{m_2}\left(\frac{t_+}{z_+}d\mu_+ + \frac{t_-}{z_-}d\mu_-\right) \tag{10.67}$$

$$\Delta\varphi_{diffusion} = -\frac{RT}{F}\int_{m_1}^{m_2}\left(\frac{t_+}{z_+}d\ \ln m_+\gamma_+ + \frac{t_-}{z_-}d\ \ln m_-\gamma_-\right) \tag{10.68}$$

For thin transition layers, the coefficients $t_\pm$ can be assumed as constant and independent of the concentration leading to:

$$\Delta\varphi_{diffusion} = -\frac{RT}{F}\left[\left(\frac{t_+}{z_+} + \frac{t_-}{z_-}\right)\ln\frac{m_2}{m_1} + \frac{t_+}{z_+}\ln\frac{\gamma_+^2}{\gamma_+^1} + \frac{t_-}{z_-}\ln\frac{\gamma_-^2}{\gamma_-^1}\right] \tag{10.69}$$

The activity coefficients $\gamma_\pm^{1,\,2}$ in the partitions 1, 2 are experimentally not directly accessible. Only for highly diluted solutions it can be calculate using $t_\pm = const.$; $\gamma_\pm = 1$:

$$\Delta\varphi_{diffusion} = -\frac{RT}{F}\left(\frac{t_+}{z_+} + \frac{t_-}{z_-}\right)\ln\frac{m_2}{m_1} \tag{10.70}$$

For a 1–1 electrolyte ($z_+ = -z_- = 1$) Eq. (10.70) further simplifies:

$$\Delta\varphi_{diffusion} = -\frac{RT}{F}(t_+ - t_-)\ln\frac{m_1}{m_2} = -\frac{RT}{F}(t_+ - t_-)\ln\frac{c_1}{c_2} \tag{10.71}$$

From Eq. (10.71) it is obvious that the diffusion potential depends on the difference in Hittorf's transportation numbers (e.g., the difference in mobility of both ions). Table 10.4 lists some examples for pairs of transport numbers. From these examples it becomes also evident why KCl is a favored electrolyte in electrochemistry as K^+ and Cl^- contribute equally to the conductivity of the solution and diffusion potentials are minimized.

Table 10.4 Examples of Hittorf transportation numbers of some combinations of diluted 1–1 binary electrolytes at room temperature (25°C).

	t_+	t_-
KCl	0.4906	0.5094
HCl	0.821	0.179
KOH	0.274	0.726
NaCl	0.3962	0.6038
CH_3COONa	0.5507	0.4493
CH_3COOK	0.6427	0.3573

An example that illustrates the differences between the Ag/AgCl electrode and the reference electrode in a more complex situation with a semipermeable membrane is shown in the following.

Donnan potential

Ion exchanger membranes are polymers that are permeable for water and have charged groups fixed to the three-dimensional network of the polymer (Fig. 10.16). Pores allow water to enter the polymer network. The fixed charges are compensated by mobile counter-ions of opposite charge in the fluid. However, besides the fixed charges the solution may contain mobile ions of the same charge as the fixed groups that are mobile and called co-ions. When brought into contact with a solution the counter-ions can be exchanged against ions with the same charge from the solution and thus the ion exchanger membrane can be permeable for ions of opposite charge to the fixed charges.

When brought into contact with a solution of lower concentration than in the membrane, mobile counter- and co-ions will leave the membrane. However, the counter-ions can leave the exchanger only to a degree that they are not needed to compensate the fixed charged groups. The membrane depletion of co-ions will be larger the greater the concentration of fixed charges is compared to the concentration of the outside solution. Hence, below a certain concentration these membranes are selectively permeable for ions having the opposite charge of the fixed groups but not for ions with

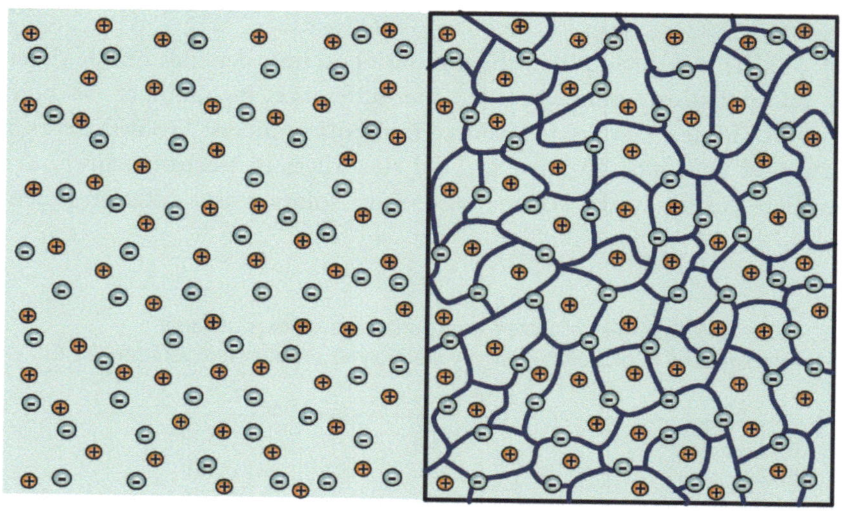

Fig. 10.16 Schematic of a cation exchanger membrane *(right)* in contact with a fluid *(left)*. Negatively charged groups are fixed to the polymer network and immobile in contrast to the co-ions with the same charge that are mobile in the solution inside and outside of the ion exchanger membrane. For simplicity, only one type of ion for each charge is depicted.

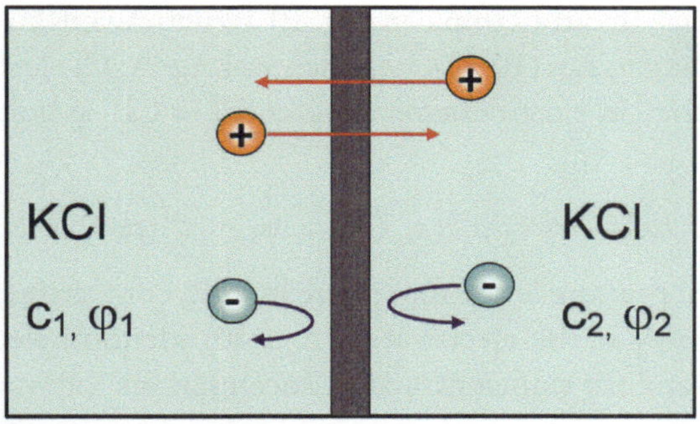

Fig. 10.17 A cation exchanger membrane between two solutions of KCl of different concentrations c_1 and c_2. The exchanger membrane will be permeable for cations, in this case for K^+ but not for Cl^-. Left compartment with index 1, right with index 2.

the same charge. This is the case if no co-ions are in the ion exchanger membrane any more. However, the counter-ions will still be inside the membrane in sufficient concentration to ensure electroneutrality and will enable permeation of ions of the same charge.

As an example, we take a cation exchanger membrane having different concentrations c_1 and c_2 of the same salt on both sides (Fig. 10.17). At sufficient low concentrations, the cation exchanger membrane is only permeable for cations and in our example K^+ can migrate from the higher concentration to the lower. For $c_1 < c_2$, K^+ will flow from the right to the left compartment (with index 1) carrying positive charges and the originally identical electrical potentials will become $\varphi_1 > \varphi_2$ until the electrostatic force balances the osmotic force given by the ratio of concentrations.

The equilibrium (in case of flowing co-ions a steady state) of K^+ that is established can be given at constant temperature and pressure according Eq. (10.46) as the equivalence of the electrochemical potential of the permeating ion:

$$\Delta\eta_+ = \eta_+^1 - \eta_+^2 = 0 \tag{10.72}$$

For low concentrations, the electrochemical potential can be given by Eq. (10.47). From this the electrical potential difference $\Delta\varphi = \varphi_1 - \varphi_2$ between the two reservoirs, the **Donnan-Potential** E_{Donnan} follows as:

$$\Delta\varphi = \varphi_1 - \varphi_2 = \frac{1}{e_+}\left(\eta_+^1 - RT\ln c_1 - \eta_+^2 + RT\ln c_2\right) \tag{10.73}$$

$$E_{Donnan} = \frac{RT}{e_+}\ln\frac{c_2}{c_1} = \frac{RT}{e_+}\frac{1}{\log e}\log\frac{c_2}{c_1} \tag{10.74}$$

Ag/AgCl electrodes, as mentioned (see "Ag/AgCl electrode" section), measure the difference in the electrochemical potential of Cl^- by providing the reversible reaction

$AgCl + e^- \Leftrightarrow Ag + Cl^-$. In our example in Fig. 10.17 with two KCl solutions of different concentration according to Eq. (10.57), two identical Ag/AgCl electrodes in reservoirs 1, 2 measure the difference in electrochemical potential of Cl^- as voltage ΔE between the electrodes:

$$\Delta E = \eta_-^1 - \eta_-^2 = \mu_1^\infty(p, T) + e_-\varphi_1 - \mu_2^\infty(p, T) - e_-\varphi_2 \tag{10.75}$$

In the case of identical pressure and temperature in both compartments the electrochemical potential differs only in the electrical term, as for identical electrodes the chemical potential is identical and for sufficient small concentrations follows:

$$\Delta E = \frac{1}{e_-}\Delta\eta_{Cl^-} \tag{10.76}$$

In contrast if we use **reference electrodes** (see paragraph Reference electrode) to measure in compartments 1, 2, we will measure the difference in electrical potential. For the cation exchanger membrane in our example the electrochemical potential of the permeating cation is $\Delta\eta_+ = 0$. The chemical potential $\mu_S$of a 1–1 salt can be given as:

$$\begin{aligned} \mu_S &= \eta_+ + \eta_- \Rightarrow \Delta\mu_S = \Delta\eta_+ + \Delta\eta_- \\ \Delta\mu_S &= \Delta\mu_- = e_-(\varphi_1 - \varphi_2) = e_-\Delta E \end{aligned} \tag{10.77}$$

In case of a sufficiently diluted 1–1 salt solution the chemical potential is given by:

$$\mu_S = \mu_\infty^S(p, T) + 2RT\ \ln c_S \tag{10.78}$$

From Eqs. (10.77), (10.78) it follows that the difference in electrical potential (measured with a pair of reference electrodes) can be calculated from the salt concentrations as:

$$e_-\Delta E_{ref} = 2RT\ \ln\frac{c_S^1}{c_S^2} \tag{10.79}$$

In a salt solution the number of positive charges equals the number of negative charges and the difference in charges that is needed to create an electric potential difference is negligible compared to the salt concentrations. From electroneutrality $c_S = c_- = c_+$ and $e_+ = -e_-$ it follows that the difference in electrical potential ΔE_{ref}measured with reference electrodes is:

$$\Delta E_{ref} = 2E_{Donnan} \tag{10.80}$$

This comparison between the reference and the Ag/AgCl electrode nicely illustrates that two different qualities and quantities can be measured using different electrodes. Although both types of electrodes use Ag/AgCl electrodes to measure the difference in electrochemical potential of chloride ions $\Delta\eta_{Cl^-}$, reference electrodes compensate the concentration term in the chemical potential by using a defined environment with equal concentrations at both electrodes. By this, only the difference in electrical potential in the reference electrode is measured. As the reference electrode volumes are electrically connected to the environment by diaphragms, consequently the difference in electrical potential is measured if diffusion potentials are minimized (e.g., by the use of KCl).

Finally, we now illustrate the use of different electrode combinations from the preceding examples of different electrodes and their properties. The broad range of different electrodes to interact electrically and chemically with their environment offers multiple possibilities to measure different qualities of the surrounding tissue with specifically designed electrode combinations as sensors. On one hand, the Clark oxygen electrode illustrates how the current across a polarizable electrode can be employed to determine the concentration of oxygen in tissue. On the other hand, the pH electrode serves as an example of how the electric potential created by a surface exposed to a medium can be measured and, by this, the concentration of hydronium ions [H_3O^+] can be determined. Both examples rely on a return path through a reference electrode composed of an Ag/AgCl electrode and a diffusion barrier as described before.

Clark electrode

The Clark electrode uses a combination of a polarizable electrode consisting usually of platinum in combination with an Ag/AgCl electrode shown in Fig. 10.18. In contrast to the electrode configurations shown before an adjustable voltage can be applied to the pair of electrodes while the voltage and current are measured. The voltage-current

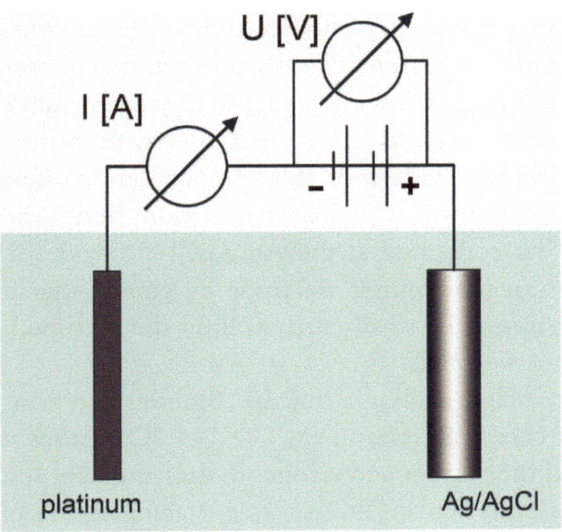

Fig. 10.18 Schematic of a Clark oxygen electrode. Between a polarizable platinum electrode and an Ag/AgCl electrode in a solution, a variable voltage can be applied and the current can be measured.

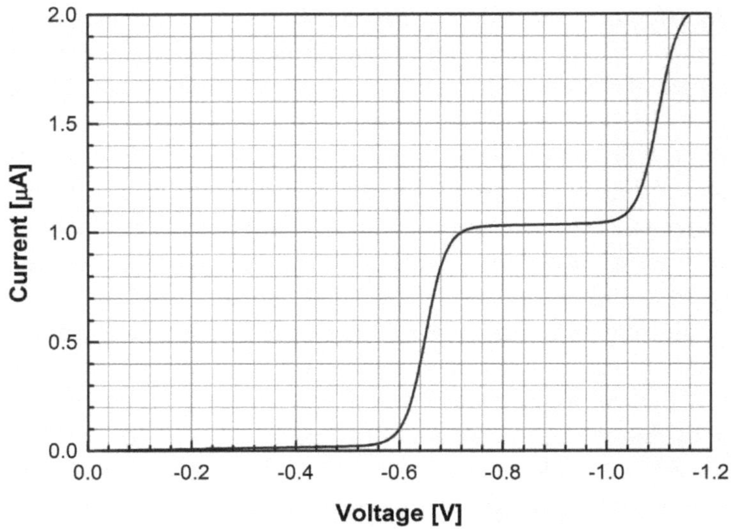

Fig. 10.19 Voltage-current relationship if a voltage is applied to the electrode configuration in Fig. 10.18.

characteristic obtained is depicted in Fig. 10.19. When negative low DC voltages are applied to the platinum electrode the polarizable electrode double layer acts as a capacitor and no major Faraday currents are measured. At around −0.6 to −0.8 the current increases and reaches a plateau at around −1 V. In this voltage range, the chemical reaction $O_2 + 4e^- \rightleftharpoons 2O^{2-}$ of O_2 dissolved in the solution can take place and generates a Faraday current. Each O_2 molecule at the electrode generates four electrons in the electrode that can be measured as current, directly proportional to the amount of oxygen in the solution. Hence, applying a constant voltage in the plateau range to the platinum-Ag/AgCl electrode combination results in a current directly proportional to the concentration of oxygen in the solution. However, this system differs in one significant aspect from the previous ones, as it requires a DC voltage application. Beside the generation of O^{2-} at the Pt electrode, Cl^- is converted at the Ag/AgCl electrode to AgCl, changing the chemical composition of the counter electrode by consuming silver. Although stable and usable over long times, the small currents limit the lifetime by the finite reservoir available at the counter electrode.

Additionally the principle shown in Fig. 10.18 suffers also from another problem. In an acidic solution the chemical reaction $O_2 + 4e^- \rightleftharpoons 2O^{2-}$ stops at $2H^+ + O_2 + 2e^- \rightleftharpoons H_2O_2$ resulting in half the current and erroneous measurement results. Technically, this is handled by using a buffer at the Pt electrode, stabilizing the pH. As this requires a well-defined additional solution, the configuration shown in Fig. 10.20 is used in

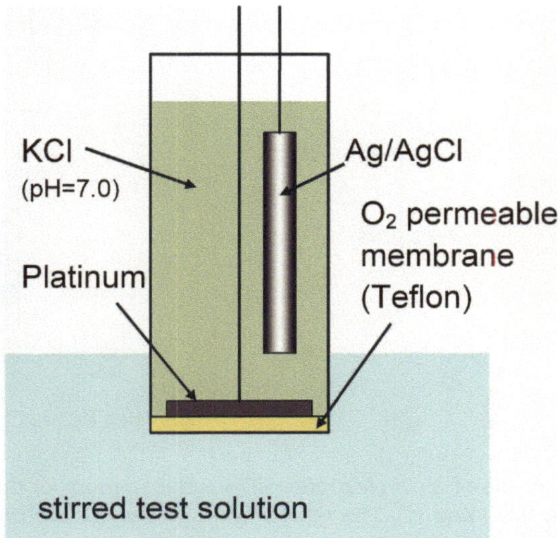

Fig. 10.20 Schematic of a Clark electrode measuring oxygen concentrations. The polarizable Pt electrode is in an oxygen-free buffer solution separated from the test solution by a thin Teflon membrane. An Ag/AgCl electrode serves as return electrode when a voltage of approx. −0.8 to −1.0V is applied.

technical applications; the Pt electrode is exposed to an oxygen-free buffer solution but separated by a membrane that is permeable for oxygen from the test solution (e.g., a thin Teflon membrane). In this case, oxygen can diffuse from the test solution to the Pt electrode, and by a defined redox reaction, a current proportional to the oxygen concentration can be measured. However, by the chemical reaction $O_2 + 4e^- \rightleftharpoons 2O^{2-}$ oxygen is removed from the layer close to the Pt electrode and in the absence of convection can be replenished by diffusion only. As a result, an O_2 concentration gradient will be established having a steady state when the O_2 reaction rate at the electrode equals the diffusive flow from the bulk concentration. To avoid erroneous measurements of the steady-state concentration at the Pt electrode a convective flow is required providing fresh test solution with the oxygen bulk concentration by stirring the test solution.

pH electrode

Another example of combining different electrodes to measure specific properties is the pH electrode. Here a glass with a surface consisting of SiOH is used to measure the pH (concentration of H^+) of a test solution (Fig. 10.21, left panel). When the glass is brought

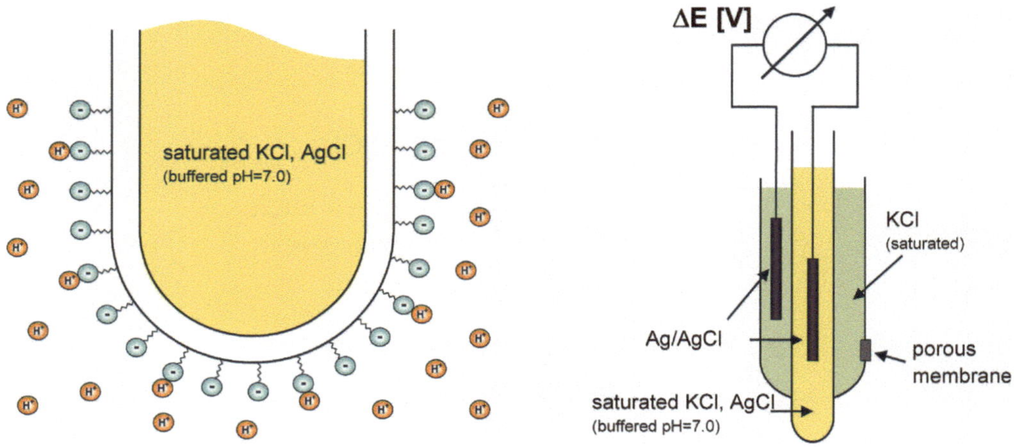

Fig. 10.21 *Left panel*: Principle of a pH electrode. SiOH surface groups of the glass dissociate in an aqueous test solution in SiO^- and H^+. The equilibrium and the surface potential will depend on the H^+ concentration of the test solution, i.e., the pH. *Right panel*: Schematic of a pH-measuring electrode. The glass electrode from the upper panel filled with a buffer solution is connected with an Ag/AgCl electrode. A surrounding reference electrode electrically connected to the test solution by a diaphragm is used as return electrode.

in contact with an aqueous test solution, the surface groups will dissociate according to the law of mass action:

$$\frac{[H^+]\cdot[SiO^-]}{[SiOH]}=\text{const.} \tag{10.81}$$

As the equilibrium in Eq. (10.9) depends on the concentration of H^+ (better H_3O^+), the surface potential can be used to measure the pH of the test solution. Equally on the inside the same reaction takes place and there the surface charges are dissociated according to the pH of the buffer inside, here in our example a pH = 7.0 as reference. In analogy to Eq. (10.74) it follows from this a voltage measured between the reference electrode and the pH sensitive electrode of:

$$\Delta E=-0.059\,V(pH_{outside}-pH_{inside}) \tag{10.82}$$

In practice, the zero-point of a pH electrode will depend on the electrochemical identity of the Ag/AgCl electrodes and the equivalence of the KCl concentrations on the inside and outside. Furthermore, the slope will be not be ideal as diffusion potentials at the diaphragm may depend on the outside concentration and on the less than infinite input resistance of the voltmeter amplifier. Hence, pH electrodes have to be calibrated using pH standard solutions in the range to be measured, to adjust the zero point and slope.

In contrast to electrical conduction in metals, conduction of current in electrolytes is a complex process. As shown here, it has to be considered that current in aqueous solutions decomposes into separate components carried by different types of ions present in the solution. Each of them and its contribution to the bulk conductivity of the solution has a complex dependency on its own and the overall concentrations. In addition, ions may interact chemically and can be quasi-immobile if they are fixed to cells as surface charges contributing to a pronounced spatial dependence of the local conductivity. For example, the spatial distribution of conductivity in tissue matrices will contribute to anisotropies on a cell-size scale and to dispersion and frequency specific conductivity on a bulk-size scale. Moreover, the transition of charges across the boundary layer of electrodes is no less complex. While the examples treated here were limited to simple and well-defined situations, electrodes in tissue are exposed to mixtures of ions with local concentrations that can be difficult or impossible to quantify and that may vary substantially over time. Nevertheless, the complexity of currents, potentials, and electrode processes give rise to a multitude of specific applications if properly understood. The pH and Clark electrodes may serve as examples for the use of current or surface potential here, but more sophisticated application are used or under development. A better in-detail understanding of the mechanisms underlying the stimulation of neurons by electric currents will help to improve recording of neuronal activity as well as stimulation of selected neuronal populations and substructures such as axons or cell bodies.

Brief summary

- In electrolyte solutions, ions are the carrier of the current.
- Each type of ion in an electrolyte carries a current that is distinguishable from other ion currents. The sum of all ion currents in the solution is the total current.
- Strong electrolytes are fully dissociated and the molar conductivity is proportional to $1/\sqrt{c}$ following Ostwald's dilution law. Weak electrolytes are not fully dissociated and the amount of ions is given by the law of mass action.
- The mobility of an ion determines the speed of movement in an electric field. It is directly related to the molar conductivity of this type of ion.
- The double layer at an electrode interface to a solution can be modeled as a "rigid" Helmholtz layer at high concentrations or as a "diffuse" Gouy-Chapman layer at low ion concentrations.
- An ionic double layer can be generated either by an electric potential difference or by a chemical surface charge by dissociable groups at the surface.
- Electrically the interface between a solution and an electrode can be modeled by a circuit of resistors and capacitors as an approximation.
- In a real solution-electrode interface the capacity and the resistivity will depend on frequency.

Key literature and further reading

Atkins, 1990. Physical Chemistry, fourth ed. Oxford University Press, Oxford, Melbourne, Tokyo.

Lide, D.R. (Ed.), 1995. CRC Handbook of Chemistry and Physics. Seventy sixth ed. CRC Press.

Faraday, M., 1834. VI. Experimental researches in electricity.-Seventh Series. Philos. Trans. R. Soc. Lond. 124, 77–122.

Hille, B., 2001. Ion Channels of Excitable Membranes, third ed. Sinauer Associates Inc.

Hunter, R.J., 1988. Zeta Potential in Colloid Science. Academic Press Ltd., San Diego.

Kohlrausch, F., 1897. Ueber platinirte Electroden und Widerstandsbestimmung. Ann. Phys. 296, 315–332.

Leber, M., Bhandari, R., Mize, J., Warren, D.J., Shandhi, M.M.H., Solzbacher, F., Negi, S., 2017. Long term performance of porous platinum coated neural electrodes. Biomed. Microdevices 19, 62.

Schwan, H.P., 1992. Linear and nonlinear electrode polarization and biological materials. Ann. Biomed. Eng. 20, 269–288.

Warburg, E., 1901. Ueber die Polarisationscapacität des Platins. Ann. Phys. 311, 125–135.

PART 3

Applications

CHAPTER 11

Auditory neuroprostheses

The auditory system is the model system for neuroprosthetic restoration of a sensory system. It has the largest portfolio of clinical implants used across many different brain structures, which are in successful daily use in hundreds of thousands of subjects. The level of functional restoration in hearing surpasses any other sensory restoration approach.

The auditory system stands out among the sensory systems due to its tight relation to language. While other organisms have developed complex ways of communication, only humans use a symbolic communication, the language. Children acquire language capacity by means of hearing. Language is the cognitive function that most clearly differentiates humans from any other species and lies at the core of human nature.

In addition to its importance for human communication, hearing is also integral for orientation: it allows identifying and localizing sounds in space, even in situations when vision cannot provide this information (e.g., beyond the field of view—in darkness, in dense vegetation—or outside of the focus of attention). Hearing is also the sense with the greatest temporal acuity: it can provide precise phase information for stimuli up to 4000 Hz. Loss of hearing therefore impedes all these functions and affects human life in extensive ways.

The ear has a complex architecture, given by its acoustic and biological function. The cells that detect mechanical movement (the **hair cells**) are embedded in supporting tissue and surrounded by bodily fluids. Since the mechanical compliance of the fluid is much less than that of the air, more than 99% of sound is reflected at the surface of fluid. It is thus not trivial to "inject" sound into a fluid-filled space, such as the mammalian inner ear. The transition of sound in air to a corresponding mechanical movement of fluids near the hair cells requires a mechanical impedance transformation.

Anatomically, the peripheral auditory organ (Fig. 11.1) can be differentiated into three parts: the outer, the middle, and the inner ear. The *outer ear* consists of the pinna and outer ear canal, and is separated from the middle ear by the tympanic membrane. The *middle ear* is in principle a cavity that houses the middle ear ossicles (the smallest bones of the human body): the malleus, the incus, and the stapes. The stapes footplate is attached to the oval window that represents the border to the inner ear. The middle ear cavity, to provide pressure adaptation (e.g., in an airplane with changing atmospheric pressure), is connected through the Eustachian tube to the pharynx and thus the upper airways. While this is essential for appropriate function of the middle ear, it is also a connection to a

Prostheses for the Brain
https://doi.org/10.1016/B978-0-12-818892-7.00001-8

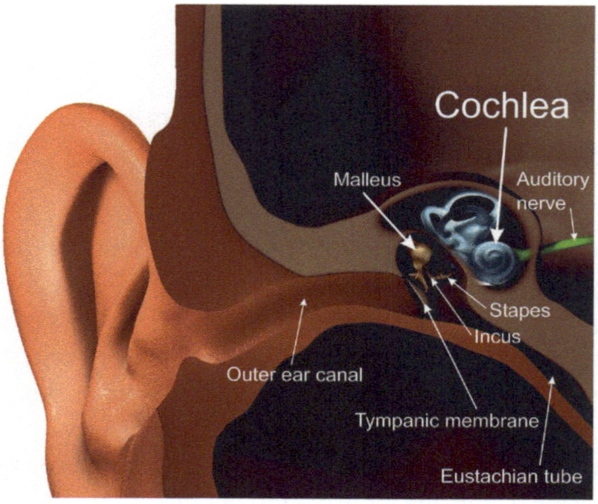

Fig. 11.1 The structure of the human peripheral auditory organ. The entrance of the middle ear is defined by the tympanic membrane that separates it from the outer ear canal. The malleus, one of the ossicles of the middle ear, is attached to the tympanic membrane to effectively pick up the vibrations and transfer it to the incus and the stapes. The stapes footplate is in the oval window of the inner ear. The inner ear (the cochlea) and the vestibular organ are printed in *blue*, the vestibulocochlear nerve in *green*. The cochlea is embedded in a very solid bony structure called petrous bone.

non-sterile ventilation apparatus (upper respiratory tract) that can be a pathway for microbes and thus a pathway for middle ear infections, particularly in children.

Functionally, the outer ear preserves and shapes the energy and the spectral content of sound. First, the pinna adds spectral information about the sound source position in space, particularly along the elevation (vertical direction). This, however, works only for broadband sounds that the brain has experienced previously and has stored it in memory. Subsequently, the outer ear canal (a tube that is open on one end and closed on the other end) amplifies frequencies near 3kHz (its resonant frequency). The middle ear provides the required impedance adaptation, since it transforms a small force at a large tympanic membrane to a large force at a small stapes footplate in the oval window. There is an additional lever effect involved that increases the vibration amplitude. This counteracts the reflection of sound waves on the surface of a fluid and provides approximately a 24-dB increase in pressure delivered into the inner ear . An additional ~22-24dB comes from compliance adaptation.

The sensory organ itself is located in the **inner ear** which has a spiral shape similar to a see mollusk (therefore the Greek name "cochlea," Fig. 11.2A). It has a small tip, the apex, and a broad base. The auditory nerve leaves the cochlea and connects it to the brain (Fig. 11.2B). When reoriented and cut through the middle (Fig. 11.2B) it reveals a central bony pyramid (modiolus) with a bony lamina (osseus spiral lamina; Fig. 11.2C) curving

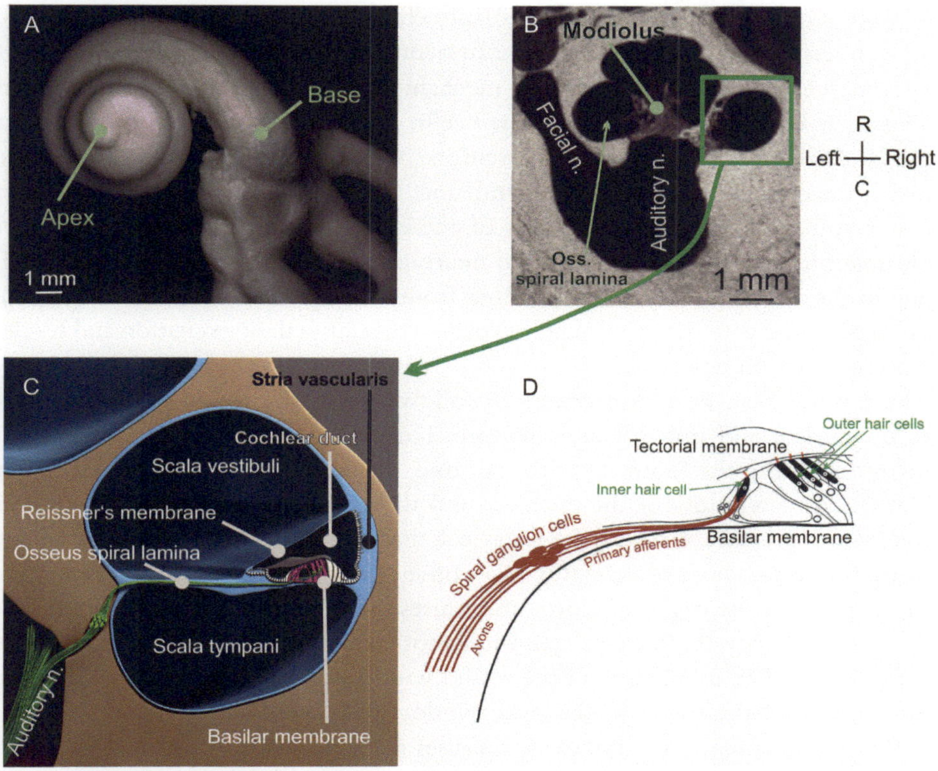

Fig. 11.2 Anatomy of the human inner ear. (A) A corrosion cast obtained after the inner space of the cochlea was filled with a resin and the bone surrounding it was chemically corroded. This allows us to see the cochlear spaces in totality. Lower right corner of the corrosion cast shows the connected vestibular organ with the semicircular canals. (B) A μCT allows us to see the inner spaces inside of the cochlea. It reveals a central bony structure called the modiolus. *R*, rostral; *C*, caudal direction. (C) A schematic view of one turn of the cochlea with the scala tympani, scala vestibuli, and the cochlear duct with the organ of Corti *(pink color)* on the top of the basilar membrane. (D) Schematics of the organ of Corti with three rows of outer and one row of inner hair cells, contacted by the primary afferents of the bipolar spiral ganglion cells. Their axons constitute the eighth cranial nerve (vestibulo cochlear nerve). Cilia of hair cells are shown in *red*. *(Data taken from Pietsch et al. (2017).)*

around the modiolus in 2.5 turns (in humans). Attached to it is a membranous tube, the cochlear duct (Fig. 11.2C), which follows the course of the spiral lamina. It is connected to the vestibular organ and filled with endolymph, a fluid with a specific composition that leads to a high electric potential of +80 mV relative to the scala tympani and scala vestibuli (Fig. 11.2C). This endocochlear potential favors the transduction of vibration into neuronal excitation. The endolymph is produced in a special organ in the cochlear duct called stria vascularis (Fig. 11.2C). On the basilar membrane is the **organ of Corti** with three rows of outer and one row of inner hair cells (Fig. 11.2D). The hair cells are contacted by fibers of spiral ganglion cells, bipolar neurons whose central axons constitute the auditory nerve. The hair cells transform mechanical energy into a receptor potential.

The organ of Corti contains 16,000 hair cells: 12,000 outer hair cells and 4000 inner hair cells. All hair cells are mechanical sensors. When their tiny hair-like protrusions located at the contact to the tectorial membrane, the *stereocilia*, are tilted, ionic channels in their membranes open and the inflow of potassium depolarizes the hair cells. Such a transformation of a physical stimulus into neuronal excitation is called *transduction*. The change in the membrane potential resulting from the depolarization leads to glutamate release at the synapse to the spiral ganglion cells. This causes their excitation and results in generation of action potentials.

The transduction process proceeds as follows. First, the sound reaches the tympanic membrane and initiates its vibration. This is conducted by the three ossicles of the middle ear to the footplate of the last one, the stapes. The footplate of the stapes rests in the oval window of the cochlea, and thus a vibration of the stapes is transformed into a pressure wave in the inner ear that sets the structures inside the inner ear into motion. The pressure wave is conveyed from the scala vestibuli to the cochlear duct and the organ of Corti, and causes movement of the basilar membrane. This is possible since the scala tympani has another opening into the middle ear, the round window. The membrane of the round window allows for the compensation of the movement of the stapes in the oval window.

When sound reaches the inner ear, it causes a characteristic vibration of the basilar membrane that starts near the cochlear base and proceeds to the apex. This **traveling wave** has a remarkable property: depending on the spectrum of the stimulating sound, it has different maximal amplitudes along the cochlea. If the sound contains high frequencies, the amplitude is large at the base. If it contains low frequencies, it has high amplitudes at the apex. If both low and high frequencies are present, the amplitude is large at both the base and the apex. There is a strict topological order of the sound frequencies that cause the maximum vibration on the basilar membrane from base to the apex. This topological order is called **tonotopy**. In other words, the basilar membrane, due to its mechanical (physical) properties, performs a frequency analysis of the sound. The frequency analysis is transduced into neuronal excitation in the auditory nerve. Each auditory nerve fiber contacts only one inner hair cell, preserving the tonotopy. The tonotopic principle is further preserved in most nuclei of the central auditory pathway. Consequently, the brain receives the excitation corresponding to the sound frequency spectrum. The operation of the basilar membrane and the organ of Corti can be best compared to a Fourier transform in signal analysis. This takes place instantaneously in the ear based on passive physical properties of the basilar membrane (its stiffness and the mass that is moved by it).

The vibration of the basilar membrane causes a shear force between the hair cells and the tectorial membrane that covers them (Fig. 11.2D). This tilts the tiny hairs of the cells (the stereocilia) and opens the mechanically sensitive ionic channels on their tips. A receptor potential emerges. As such, hair cells are functionally very sensitive sensors for movement. There is an additional code for sound frequency that is revealed if the receptor potential of hair cell is recorded: for frequencies less than 4000 Hz, the receptor potential follows the time structure of the basilar membrane movement and thus the time structure of the sound (similar to a microphone signal). This information is then conveyed to the auditory nerve through the hair cell-auditory nerve synapse. Therefore, in addition to tonotopy, the timing of neuronal activity can code sound frequency for low-frequency sounds.

In summary, there are two codes used in the cochlea:

(1) A place code, corresponding to the spectral analysis by the basilar membrane. This code is reflected by the responsiveness of a given fiber to sound, as shown in Fig. 11.3 for three different fibers innervating the apex, middle, and base of the cochlea. Under acoustic stimulation, each auditory nerve fiber responds to a certain combination of frequencies and sound pressure levels (the *receptive field*). Since the range of frequencies to which the fiber responds at low sound pressure levels is rather limited, it is reminiscent of an electronic bandpass filter tuned to a certain frequency range. The border of the receptive field is therefore called the **frequency tuning curve**. The frequency for which the neuron shows the greatest sensitivity (and where the tuning is also sharpest) is called the **characteristic frequency (CF)**. The frequency tuning curve shows a systematic shift in the frequency sensitivity towards higher frequencies when progressing from a fiber innervating the apex of the cochlea to a fiber that is innervating a more basal portion of the cochlea.

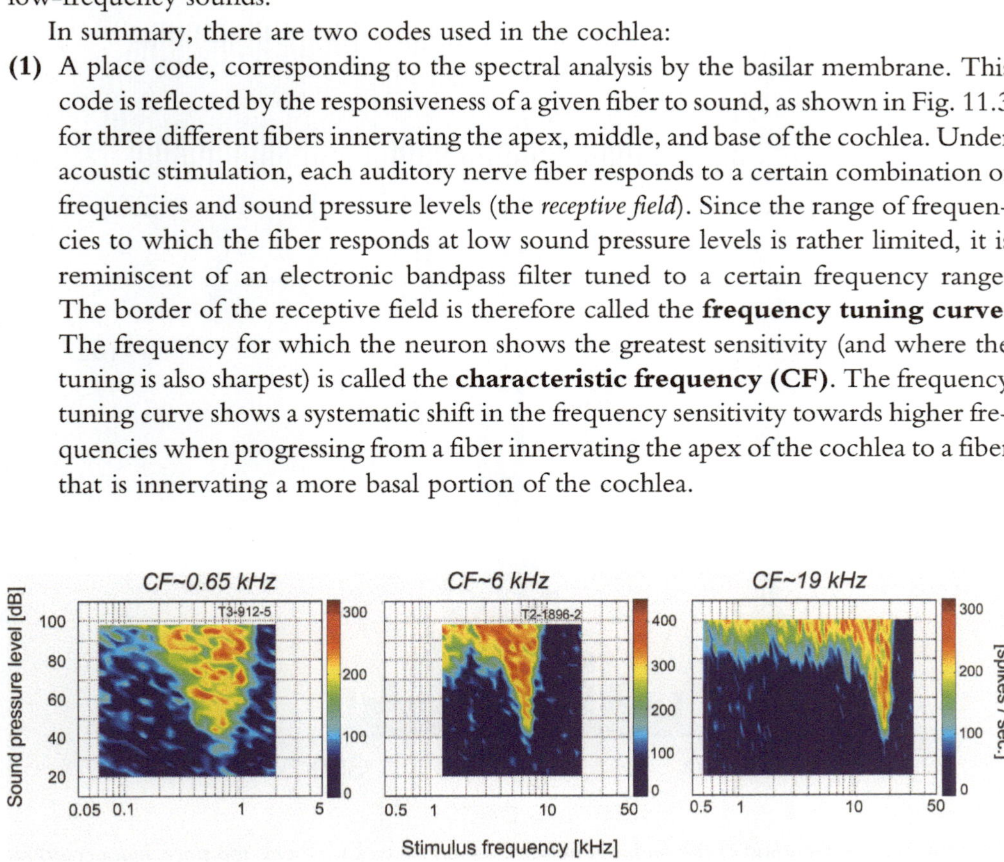

Fig. 11.3 Spiking activity of single auditory nerve fibers under acoustic stimulation. Shown is the color-coded evoked firing rate as a function of sound pressure level and frequency. An island with increased firing rate defines the receptive field of the neuron (the stimulus range that activates the fiber). The frequency that evokes a response at the lowest sound pressure level is called the "characteristic frequency" (CF), since it characterizes the place in the cochlea that the fiber innervates. Three fibers are shown with a different characteristic frequency. The tuning of each fiber to a given frequency (defined by the border of the receptive field) is called frequency tuning curve. *(Data from Tillein et al. (2015).)*

(2) A temporal code, which codes the frequency of the acoustic stimulus by the timing of the action potentials. When inspecting a trace with action potentials recorded in one auditory nerve fiber one can observe that they are coupled to the phase of the acoustic stimulus presented (Fig. 11.4), even though they are not capable of responding to every period of the stimulus. To quantify this phase coupling, the recorded signal trace is folded in time relative to the period of the tone to obtain a "period histogram." Such histogram reveals a peak around a certain phase angle, showing that the fiber phase-locks to a certain phase of the period of the acoustic stimulus.

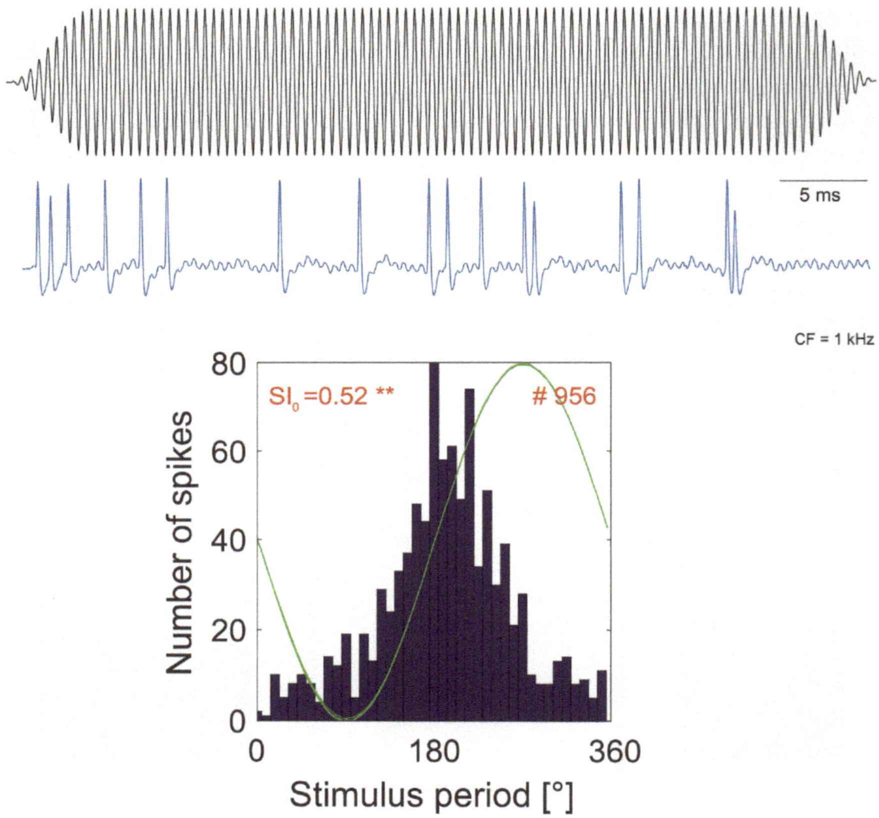

Fig. 11.4 Temporal coding of the auditory nerve. In response to a tone pip *(top trace, black color)* an auditory nerve fiber generates a series of action potentials that are phase-locked to the acoustic stimulus *(middle trace, blue color)*. For frequencies above 300 Hz the fiber cannot generate action potentials at each stimulus period, but the phase locking can be revealed using a period histogram: the distribution of action potentials as a function of stimulus phase reveals that the action potentials are "locked" to a phase, in this case near 180 degree *(lowest panel)*. *Green line* shows the stimulus period, histogram of action potentials shown in blue (956 action potentials evaluated). Synchronization index (SI), a value between 0 and 1, quantifies the phase locking. *(Data from Tillein et al. (2015).)*

Fibers with characteristic frequencies below 4000–5000 Hz show such phase-locking. This limit is related to the capacitive properties of the hair cell membrane. Since the membrane capacitance represents a short circuit for high frequencies, the alternating component of the receptor potential is lost for frequencies greater than 4000–5000 Hz, and the temporal code in the auditory nerve is consequently absent for frequencies greater than 4–5 kHz.

The sound pressure level is coded by the number of action potentials generated by the stimulus in all active auditory nerve fibers. For each fiber the firing rate increases with increasing level, with a dynamic range (the range over which firing rate increases) of 40–80 dB. Furthermore, at increasing sound pressure levels additional auditory nerve fibers are recruited by the acoustic stimulus due to their wider receptive fields at higher sound pressure levels. These two pieces of information convey the psychophysical loudness.

However, the situation is more complex; while the main function of inner hair cells is to transduce sound into neuronal excitation, the main function of the outer hair cells is to amplify the vibration of the basilar membrane. The molecular mechanism is beyond the scope of this book, but a dedicated membrane protein, prestin, allows the membrane to contract extremely quickly, much faster than muscle (up to 80,000 Hz in some species!). Via this mechanism, outer hair cells, similar to gymnasts on a trampoline, increase or decrease the vibration amplitude of the basilar membrane and thus amplify and sharpen the profile of the traveling wave. This mechanism has been called the cochlear amplifier. This is an active process since the driving force (the battery) is the endocochlear potential that is actively generated by the stria vascularis. But why do the outer hair cells themselves not extract the energy for the process? Why is this complicated mechanism of the driving energy detached from the hair cells?

The reason might be that biological energy requires oxygen and glucose, and that requires blood supply. The organ of Corti is so sensitive that it operates just above the level of Brownian motion (the thermally determined movement of molecules; we can nearly hear this). An artery located close to this organ would disturb it; we could hear the blood flow. Therefore the energy is provided to the hair cell by the endocochlear potential, but is generated at the (more distant) stria vascularis.

After the sound has been translated into a receptor potential of an inner hair cell, the next stage is the transfer of this information to the auditory nerve fiber. This is performed chemically, using the neurotransmitter glutamate. Each inner hair cell is innervated by a number of "type I" primary afferents. These are peripheral axons of the bipolar spiral ganglion cells that are located in the modiolus and form 95% of ascending fibers (connecting the cochlea to the brainstem). The action potentials are generated right at the synapse and travel into the brainstem. The remaining few percent of afferents ("type II") carry information from the outer hair cells. It is not well understood what this information is and how it contributes to the perception of sound. There are also thinner efferent fibers that innervate type I primary afferents near the synapse and outer hair cells.

They become involved in noisy conditions with a lot of background noise and suppress portions of sound representation in the cochlea and in the auditory nerve.

The coding of sound by the cochlea has been explored in detail since the 1960s, when computers could be used to analyze the recorded data. Today it is largely understood, and despite some remaining unanswered questions in cochlear micromechanics, modern computer models mimic cochlear function well. In other words, we can make use of the knowledge we have gained and use it for stimulation with neuroprosthetic devices.

The central auditory system is a rather complicated structure, as shown in Fig. 11.5. The first nucleus (the cochlear nucleus) is located at the place where the auditory nerve enters the brainstem. It consists of three compartments that each receive a collateral of one of the auditory nerve fibers. In addition, they preserve the tonotopic organization with different frequencies represented at different places. Its anatomy will be of central importance later.

The first structure that is dedicated to processing binaural information is the superior olivary complex. It receives (directly and through the medial nucleus of the trapezoid body) timing and intensity information from the cochlear nucleus of both sides (right and left) and extracts interaural timing and level differences. These are essential for localization of sound sources.

The next large structure is the inferior colliculus, an obligatory stage of auditory processing; all afferent information has to pass it. A lot of research has been done on this nucleus due to its central position, small size, and relatively easy access. The inferior

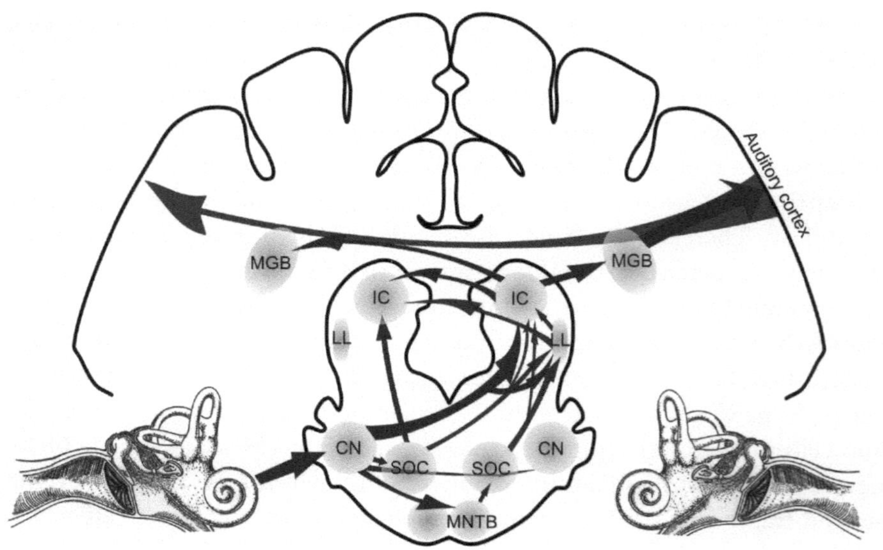

Fig. 11.5 The simplified central auditory pathway. Shown are only afferent (in the direction from the ear to the cortex) but not the efferent (in the reverse direction) connections. *CN*, cochlear nucleus; *SOC*, superior olivary complex; *MNTB*, medial nucleus of the trapezoid body; *LL*, lateral lemniscus; *IC*, inferior colliculus; *MGB*, medial geniculate body (part of the thalamus).

colliculus has three subnuclei. However, for the first time in the central auditory pathway here a functional difference can be observed. While in one nucleus the responses have features similar to the auditory nerve (fast responses with short latencies, tonotopy with sharp tuning of neurons to stimulus frequency, neurons are driven only by sound), the others have less clear tonotopy, long latency responses, and often respond to several different sensory modalities. The former gives rise to the lemniscal pathway, the latter to the extralemniscal pathway. It is preserved in the thalamus and innervates differentially the cerebral cortex. The cerebral cortex is the highest auditory center where conscious perception originates, and it controls auditory learning.

The receptive fields in the auditory pathway demonstrate similar frequency sensitivity as described for the auditory nerve. Additionally, the olivary complex extracts, for example, binaural properties of the input (interaural time and level differences) that are key for determining sound source location. Neurons in the inferior colliculus and the cortex inherit this sensitivity to binaural cues. Some neurons in the auditory pathway show sensitivity to peaks in sound in time (onsets), some to gaps in the spectrum, and some to synchronized activity over the spectrum. In the inferior colliculus, some neurons show sensitivity to movement direction. Neurons from portions of the inferior colliculus to the cortex show adaptation to the repeated presentation of the same stimulus ("stimulus-specific adaptation"), which is a sign of sensitivity for change, particularly prominent in the extralemniscal pathway. In addition, non-auditory information is integrated into auditory processing from the cochlear nucleus onwards; again most prominent in the extralemniscal pathway.

The cerebral cortex is the structure that is responsible for auditory learning, conveys conscious perception, and allows the directing of attention towards portions of the visual scene. The auditory cortex contains two to three primary areas, showing high sensitivity to sound frequency and sharp tuning, and often only few action potentials in response to the auditory stimulus (this is called "sparse coding"). The higher-order areas show broader tuning and more complex response properties. It is generally assumed that this indicates a change from feature sensitivity to sensitivity to complex relations between features characterizing certain objects in the auditory scene. As such, potential targets for therapeutic intervention with a neuroprosthetic device are the auditory pathway and potentially the primary areas of the auditory cortex, where the representation of sound relies on features that can be more easily identified and conveyed to the known code in these structures.

Hearing loss

Hearing loss is common, even in newborns. With an incidence of 0.1%, it is one of the three most frequent inherited human diseases. Incidence increases with age; in people older than 70 years, nearly every second subject has significant hearing loss. Hearing loss has extensive impact on society by affecting speech understanding and thus social interaction.

Hearing loss can be caused by disturbance of sound conduction to the inner ear (conductive hearing loss) or by disturbances in the organ of Corti (sensory hearing loss). Sometimes two or more causes combine (mixed hearing loss). Only extremely rarely is there a central cause responsible for hearing loss, for example, in the case of stroke. This is due to the way in which the blood supply is guaranteed in the auditory system as well as the overlapping complete representation of both ears in both hemispheres of the brain, which is different from how the visual system works.

Conductive hearing loss is often caused by diseases of the middle ear that lead to increased acoustic impedance of the middle ear, reducing the efficacy of the transfer of sound to the inner ear. As an example, infections can lead to inflitration of fluids into the middle ear and cause tissue reactions. This not only affects the acoustic compliance of the tympanic membrane, but also affects the transmission of the middle ear. Some genetically transmitted diseases lead to ossification of the middle ear ossicles (otosclerosis). This limits the motion of the middle ear and causes hearing loss. There are inborn (genetic) causes of hearing loss that can manifest at birth, but also during childhood and even in adulthood. They can be progressive and may lead to loss of hair cells and spiral ganglion cells.

Sensory hearing loss involves damage to the organ of Corti. Since the organ operates at the lowest imaginable energetic threshold, it can be easily affected. For example, loud sound, like at a rock concert, can easily damage hair cells, resulting in noise-induced hearing loss. The mildest change to the delicate hairs on the top of the hair cells can shift or break the tiny protein links between them, changing their mechanical properties. The tectorial membrane can also lose attachment to outer hair cells, the hairs (the cilia) can break or fuse with neighboring ones, and the hair cells may die. Since the organ of Corti is a highly differentiated structure, there is no regeneration in this organ; we have our hair cells for our whole lifetime, and their loss is permanent. In some conditions, both conductive and sensory hearing loss combine (e.g. in the case of otosclerosis that also causes a loss of hair cells and auditory nerve fibers), resulting in **mixed hearing loss**.

With respect to severity we differentiate mild (<40 dB), moderate (<70 dB), severe (<90 dB), and profound (≥90 dB) hearing loss. The reasons for profound hearing loss (etiology) can be different. They can be either inborn (mainly genetic, due to mutations in one or several genes, but also due to intoxication, perinatal infections, and traumata) or acquired (due to infections, trauma including loud sound, ototoxic drugs, or genetics but with slow progression, etc.). Regardless of the etiology, profound hearing loss is not due to middle ear disease only, and thus must include the loss of hair cells (a sensory component). The middle ear improves hearing thresholds by ~55 to 60 dB, but would not make the subject deaf.

The deaf ear (cochlea and cochlear nerve)

Complete deafness has downstream consequences on the spiral ganglion and the auditory nerve. This is caused by the fact that hair cells are completely absent in complete deafness

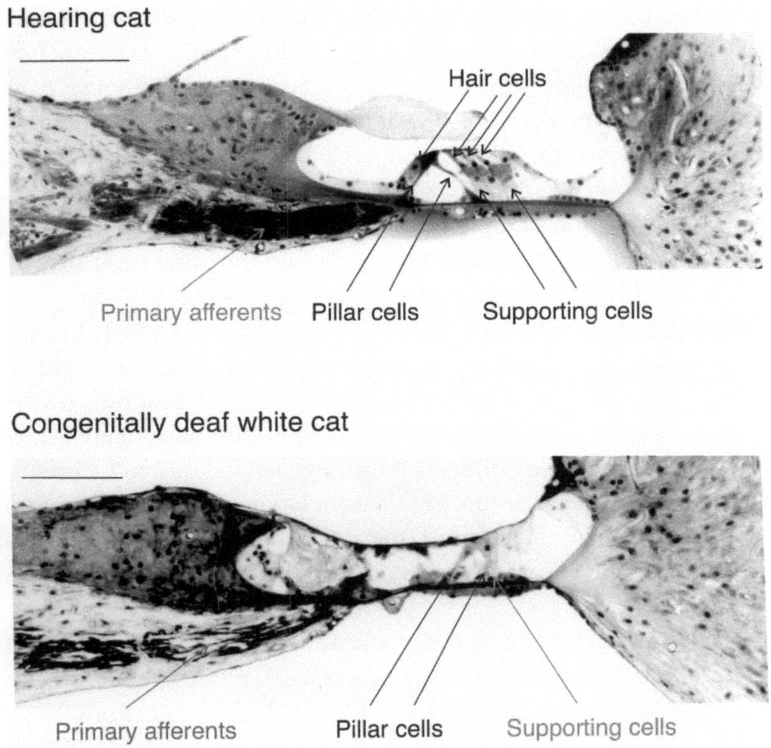

Fig. 11.6 The organ of Corti of a hearing cat and a congenitally deaf cat (2 years age), a natural model of congenital deafness, in the basal turn of the cochlea. In the hearing cat, three rows of outer and one row of inner hear cells are discernible. In the deaf cat hair cells are absent, but residual supporting cells are discernible on the basilar membrane, including pillar cells. Primary afferents and correspondingly the spiral ganglion cells are reduced at this age (visible by less dense packing of the dark-stained primary afferents), but still preserved in high numbers despite two years of complete deafness (a long time for a cat that is adult with 6–8 months of life). Scale bar: 100 μm. *(Modified with permission from Heid et al. (1998).)*

(Fig. 11.6). Hair cells not only activate primary afferents of spiral ganglion cells and cause them to generate action potentials, but they also provide neurotrophic factors for the spiral ganglion cells. Their loss therefore compromises the spiral ganglion cells. How much also depends on the other cells in the organ of Corti that also provide trophic input for spiral ganglion. Finally, auditory nerve fibers in absence of stimulation have a spontaneous activity (up to around 100 spikes per second) driven by spontaneous transmitter release from hair cells. This normal spontaneous activity is completely abolished if hair cells die.

Other cells in the organ of Corti (the supporting cells) are also compromised in hearing loss to an extent heavily dependent on the etiology. Their number is particularly reduced in deafness caused by ototoxic substances that damage hair cells and supporting cells directly. This is also the case in many experimental models of deafness. Fortunately, in other etiologies, and most frequently in human deafness, the loss of supporting cells is not as severe as with ototoxic substances.

Thus, loss of hair cells, particularly if combined with loss of supporting cells, leads to a degeneration of the auditory nerve. This degeneration can be extensive: deaf subjects have on average only about 10,000 spiral ganglion cells, and some have less than 3000. This means that typically nearly 70% of the neurons of the auditory nerve are degenerated and lost over time in a deaf subject. This requires consideration and affects therapeutic options. However, complete loss of spiral ganglion cells nearly never occurs, and thus electrical stimulation of surviving spiral ganglion cells is an excellent therapeutic option for deafness. The state of the auditory nerve and the other cellular structure of the hearing-impaired cochlea has been recently called *cochlear health*.

The human spiral ganglion does not extend throughout the whole cochlea, but only covers 1.6–2.0 turns of the cochlea. The remaining portion of the cochlea is normally innervated by primary afferents reaching out into the most apical turn from the second turn. This is an important factor, since the cell bodies of the spiral ganglion cells, particularly in cases when the primary afferents have degenerated due to hearing loss, are the targets for the electric field in neuroprosthetic stimulation. This is a fortunate factor, since the size of the scala tympani in the most apical turn is so small that implantation there would inevitably damage the remaining cochlear structures there and induce further degenerative processes.

Fortunately, complete deafness does not affect the scala vestibuli and scala tympani in any significant way in most cases. This means that the scala tympani remains open and fluid-filled and is available for cochlear implantation. Only following infections (like those when inner ear infection accompanies meningitis and is caused by bacteria) can these spaces ossify (fill with connective tissue that turns into bone) and complicate therapeutic options.

The cochlear implant

Three fortunate circumstances favor neuroprosthetic therapy of hearing loss:

1. The loss of hair cells is not connected with total loss of auditory nerve fibers. While the survival of spiral ganglion cells depends on signals from hair cells, they are also supplied by trophic factors from supporting cells in the organ of Corti. These survive the loss of hair cells. Therefore, even in cases of years-long deafness we can still find more than 30% of surviving spiral ganglion cells in the auditory nerve.
2. The space underneath the cochlear duct, the scala tympani, forms a natural channel for introducing a neuroprosthesis. It still requires an operation, but the position of the prosthetic device within the scala tympani is well secured and is located along the tonotopic gradient of the cochlea. While the first ideas for cochlear stimulation involved the direct stimulation of the auditory nerve, it soon became clear that implantation within the scala tympani is easier and less complex surgically. Also, it carries much less risk of damage, since the scala tympani is a channel that is normally free, filled only with a fluid (perilymph), and the main damage comes from mechanical interference with the bony walls of this channel or the basilar membrane. This can

be much better controlled than the damage caused by inserting a technical device into a soft nerve.

3. The spiral ganglion is relatively homogeneous both in anatomical features (location, orientation, etc.) as well as in functional features (type of information the fibers carry). While the stimulating electrode in the scala tympani is at some distance from the spiral ganglion cells, and thus requires slightly higher currents to reach threshold compared to an electrode deeply immersed into the auditory nerve, there are no diverse sub-populations of fibers that need to be differentially targeted by the implant. This is very different from central prostheses where an electrode is in intimate contact with a highly diverse population of neurons.

We can use a simple device (e.g., a linear array of electrodes inserted into the scala tympani) that electrically stimulates the surviving auditory nerve, and can make use of the natural coding principle in the normal hearing cochlea: the tonotopy. This requires several electrodes arranged longitudinally along the scala tympani. Indeed, the cochlear implant is designed as a linear array of electrodes that are placed on a silicone carrier and inserted into the scala tympani, underneath the organ of Corti and the primary afferents (Fig. 11.7).

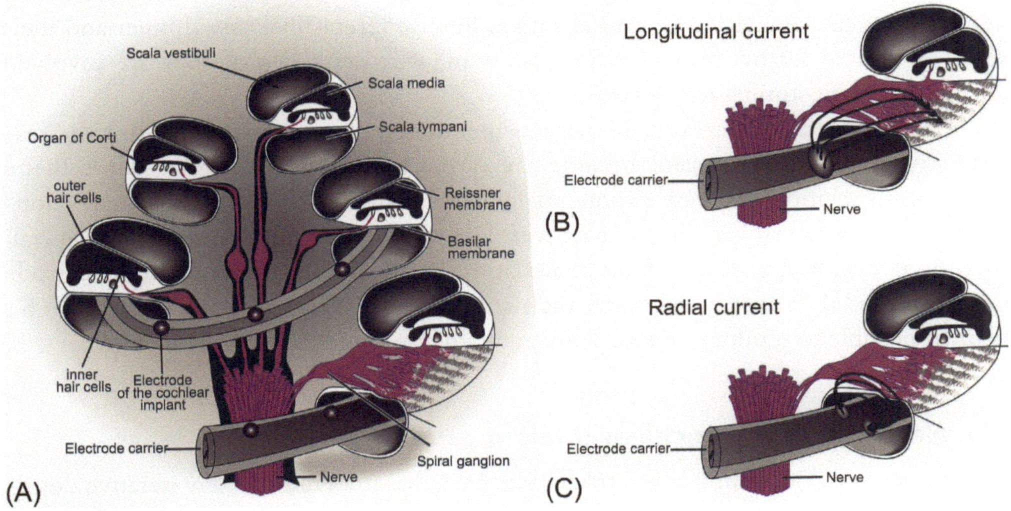

Fig. 11.7 Location of a cochlear implant in the cochlea of a deaf subject. (A) The cochlear implant is a linear array of electrodes *(black circles)* placed on a silastic carrier. The electrodes are contacted with lead wires that run in the silastic carrier. As a rule, the implanted ear has a degenerated organ of Corti. (B) In case of a longitudinal arrangement of electrodes, particularly in bipolar configuration, current flows longitudinally in the scala tympani and hits the primary afferents in perpendicular (unfavorable) direction. (C) If electrodes are placed radially on the silastic carrier, radial currents can be generated by bipolar configuration. These show a much more favorable current direction. In monopolar configuration, both radial and longitudinal currents are present. Also, the trunk of the nerve is another place of excitation with cochlear implants.

One problem for this stimulation, however, is the large spread of excitation in the electrically conductive scala tympani. Therefore several attempts have been made in the past to limit the current spread. One obvious approach is to use bipolar configuration of electrodes in the stimulation. This, however, has the disadvantage that with a linear array of electrodes oriented longitudinally in the scala tympani, current direction is in fact perpendicular to the course of the spiral ganglion cells, and thus, as discussed in **Chapter 7**, provides the unfavorable direction for electrical stimulation (Fig. 11.7B). Therefore, attempts have been made to orient the electrical field by 90 degrees, rotated using radially arranged electrodes on the silastic carrier (Fig. 11.7C). Theoretically, this should provide much more focused excitation; the problem with cochlear implants, however, is the small distance between the working and return electrodes limited by the size of the silastic carrier. Thus a lot of energy is wasted on currents that flow between the electrode within the scala tympani and never reach neurons. In practical application, the induced perceptions were faint and required large currents to be perceptible.

Since the most important targets of the nerve, the type I ganglion cells, are also large cells, they are most likely the ones that are predominantly activated by current (**Chapter 7**). Only at high current levels might other fibers get involved. However, it is unclear how much of these targets for the electric field are preserved in the deaf cochlea of the given hearing-impaired subject. Likely it is the soma (or the axons near the soma) where electrical stimulation is most effective. Since efferent fibers are thinner and their soma us located further away (in the brainstem) it is unlikely that they are involved cochlear implant stimulation effects.

Nonetheless, the three favorable aspects mentioned previously are probably the reason why the cochlear implant became the most clinically successful neuroprosthetic device. Implantations increase exponentially every year. It also promoted the development of central prostheses that in part were dependent on the (commercial, financial) success of cochlear implants. Companies introduced modifications on the electrode design, but used the same processors and medical device manufacturing structure. This made it possible to produce and sell less frequently used, and thus less profitable, devices.

The electrode of the cochlear implant

The modern cochlear implant electrode (Fig. 11.8) has undergone many iterative developmental steps during the last three decades. The first experiments started with simple platinum wires placed in the auditory nerve, isolated by a silicone carrier. Later the electrodes became larger, indented into the silicone to prevent high current densities near the edge of the electrode (as discussed in **Chapter 6**). The shape changed from rings circumventing the electrode carrier to somewhat smaller ellipsoid plates. The material did not change: the implant consists of platinum electrodes each contacted by a platinum wire and placed on a silicone carrier. The original size covered only part of the basal turn of the cochlea, but as success became apparent, longer cochlear electrode carriers have

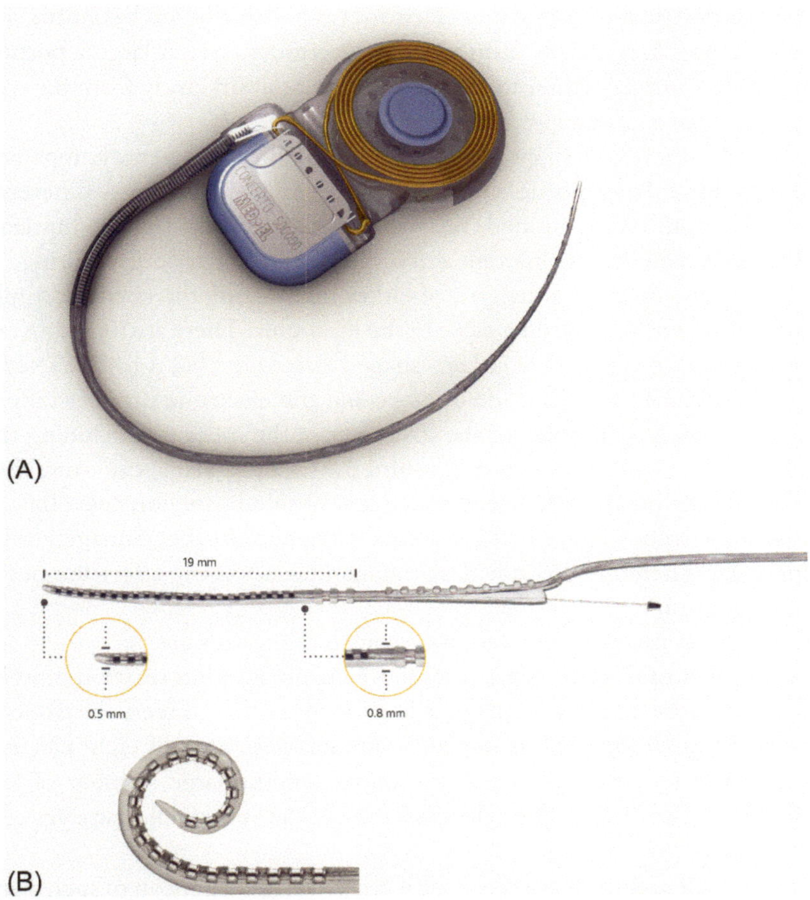

Fig. 11.8 Modern cochlear implant. (A) The internal part of the cochlear implant is completely in the body of the recipient. It is a purely passive equipment. The receiver coil receives the energy and the control signals via electromagnetic fields, while the electronics in the hermetic housing transforms it and leads it to the lead wires that contact the individual electrodes. (B) Detail of an electrode tip from another manufacturer. The electrode shown is initially implanted in the straightened form, kept in shape by a stylet. After some insertion has been achieved, the stylet is removed while the electrode is pushed further into the cochlea. By this, the electrode can hug closer to the modiolus. (C) The pre-curved shape shows up after stylet removal. Note the recessed design of the electrode contacts below the surface of the silicone carrier. *((A) Copyright © MedEl Comp., Innsbruck, Austria. (B,C) Copyright © Cochlear Ltd., Sydney, Australia. Similar designs of cochlear implants are also in clinical use from Oticon Medical, Kopenhagen, Denmark and Advanced Bionics, Valencia, USA.)*

been designed that can cover the basal and the middle turn of the cochlea. The apical portions of the cochlea are still out of reach of an implant because the space in the scala tympani is too small. Nonetheless, the spiral ganglion itself covers only 1.6–2.0 turns of the cochlea. With regard to *cochlear coverage* by the implant, device companies follow different strategies. Some pack as many electrodes as possible in the basal turn, as close to the modiolus as possible. Others distribute the electrodes over as large a portion of the cochlea as possible and stay closer to the abmodiolar position (away from the modiolus). Both approaches have advantages and disadvantages.

Consequently, the exact shape of the electrode differs between companies. Some companies provide a large portfolio of electrodes, each design for a different subject group and indication. As mentioned, the size and detailed shape of the human cochlea is highly variable, and given different etiologies including residual hearing, different approaches have emerged with the goal of either minimizing the cochlear implantation trauma or positions of the electrodes close to the modiolus. There are long thin electrodes (Fig. 11.8A), short thin electrodes, and pre-shaped electrodes (Fig. 11.8B,C), some with a guide (Fig. 11.8B); the interelectrode distance and the electrode number differ as well.

Cochlear trauma (i.e., damage to the structures of the inner ear including the basilar membrane, the spiral lamina, the modiolus, and the stria vascularis) can cause tissue reactions, including inflammation and accelerated loss of spiral ganglion cells. Inflammation may increase impedance of the electrode contacts as well as further damage surviving spiral ganglion cells. Therefore any cochlear trauma may adversely affect the outcomes of cochlear implantation.

The factors to consider in the design of cochlear implants are:

1. A larger number of electrodes provides more channels of information; however, due to the current spread, the advantage is less for more than fifteen electrodes. Speech perception in quiet in cochlear implants saturates with around eight electrodes.
2. A larger number of electrodes and the corresponding large number of lead wires increases the stiffness of the electrodes and the potential damage caused by implantation.
3. Thin and flexible electrodes may also be a disadvantage. Insertion of such electrodes is more tricky, since when inserted they can lead to buckling of the electrode (Fig. 11.9) in the attempt to push it further into the cochlea. Electrode buckling is a frequent cause of cochlear damage. Furthermore, buckling prevents the surgeon from

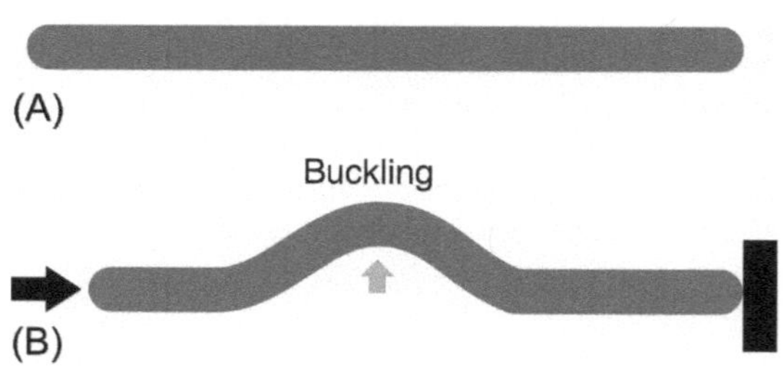

Fig. 11.9 Electrode buckling when attempting to push the electrode (A) against a resistance *(black block in B)*. In that case somewhere in the course of the electrode the corpus starts to move away *(light gray arrow)* from the push direction *(black arrow)*, damaging typically the basilar membrane.

"feeling" resistance, since the compliance of the buckled electrode is usually greater than that of a straight electrode.

This makes clear that electrode design requires the consideration of many factors: not only the way it stimulates neurons, but also the mechanical factors that play an essential role during surgery and affect outcomes following implantation.

Neurophysiological background of cochlear implants

The idea that electrical stimulation of the auditory nerve might lead to auditory sensations dates back to Volta who used an electric "shock" applied to the outer ear canal. This created sounds that reminded him of a boiling paste. As outlined in **Chapter 2**, this idea has repeatedly come up during history, but could not be translated into practically usable concepts due to insufficient technical development. The first attempts to implement a medical device that could be implanted into the modiolus took place in the 1960s. One of the pioneers of this development, Blair Simmons, named the device "cochlear implant." It consisted of six electrodes that were probably inserted into the basal portion of the auditory nerve. Using a transcutaneous direct connection, these electrodes could be contacted to a source of electric current. Using electrical stimulation, it was possible to evoke auditory sensations in the deaf subject, and these could be studied in detail. The lowest thresholds were 1 μA, with an electric dynamic range of 15 dB. Place pitch and temporal pitch, as well as temporal pitch limit of 300 Hz were reported on the one implanted subject. The results suggested that unprocessed speech signals would not be understood, and indeed while they were identified as speech, it remained unintelligible.

These first attempts were accompanied by a lot of skepticism from auditory anatomists and physiologists who could not believe that such a simple device would replace the intricate physiology of the inner ear with sensitivities approaching the thermal motion of molecules, with 16,000 hair cells and up to 38,000 auditory nerve fibers. However, what these physiologists had forgotten was that speech, while being an extremely complex signal, is also highly redundant, and its discrimination rests on many features that do not always have to be present to allow discrimination. Furthermore, our decoding of language not only rests on the acoustic signal, but also on the context, and that grammar, once mastered, supports the decoding of acoustic signals.

Indeed, subsequent studies with one-channel stimulation placed on the round window lead to better success and these systems were used in Austria and the United States in some patients, including deaf-born children. In the 1980s, multichannel devices were introduced that substantially improved performance. The first attempts for electric stimulation in single-channel implants were performed with compressed analogue signals (thus an electrical current derived from the microphone signal). Later, particularly with multichannel systems, pulsatile stimulation with biphasic charge balanced pulses was used (typical phase durations today are <50 μs/phase).

Modern cochlear implants consist of a silicone carrier and 12–22 electrode contacts (Fig. 11.8) inserted into the scala tympani through the round window, or, in some cases, through a drilled opening underneath of it. Due to the position within the scala tympani, the individual electrodes come to lie at different places in the cochlea. This means that the electrode array follows the tonotopic organization of the cochlea. This gives it the possibility to mimic the place code by activation of different electrodes of the implant. Indeed, auditory neuroscientists were interested in to what extent the tonotopy can be coded by electric stimulation, and how much further it can be focused. Recordings from the auditory nerve in cats have shown that the spread of excitation of the electric field was extensive with monopolar configuration of electrodes. Using bipolar and tripolar configurations, as outlined in **Chapter 7**, could improve the current focusing substantially, and narrow the excitation to an extent necessary for discrimination of complex acoustic stimuli (one critical band, Fig. 11.10). Compared to acoustic stimulation, this was possible only for current levels within a few dB above the stimulation threshold (see red curve in Fig. 11.10), whereas in acoustic stimulation this is observed for 20–30 dB. Also the loudness evoked by tripolar stimulation was low, most likely due to its effectively reduced current spread. Due to small number of active channels this caused faint perceptions that precluded to make use of the improved channel separation. Furthermore, the degeneration of the auditory nerve in deaf ears, which is not uniform along the cochlea, causes stimulation thresholds to vary along the cochlea in many subjects when tested with tripolar stimulation. This means that different electrodes require different stimulation current to reach threshold, and this complicates the adjustment of the three electrodes required for tripolar stimulation. Furthermore, increasing stimulation currents increases current spread for the given individual electrodes. This means that the spatial precision varies with stimulation channel. This and other reasons do not allow us to take pragmatic advantage of this useful technology in deaf subjects. Monopolar stimulation, however, can reach the surviving auditory nerve fibers even if they are not close to the active electrode. Therefore threshold profiles are more uniform and thus better with monopolar stimulation.

In conclusion, this means that electric stimulation cannot make such an efficient use of the place code as normal hearing ears. This is one limiting factor of cochlear implants, since less precise place code will smear the spectral information (and reduce the number of independent channels of information) that is critical in complex hearing situations. If different complex stimuli are presented at the same time, individual spectral peaks can be associated with one or the other stimulus based on their temporal fluctuations (related to pitch). If spectral peaks are overlapping, peaks from different stimuli can fuse at the level of the auditory nerve and become no longer separable by this principle.

As discussed in **Chapter 7**, phase-locking to electric stimulation is artificially high compared to activity caused by transmitter release on a synapse. This is also the case

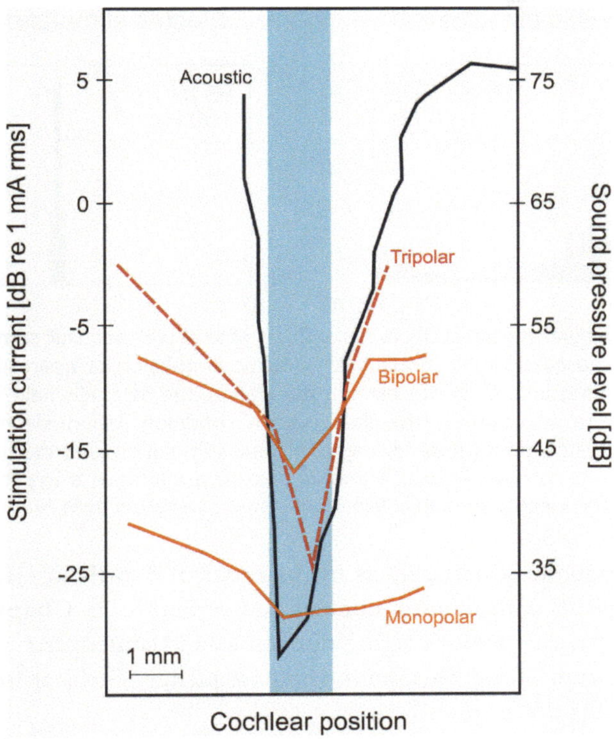

Fig. 11.10 Electrical tuning curves for single auditory nerve fibers of a cat. Shown is threshold in dB as a function of cochlear position. For comparison, an acoustic frequency tuning curve of a hearing ear for the approximate CF region is shown in black (note the cochlear position from base is shown on the abscissa, thus X-axis is reversed compared to Fig. 11.3). *Blue region* corresponds to one critical band of a normal hearing ear in this frequency region. Electric tuning curves obtained in the same auditory nerve fiber in the region of the nerve with CFs in the range of 8–10 kHz. Monopolar configuration shows only a weak positional specificity, bipolar shows higher specificity, and the best place specificity with clear minimum threshold is found in tripolar *(dashed red)* configuration. The lowest thresholds vary by more than 10 dB for the different configurations, with best thresholds observed in monopolar configuration. *(Data from Kral et al. (1998).)*

for cochlear implants. Therefore the temporal code is highly precise with electric stimulation, and phase-locking is greater in the ear than with acoustic stimulation (Fig. 11.11). This leads to hyper-synchronization of auditory nerve activity to the electric stimulus. While this provides the opportunity to convey highly reliable timing information to the brain, it comes also with a disadvantage. Since the auditory nerve fiber can only generate one or two action potentials to each stimulus period or pulse with electric stimulation, the stochasticity of the responses is low and correspondingly so is the range of intensities (currents) that can be coded by the stimulus. The consequence is the reduced

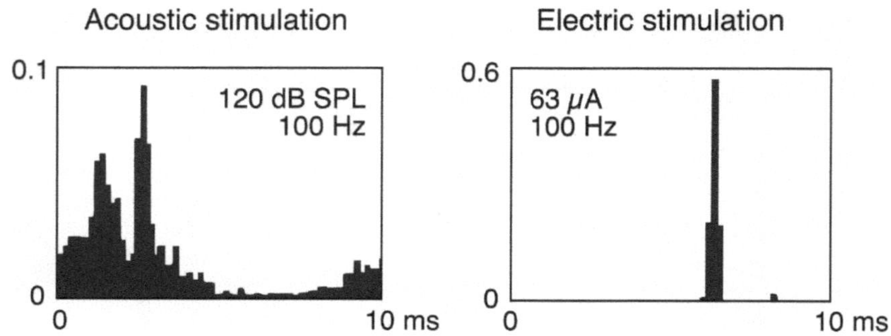

Fig. 11.11 Period histograms from auditory nerve fibers of a cat with acoustic stimulation and electric stimulation using a sinusoidal 100 Hz stimulus (for acoustic stimulation, compare also Fig. 11.4). Period (abscissa) shown in time units (ms). For electric stimulation, the hair cells have been destroyed by ototoxic substances to approximate the deaf human condition. Using electric stimulation, the period histogram reveals a tight phase locking in electric stimulation with the occurrence of action potential only within a narrow range of stimulus phases, resulting in a hyper-synchronization of neuronal activity to the electric stimulus. *(Reproduced with permission from Hartmann et al. (1984).)*

dynamic range of auditory nerve fibers in the order of 3–6 dB in electric stimulation, compared to 40–80 dB with acoustic stimulation (see Fig. 7.7 in **Chapter 7**). However, speech is a highly dynamic acoustic signal with louder and fainter parts, all of them important for discrimination of speech sounds. In consequence, cochlear implant processors must compensate for this issue.

Fortunately, different auditory nerve fibers show different thresholds to stimulation through the same electrode of the implant. This can be concluded from Fig. 11.10, where the response of one fiber to different implant electrodes is shown. Each of the electrical tuning curves, particularly the one for tripolar configuration, shows a larger range of threshold currents. The same applies in the reversed situation: different fibers show different thresholds for stimulation with the one given electrode. This increases the electric dynamic range to 20 dB. It is still low, but much more than the range predicted by one fiber alone.

The chronaxies measured in the auditory nerve vary substantially depending on species and status of the auditory nerve, and usually fall in the range 60–300 μs. Models of auditory nerve usually rely on small chronaxie; however, it remains unclear if this is the correct approach. There is some discrepancy on the effect of loss of spiral ganglion cells on strength-duration functions, where experimental evidence paradoxically suggests both decrease in steepness as well as increase in steepness. Conceptually, loss of myelin is supposed to lead to decrease in steepness of strength-duration curves.

There is still research on the sensitivity with regard to polarity of the electric stimulus in cochlear implants. While in animal models, consistent with other neuronal structures, lower thresholds were observed with cathodic leading bipolar pulses, some observations suggest that in humans anodic-leading stimuli might be more favorable. This may depend on the 3D orientation of the neuronal elements relative to the implant and a degeneration of primary afferents. The reader is referred to Figs. 7.3, 7.4, and 7.5 and the related text in **Chapter 7**.

Cochlear implant stimulation is also the area with the most detailed information on the properties of electrical responses. Over decades, scientist related the physical properties of the stimulus to neuronal excitation patterns and to perceptions in animals and humans in parallel. Thus we learned that with sinusoidal stimulation of increasing frequency, the thresholds increase by 4 dB/octave (comp. Fig. 6.1). Similarly, with pulsatile stimulation the increase in phase duration decreases the thresholds by approximately the same amount (Fig. 11.12). Since the change of threshold is less than 6 dB/octave, as would be expected if deposited charge per period alone would define thresholds, the neurons indeed electrically behave like leaky integrators, as described in **Chapter 4**. When threshold is expressed in units of charge one can indeed observe an increase in threshold with increasing phase duration. However, beyond 0.8–1.0 ms, the steepness further changes in the other direction (the threshold drops), probably as a consequence of multiple spikes that are evoked per phase.

These data document that stimulation with long phase durations is not particularly efficient with respect to consumed electric energy. This is one reason why today cochlear implants use charge-balanced pulsatile stimulation with phase durations less than 100 μs.

Impedance of the implanted electrodes typically increases during the first 3–4 weeks after implantation from ~ 4 kΩ to ~ 7 kΩ (depending on the make of the implant), and subsequently show a slow decrease in impedance. Impedances less than 10–15 kΩ are considered within compliance limits in clinical cochlear implants. However, if impedances increase significantly above the compliance limit, the current sources no longer

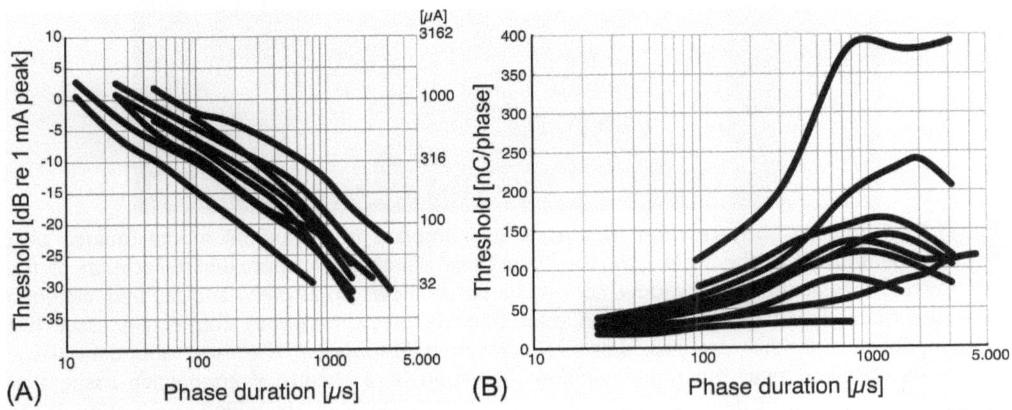

Fig. 11.12 Thresholds depend on the duration of the stimulus phase. Data from human subjects. (A) Current threshold as a function of pulse duration. (B) Charge threshold as a function of phase duration. *(Reproduced with permission from Moon et al. (1993).)*

can supply the requested current and reprogramming is required (either switching off the high-impedance electrodes or increasing the pulse duration on these electrodes). Very likely, the first increase in impedance after implantation is related to acute reaction to implantation, as outlined in **Chapter 8**. The subsequent slight decrease of impedances is likely related to changes in the electrode surface, including the increase in effective electrode area due to chronic stimulation. The implant is very often covered by a sheath of connective tissue, as animal studies have revealed (Fig. 11.13). This tissue is often largest at the round window, and a source of this tissue is most likely at the middle ear. While the opening of the round window membrane heals within a few weeks and thus closes the

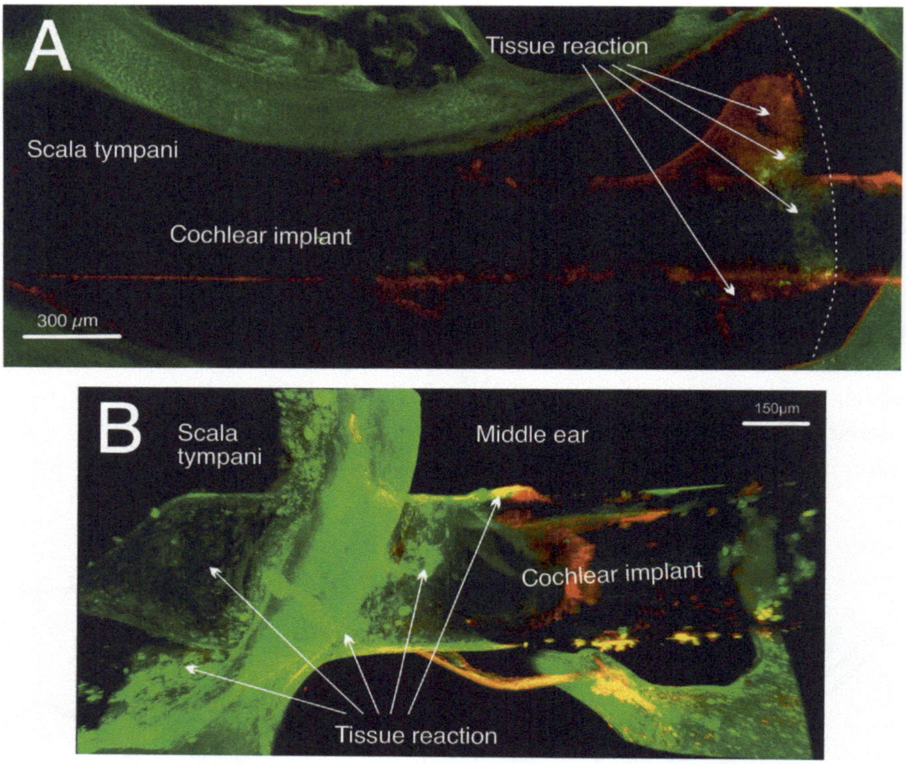

Fig. 11.13 A foreign body reaction to the cochlear implant in an animal model (guinea pig). (A) Cochlear implant in the scala tympani. *Dotted line* denotes the approximate location of the round window. Near the round widow, connective tissue shows up as *green* and *red* (*red*: vimentin molecules marked with an antibody; *red color* thus denotes amorphous connective tissue like collagen fibers and other proteins, *green color* includes fibroblasts). The most abundant tissue reaction is observed near the round window, but there is a sheath of connective tissue that encapsulates the implant deeply into the scala tympani. (B) Detailed, magnified penetration at the round window. Connective tissue is discernible at both the middle ear and in the scala tympani side of the round window. *(Data from Wrzeszcz et al. (2015), figure courtesy of Prof. G. Reuter, Institute of AudioNeuroTechnology.)*

opening, the tissue that entered the scala tympani continues to grow along the electrode. Application of corticoids can reduce this tissue growth and reaction to the implant. Cochleostomy (an artificial access to the cochlea formed by drilling the wall of the scala tympani) has been shown to induce stronger tissue growth and even ossification, very likely due to the material that enters the scala tympani during drilling. Fibrous tissue may be responsible not only for an increase in impedance, but also for an additional spread of the electrical field due to electric inhomogenities within the scala tympani. Currently, approaches are tested that allow a deposition and a slow release of dexamethasone after implantation from the silicone of the implant to reduce the foreign body reaction. In some centers the implant is covered with corticoids prior to implantation and subjects receive corticoids systemically after implantation.

Subjects with cochlear implants seem to perceive pitch based on the tonotopy (i.e., different electrodes evoke different pitch consistent with the tonotopic organization of a hearing cochlea, place pitch) and based on temporal code (temporal pitch, saturating, however, at around 200–400 Hz, the pitch saturation limit of electric hearing). Place pitch is rather weak (discernible differences need to be greater than one octave, i.e., frequency doubling) and since the implant covers a limited frequency range it is also not key to the success of cochlear implants. Temporal pitch is probably the main cue for perceiving pitch in cochlear-implanted subjects. Pitch perception is one of the ongoing issues of cochlear implants to this day.

Loudness of the perceived sound is more difficult to directly relate to the electric stimulus. Of course, loudness of the single pulse relates to the current that is applied; however, within a time window of 7 ms the perceived loudness is also the consequence of integration over the pulses presented (i.e., when more pulses are presented within 7 ms window, the louder the percept). Thresholds best relate to the distance between the implant and the stimulated neurons, whereas maximal loudness is often a function of the largest peaks in the signal over time.

Previously we discussed that the dynamic range is reduced with electric stimulation. Correspondingly, also the mapping of stimulus intensity (expressed as function of dynamic range) to perceived loudness is different between electric and acoustic stimulation. In acoustic stimulation loudness increases steeply already at low intensities, in contrast to electric stimulation that increases slowly at low-input intensities. At high intensities, characteristics for electric and acoustic stimulation invert and electric stimulation attains a steep course (i.e., it is an expansive function) while acoustic stimulation is compressive. This needs to be accounted for in the processor.

It is beyond the scope of this chapter to review all the literature that describes the detailed properties of responses to electric stimulation, but here we want to emphasize that the most extensive and comprehensive investigation on electrical responses has been performed in the auditory system using cochlear implants, in different species and in human subjects.

Another issue is the power delivery into the inner ear. Initially, cochlear implant electrodes were physically connected using a direct percutaneous connection to the processors and current sources. This percutaneous connection, by disrupting the skin integrity, required prevention of infection entering into the body along the implant. Since implants may allow biofilm formation (see **Chapter 8**), this was a subject to medical complications. A wireless connection via electromagnetic fields, as used in cortical implants by Brindley et al. in the 1960s, provided a possible solution. Currently all commercial implants use such a transcutaneous connection (through intact skin). Present-day implants therefore consist of two parts: (i) an **internal part** located in the body, consisting of a receiver coil for radiofrequency communication (a transmitter coil in the part outside of the body would communicate with the receiver coil), the necessary electronics with the current sources for addressing the individual electrode contacts, and the electrode carrier with the electrodes, and the other (ii) **external part**, located outside of the body—with batteries, speech processor and the transmitter coil (Fig. 11.14). The receiver coil is usually placed behind the auricle in the skull, where a bony bed for it is drilled during the implantation. From there, a retroauricular approach to the middle ear is used and the electrode lead is placed behind the middle ear ossicles. The entrance into the inner ear was initially through an artificial opening in the cochlea (a cochleostomy), but today most implantations are performed through one of the natural openings of the cochlea, the round window. This needs to be slightly enlarged in many patients by removing a bony overhang with a drill. The membrane of the round window is opened by a sharp instrument, and through this opening the electrode is inserted into the scala

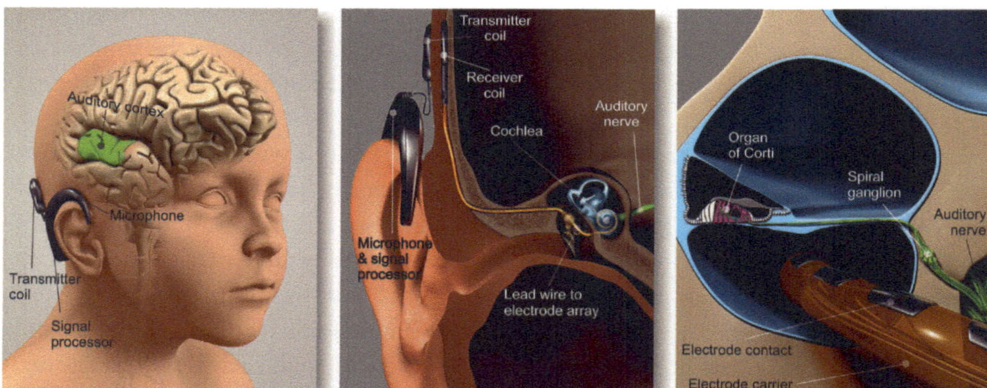

Fig. 11.14 Positioning of the cochlear implant. The implant consists of an external part, located behind the ear including the microphone, the speech processor, the batteries and the transmitter coil, and the internal part, placed in the body and shown in Fig. 11.9. The transcutaneous connection through the intact skin is achieved using radio frequency electromagnetic communication between the transmitter and the received coil. This transmits both the energy and the control signals to the electrodes in the scala tympani. *(Reproduced with permission from Kral et al. (2016).)*

tympani. The membrane heals itself within few days and closes the opening naturally. Some surgeons place muscle fascia or other material on the round window to seal it better.

Such an operation is also possible in small children, since the cochlea does not substantially change in size after birth. However, the skull grows, and therefore it is important that the implant is not dragged out of the cochlea. This can be secured by placing the electrode carrier with the lead wires into one to two loops that provide material for the increasing distance between receiver coil and the inner ear during growth of the head.

After the wounds have healed, the external processor and the transmitter coil can be placed behind the ear. The transmitter coil is held in place by a small magnet in the center that matches the opposite magnet in the receiver coil. This secures the optimal location of both coils and sufficiently small distance between the two coils.

In total, the cochlear implant can exploit the anatomic advantages in the cochlea including the scala tympani as a natural channel for housing the cochlear implant. While the place code can be exploited only rudimentary in cochlear implants, it allows for eight to twelve independent frequency channels that are sufficient for good speech understanding in quiet. A temporal code provides the possibility to convey high-precision timing information to the brain, with the disadvantage of reduced dynamic range. Given these limitations, support from signal pre-processing is required to make the implant a useful clinical device.

The processor of the cochlear implant

The speech processor of cochlear implants must take all the above differences between acoustic and electric hearing into account. For this, sound must be picked up by the microphone and transformed to an electrical signal. The microphone, together with the batteries and the processor itself is in modern implants placed in a device behind the ear. It includes all the necessary processing steps, and often also different settings for different environments, including the possibility for streaming signals directly into the device from a telephone or television.

Speech coding is an essential aspect that enabled the success of cochlear implants. It has improved substantially over the decades. Early cochlear implants were single-channel devices that in principle provided the electrical microphone signal directly into the cochlea (compressed analogue strategies). Consequently, subjects had only access to the time signal of speech. This allowed sufficient speech understanding only in a minority of the subjects, but provided awareness of sound and allowed some sound discrimination.

Subsequently, implants with several channels have been introduced. However, one difficulty was that providing two-channel compressed analogue strategies was not successful. Here, presenting two signals at neighboring electrodes led to extensive currents flowing within the scala tympani that provided a conductive short circuit between active electrodes. This means that the current applied to one electrode would be differently effective in activating the auditory nerve depending on the exact time-course of the current applied to a neighboring electrode. It was impossible to find a setting that would alleviate this issue. Only implants that could be positioned such that they directly touched the modiolus and thus involved no conductive space between electrodes could provide some success with this technology.

Multichannel coding strategies therefore relied on presentation of brief biphasic pulses that could be presented in an interleaved fashion between electrodes so that none of the channels was active if another channel of the implant was active as well. That avoided inter-channel interactions. Initial multichannel coding strategies involved heavy preprocessing and provided mainly speech-relevant cues (e.g., formant information). However, these strategies did not allow sufficient speech understanding in the majority of implanted subjects. A breakthrough in the 1990s was the use of the **continuous interleaved sampling (CIS)** strategy and its subsequent modifications (**n-of-m coding**). Here the sound was preprocessed similarly as in the normal hearing cochlea: the sound was filtered into frequency bands, then the envelope of the signal in each band was extracted (by low-pass filtering to the envelope and rectifying) and presented as an electric pulse train on the given electrode (Fig. 11.15). Before presentation it was necessary to adjust the amplitude to the reduced dynamic range of electric hearing, and therefore an automatic gain control was used to optimally adjust the stimulation current range to the range of sound pressure levels in the environment. After fitting into the dynamic range of electric hearing, the abnormal expansive function of perceived loudness, as discussed previously, had to be accounted for by a compressive function to approximate the acoustic percepts as far as possible. A sequence of stimulation was finally determined, where not all electrodes were activated, but only those that recieved the strongest input.

Speech perception with cochlear implants

Hearing subjects tolerate highly degraded acoustic speech signals without much loss of speech understanding. This underscores that speech signals include many highly redundant acoustic cues and that speech is understood through the interaction between brain expectations and sensory input, so that informational gaps in the signal can be easily filled in by the brain. This fortunate circumstance is one reason for the great success of cochlear implants.

In cochlear-implanted subjects it is thus possible to manipulate signals in real time to investigate what the brain can tolerate without significant effects on overall speech understanding.

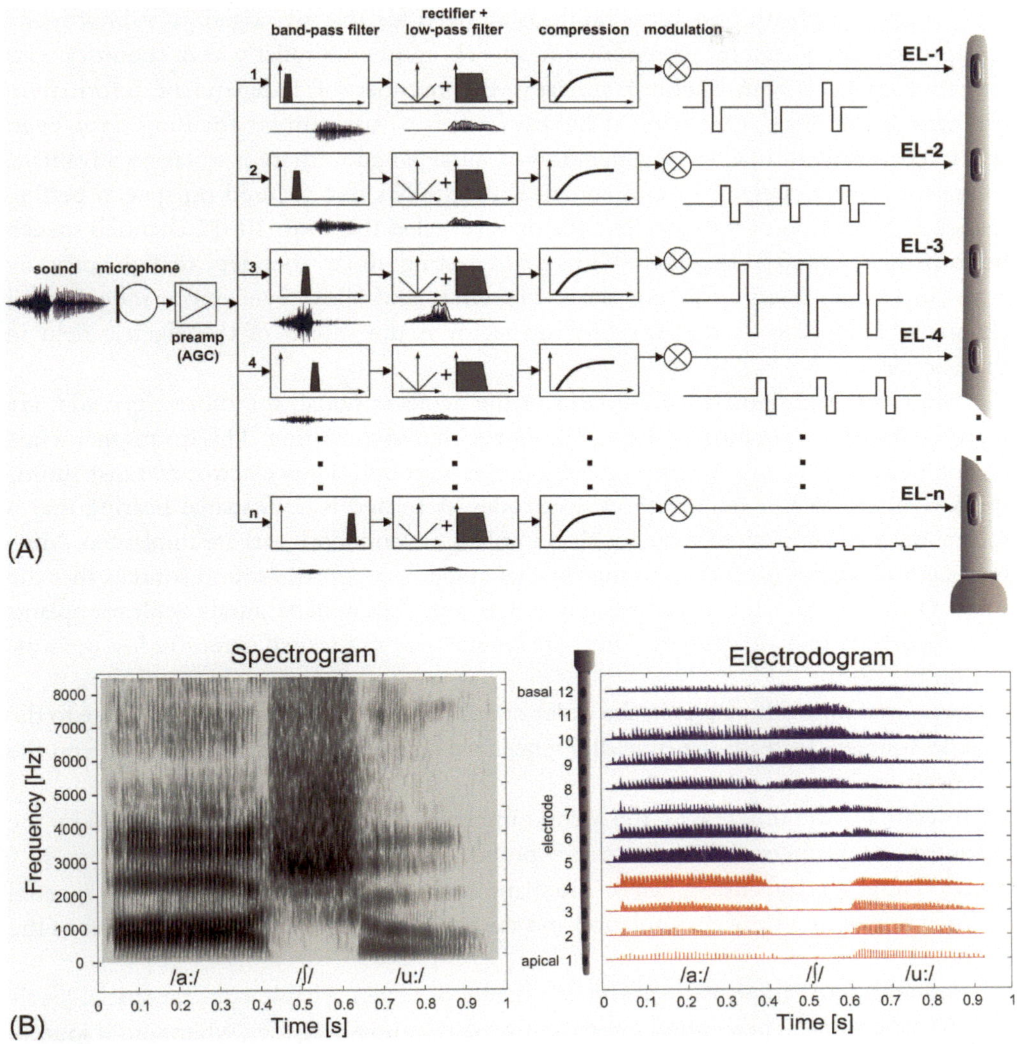

Fig. 11.15 Continuous interleaved sampling strategy. (A) The signal is first preprocessed using an automatic gain control (AGC). The sound is then decomposed into frequency channels by bandpass filtering. Subsequently, the envelope of the signal in each channel is extracted by rectification and low-pass filtering, to finally apply a compression to the dynamic range of the electric hearing. Pulsatile stimuli are presented in an interleaved fashion to prevent interference between electric fields in the cochlea. (B) Example how a sound spectrogram (pronounced "ashu") is transformed into an electrodogram. In the present example of the CIS, the apical most channels include temporal fine structure information *(red)*. *(Reprinted with permission from Kral and Tillein (2020).)*

Use of multichannel cochlear implants allowed for the investigation of how many electrodes are required for recognition of speech in quiet. Similarly as in acoustics with degraded speech, with cochlear implants the number of independent information channels is not large. One way of increasing it is to use current focusing. However, due to concomitant uneven degeneration of spiral ganglion there is so far no advantage to any of these strategies. In consequence, the studies that focused on speech performance as a function of independent channels revealed that with 10–12 channels speech performance saturates in quiet. This is interesting since vocoders that acoustically simulate electric hearing do not show this effect and allow even more independent channels. That suggests that the limiting factor is the spread of the electric field in the cochlea.

The worse the signal-to-noise ratio of the acoustic signal, the more electrodes are required to reach saturation performance in speech understanding. This means that while a good performance may be guaranteed in quiet with only a few electrodes, noisy multi-speaker environments require more electrodes. A related issue is spatial hearing that is substantially compromised with cochlear implants, even if both ears are implanted. Minimal audible angles (i.e., the minimal spatial angle between the sound sources that the subject can discriminate) are acoustically at 8 degrees, but with binaural cochlear implants they are greater than 40 degrees. There are several reasons for such extensive loss of localization precision:

1. Interaural time differences in the order of dozens of μs cannot be preserved due to the CIS strategy. Instead, the time differences are changing over time depending on the spectrum.
2. Interaural-level differences, the second important binaural cue, are destroyed by the automatic gain control of the speech processors.
3. Monaural spectral cues, given by the shape of the pinna, are destroyed by the spectral smearing of monopolar stimulation and the position of the microphone outside of the pinna.

Consequently, the implanted subject can barely use even reliable cues for spatial localization. Since speech perception improves by spatial unmasking (i.e., when sound sources are separated in space and can be resolved by the auditory system), degraded spatial hearing also complicates speech perception in multi-talker environments.

Another issue with electric hearing is the fact that exact timing between channels is affected by speech-coding strategies. Fortunately, it has been demonstrated that the brain is exceptionally insensitive to temporal shifts between channels; it can reconstruct speech even if the timing between channels is randomly varied in time (jittered) by 40–80 ms. In vocoded simulation with 16 channels, even 100 ms was tolerated and speech understanding was still possible. Remarkably, spectral compression (thus compression along the characteristic frequency dimension in the spectrum) is also very well tolerated. It appears that speech is a signal the brain is excellent in decoding and can rely on the many redundancies in the signal, resulting in high robustness of its processing.

The performance of cochlear implants, despite all these issues, is remarkable. The mean performance in single syllable recognition is around 55%–60% in modern-day implants, and mean sentence recognition is around 80%–90% (Fig. 11.16). Approximately 75% of implant users can understand speech in context-free conditions (achieve open-set speech recognition, i.e., recognition even if the words are not from a closed set of possible words used in testing). This means that these profoundly deaf subjects can integrate into hearing society, communicate acoustically with other subjects, and live a life of a mildly hearing-impaired person. Implant performance, however, decreases in background noise like in a cocktail party or a loud restaurant or bar.

Implants as recording devices

Cochlear implants have further developed into devices that can capture information from the implanted subject. Most important for the integrity check of the implant are measurements of impedance (**Chapter 8**) that provide information on the functionality of the individual electrodes. Current devices can, after presenting the stimulation pulse, record the electrical field through the other electrodes. This allows for the recording the compound action potentials of the auditory nerve and providing a correlate for haring thresholds. This is particularly important in the initial fitting of children who cannot yet communicate (**Chapter 9**). In addition, algorithms are provided that can determine the spread of excitation in the cochlea. This area is a focus of research and will likely expand in the future.

Individualization of cochlear implantations

While cochlear implants have been initially used only for subjects with profound deafness, their success has led to their use in residually hearing cochleae. Indeed the implant outcomes in these subjects, particularly if the residual hearing can be preserved, are among the best. Since most subjects preserve residual hearing in the apex of the cochlea, distant from the place where a cochlear implant is inserted, careful implantation may preserve residual hearing in many implanted patients.

The biggest issue in cochlear implantation is outcome variability. As can be seen in Fig. 11.16, performance following implantation improves over time in nearly all patients, but not all patients reach the same performance. While the means are greater than 50% in monosyllabic tests 24 months after implantation, the range covers 10%–90%; from poor to excellent performance. Since performance usually reaches saturation after the first 12 months and does not change much beyond that, this large variability represents a

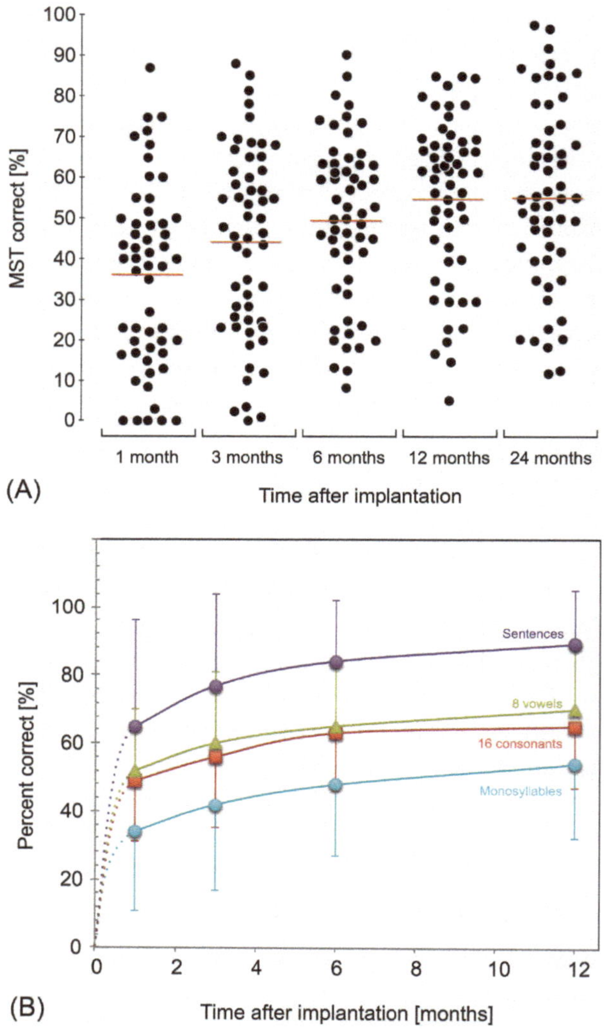

Fig. 11.16 Speech understanding with present-day multichannel cochlear implants. (A) Acoustic analysis is best assessed with a monosyllabic test (MST). Here, performance with one brand of cochlear implant and the same speech processor over time is compared. Mean is shown as an orange line. Results greater than ~45%–50% are usually sufficient to understand whole sentences in a natural setting and to interact only through acoustic input. (B) Performance of several tests conventionally used in cochlear implants. Context-involving tests, like those with sentences, and those from a very limited set of words give best results. Performance on monosyllables is usually the worst. However, they all represent a quantified measure of performance with cochlear implant. While time 0 represents the moment of implantation and thus cochlear implant data are not available, the subjects were profoundly deaf at that point and thus had 0% speech understanding. *((A) Figure reproduced with permission from Wilson and Dorman (2008). (B) Data from Helms et al. (1997), redrawn.)*

pressing clinical issue. Although implants can provide optimal benefits, these benefits are not achievable by all subjects. To understand this variability is the main goal of present day cochlear implant research.

One bottleneck is the structure that is implanted: the cochlea. The number of surviving spiral ganglion cells (the receptive tissue for the electrical field) and the homogeneity of their preservation are two main factors for this variation. The loss of spiral ganglion cells in the given subjects cannot be assessed (measured) today and, as has been mentioned already, varies greatly between patients. At present, limiting the period of deafness before implantation is a clinical goal to prevent ongoing loss of spiral ganglion cells. In the future, clinical parameters of the remaining physiological activity recorded by the cochlear implant (like cochlear microphonics from surviving hair cells or the compound action potentials of the auditory nerve) may help to detect regions with good survival or regions with pronounced loss of spiral ganglion cells in the future.

Another important aspect is individual variation of cochlear anatomy, which is a surgical issue that requires consideration. When uncoiling the cochlea and measuring the longitudinal size, the smallest human cochlea are about 36 mm in length, with the largest being about 46 mm. The microanatomy is correspondingly variable in detail. The size of the cochlea most likely relates to the size of the head, but also spatial constraints within the petrous bone shape the individual size and the morphology of the cochlea. This has obvious consequences for cochlear implants: if a small cochlea is implanted with a long cochlear implant, damage to the fragile cochlear structures is likely. Such damage leads to pronounced loss of spiral ganglion cells and loss of residual hearing in cases where residually hearing cochleae are implanted. The most recent surgical strategies therefore include cochlear imaging and use of cochlear shape models to predict the size and anatomy of the cochlea.

Finally, as discussed in **Chapter 9**, there are also indications that the central auditory adaptations to electric stimulation can be very individual, particularly in cases of pediatric cochlear implantation.

Auditory brainstem implants

There are rare cases when the auditory nerve cannot be stimulated because it has been damaged or, in even rarer cases, not formed during development (as in some cochlear malformations). In these cases, the cochlear implant is not helpful. For these subjects, auditory brainstem implants (ABIs) have been developed. These consist of the same hardware as the cochlear implant with a different electrode. The electrode is placed on the surface of the cochlear nucleus, the first station of the auditory pathway. The access to this structure is surgically complex, requiring access to the brain, thus opening the dura mater and displacing the cerebellum. This is a neurosurgical intervention with all associated risks.

A further complication is the anatomy of the cochlear nucleus. It contains three sub regions: the dorsal cochlear nucleus, the anteroventral cochlear nucleus, and the posteroventral cochlear nucleus. All these structures have a complete tonotopic representation of the cochlea. In contrast to the cochlea, they contain a high diversity of neurons, both in terms of anatomy and functional characteristics. It is still unclear which neurons can be stimulated by electric stimulation, and it remains unknown which ones are the optimal targets for such stimulation.

The first brainstem implants used only two electrodes for stimulation; only over time have surface arrays with larger sets of electrodes been developed. In addition, attempts were made to access the neurons that show temporally precise timing synchronized with acoustic stimuli (bushy cells). These are located deeply in the anteroventral cochlear nucleus, and require penetrating electrodes. Since this approach did not bring any improvement in performance, only surface electrodes are in clinical use currently.

The anatomy of the cochlear nucleus is complex in this respect, as shown in Fig. 11.17. While each segment of the cochlear nucleus contains a full representation of the cochlea and is tonotopically organized, it is interesting that in humans the innervating fibers do not twist towards the deeper parts. Thus here the tonotopic gradient may be perpendicular to that of a cat. This difference is of cardinal importance for the placement of the ABI. The electrode array is a two-dimensional grid containing up to 21 electrodes on a silicone carrier (Fig. 11.18). Only the caudal region of the dorsal cochlear nucleus is accessible for such surface grid. Here, in close proximity are low-frequency fibers and neurons. Thus, different electrodes of the implant do not have spatially specific access to different frequency representation, as in cochlear implants.

Only a small opening to the fourth ventricle, called the apertura lateralis or foramen Luschkae, is available to access the cochlear nucleus underneath the cerebellum. This opening allows the cerebrospinal fluid to circulate around the brain. It is located at the border between the pons cerebri and the medulla oblongata near the place where the IX nerve enters the brainstem. This needs to be identified and the brainstem implant inserted there. The surgeon has no real control of the exact position of the brainstem implant in this very tricky procedure. It is secured in place usually by a muscle fascia.

Fig. 11.19 shows the surgical view of the complicated access to the cochlear nucleus. Cranial nerve XII is located deep underneath nerve XI on panel A. Nerve VIII is deep underneath between nerve VII and nerve IX on panel B. The implant must be squeezed into the foramen Luschkae. Beyond this, the surgeon has limited control. Therefore, exact placement is one of the ongoing issues of ABIs.

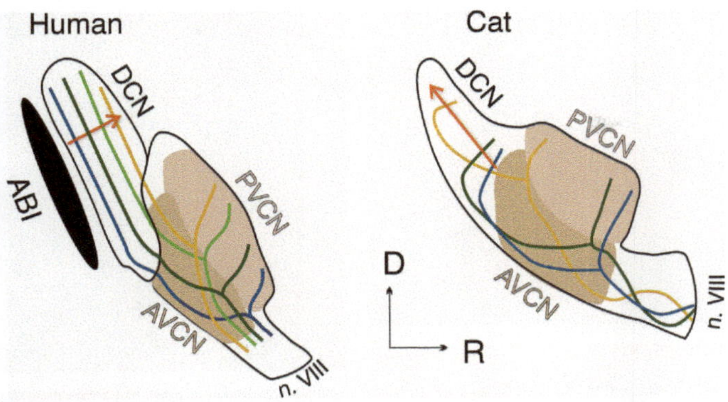

Fig. 11.17 The anatomy of the cochlear nucleus, viewed from the side (sagittal cut). Note that the course of the auditory nerve is slightly caudal shifted (i.e., to the back of the head), and the cochlear nucleus extends in caudodorsal direction. Only the dorsal portion of the cochlear nucleus is accessible via the foramen Luschkae. Fibers with low-characteristic frequency are colored blue, mid-frequency are colored green, and high-frequency are colored *yellow*. Tonotopic gradient is indicated by the *orange arrow*. While in most aspects of the function the human auditory system does match that of other mammals, including cat and mice, the tonotopic organization of the dorsal cochlear nucleus appears tilted in cats and rodents due to bending of the afferents into the depth of the DCN. This has not been observed in humans. Therefore it is assumed that the tonotopic gradient is different and that the ABI has only access to the lowest frequencies *(blue)* in humans. *DCN*, dorsal cochlear nucleus; *AVCN*, anteroventral cochlear nucleus; *PVCN*, posteroventral cochlear nucleus; *D*, dorsal; *R*, rostral. *(Figure based on data from Moore and Osen (1979), and Osen (1969).)*

The thresholds for the brainstem implants are greater than those of cochlear implants: more than 33 μA (10 nC/phase) for biphasic pulses with phase duration of 300 μs. However, they can also be substantially greater (> 666 μA, i.e., > 200 nC/phase), but still within the compliance limits of a cochlear implant processor.

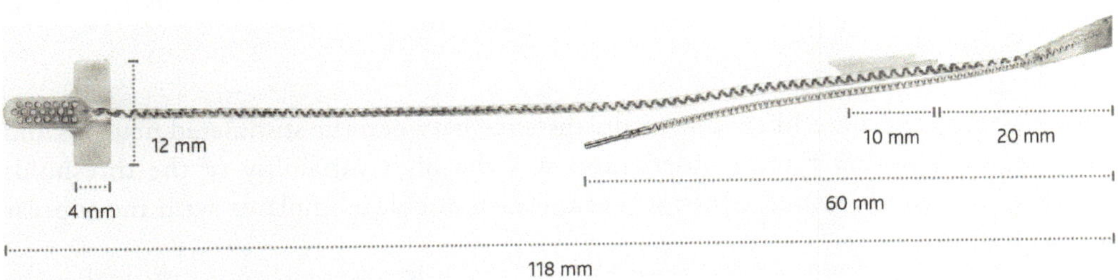

Fig. 11.18 The electrode of an auditory brainstem implant. The design of the implant receiver coil and feedthrough is identical to that of a cochlear implant. The electrode contacts are arranged in a two-dimensional grid to fit the surface of the cochlear nucleus. *(Figure courtesy of Cochlear Ltd., Sydney, Australia, with permission. A similar design from MedEl Comp., Innsbruck, Austria, is in clinical use, too.)*

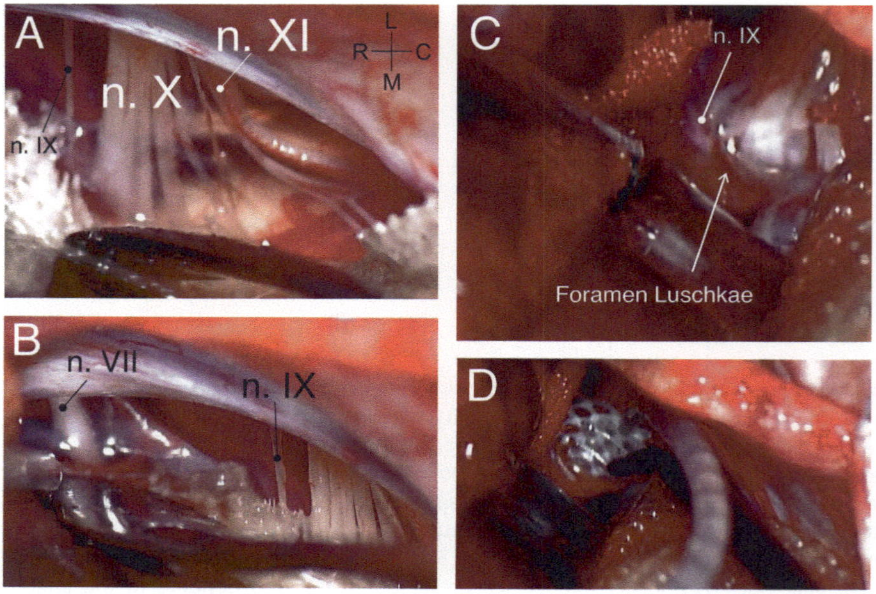

Fig. 11.19 Photographs taken through an operation microscope during an implantation of a brainstem implant at the ENT Clinics of the Hannover School of Medicine for bilateral dysplasia of the cochlea and auditory nerve, implantation on the right side, subject in lateral (lying) position. (A) Initial view underneath the cerebellum with three cranial nerves exposed. Particularly important is cranial nerve IX, which originates in the brainstem underneath the foramen Luschkae. (B) More rostral view exposing nerve VII. Vestibulocochlear (VIII) cranial nerve is not visible, but close behind n. VII (in part of their course they form one root together). Since the cochlear nerve exits the cochlea in caudal direction, the cochlear nucleus extends further caudally and thus the brainstem implant, when inserted near n. IX through the foramen Luschkae, is placed at the surface of dorsal cochlear nucleus. (C) Foramen Luschkae. (D) Situation during insertion of the auditory brainstem implant from MedEl GmbH, Innsbruck, Austria, into the foramen Luschkae, dacron mesh allows better electrode fixation. Approximately half of the electrode array is already inserted, the other half is still visible as held by the surgeon using small forceps. *R*, rostral; *C*, caudal; *L*, lateral; *M*, medial. *(Photos from surgery with kind permission of Prof. Thomas Lenarz, chairman of the ENT Clinics.)*

This higher threshold is likely due to the distance between the stimulated neurons and the implant. Another typical observation was the high variability of the thresholds between electrodes, which is not so common in cochlear implants with monopolar stimulation.

Given these factors, speech performance is significantly poorer with brainstem implants compared to cochlear implants (Fig. 11.20). Furthermore, the neurons in the cochlear nucleus show a high diversity and include inhibitory neurons. The electrical stimulation from the surface of the dorsal cochlear nucleus (DCN) cannot focus on one type of cells and is therefore assumed to have mixed effects, and generates

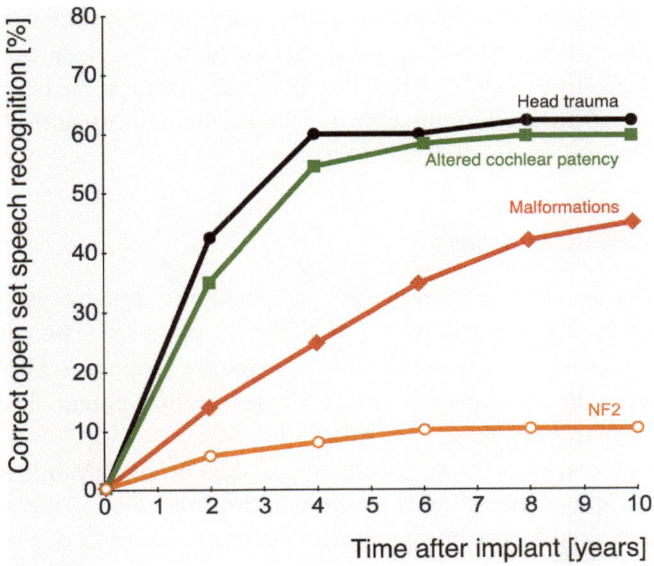

Fig. 11.20 Speech outcomes of brainstem implantation; mean performance depending on type of etiology. Brainstem implantation following head trauma provides much better outcomes than the more frequent case of neurofibromatosis 2 (NF2), a disease affecting beyond the auditory nerve as well as the central nervous system. *(Data from Colletti et al. (2009).)*

smaller cortical responses than cochlear implants. The main factor for brainstem implant underperformance compared to that of a cochlear implant is the etiology of deafness and thus the associated pathology in the auditory system. The most common disease associated with brainstem implantation is neurofibromatosis 2 (NF2). NF2 often involves tumors in the auditory nerve that damage it. Additionally, it involves damage to the central nervous system (with other tumors occurring both in the spine and in the brain). Therefore, the cochlear nucleus is likely compromised by the disease itself and/or the expansive growth of the tumor in the auditory nerve. When subjects with head trauma and thus traumatic injury of the nerve were implanted, their best performance approached the performance observed with cochlear implants (Fig. 11.20). In addition, the type of surgery is important, where a semi-sitting position provides better outcomes than a lateral (lying) position. Nonetheless, the semi-sitting position involves more risks during surgery. Unfortunately, there is not yet a clinical consensus of all these aspects.

The stimulation strategy and the speech processor are the same as in cochlear implants, thus designed for the auditory nerve and not for the cochlear nucleus. The small number of subjects using the implants (several thousand worldwide) complicates assessment of such aspects, since each (even large) clinical center implants only a limited number of such devices each year. Despite all these issues, the brainstem implant is the most successful functional prosthesis delivering information to the central nervous system (as opposed to a "pacemaker" delivering only pacing, such as in deep brain stimulation). There is a small group of deaf subjects that can only profit from brainstem implants, including some deaf-born children with developmental abnormalities of the cochlea, and some show promising results.

Auditory midbrain implants

Midbrain provides another potential target for prosthetic therapy. As mentioned, the inferior colliculus is an obligatory part of the afferent pathway. The central nucleus of it has a well-defined tonotopic organization and response properties with some temporal sensitivity (at least to the envelope of sounds). Thus, it is also a potential target for hearing restoration with neuroprostheses.

However, the access to the inferior colliculus is also complex. While it can be directly accessed, the tonotopic organization is oriented in the dorsoventral direction. Since inferior colliculus is covered by the bony tentorium cerbelli, insertion of a penetrating electrode along the tonotopic gradient is very complicated. In a first clinical trial at the ENT Clinics of the Hannover Medical University, Germany, the first three subjects have been implanted with an experimental penetrating electrode containing closely spaced 20 rings along one shaft (Fig. 11.21). The electrode contacts are smaller than in a cochlear implant.

The implanted subjects have awareness of sound with some awareness of loudness, pitch, and temporal features of sound, but their speech performance is comparable to the NF2 subjects in Fig. 11.19. Only subject AMI-3, the only one with the implant located in the central nucleus of the inferior colliculus, showed benefit somewhat greater than NF2 subjects with brainstem implants.

The result of the first clinical trial has been used to further refine the surgical approach, introduce new instruments for implantation, and refine anatomical reconstruction. Furthermore, a new electrode with two parallel shanks has been developed. The second clinical trial is ongoing in 2020.

However, several issues remain. Due to the previous high-frequency hearing loss, lasting for years, the inferior colliculus has undergone substantial plastic reorganization (see **Chapter 9**). This is in contrast to the cochlear nucleus where representation is less plastic (although some plasticity has been shown in the dorsal cochlear nucleus). Therefore, the substrate into which implantation is taking place is less uniform and clear, and thus also not the optimal stimulus-place relation. In addition, the speech coding strategy has not been adapted to the target, the inferior colliculus. In the inferior colliculus we do not find any phase-locking of activity beyond 400 Hz and, as in the cochlear nucleus, a number of functionally and anatomically diverse neurons are found. Further developments of coding strategies dedicated to the implanted structure are key for improving success of midbrain implants.

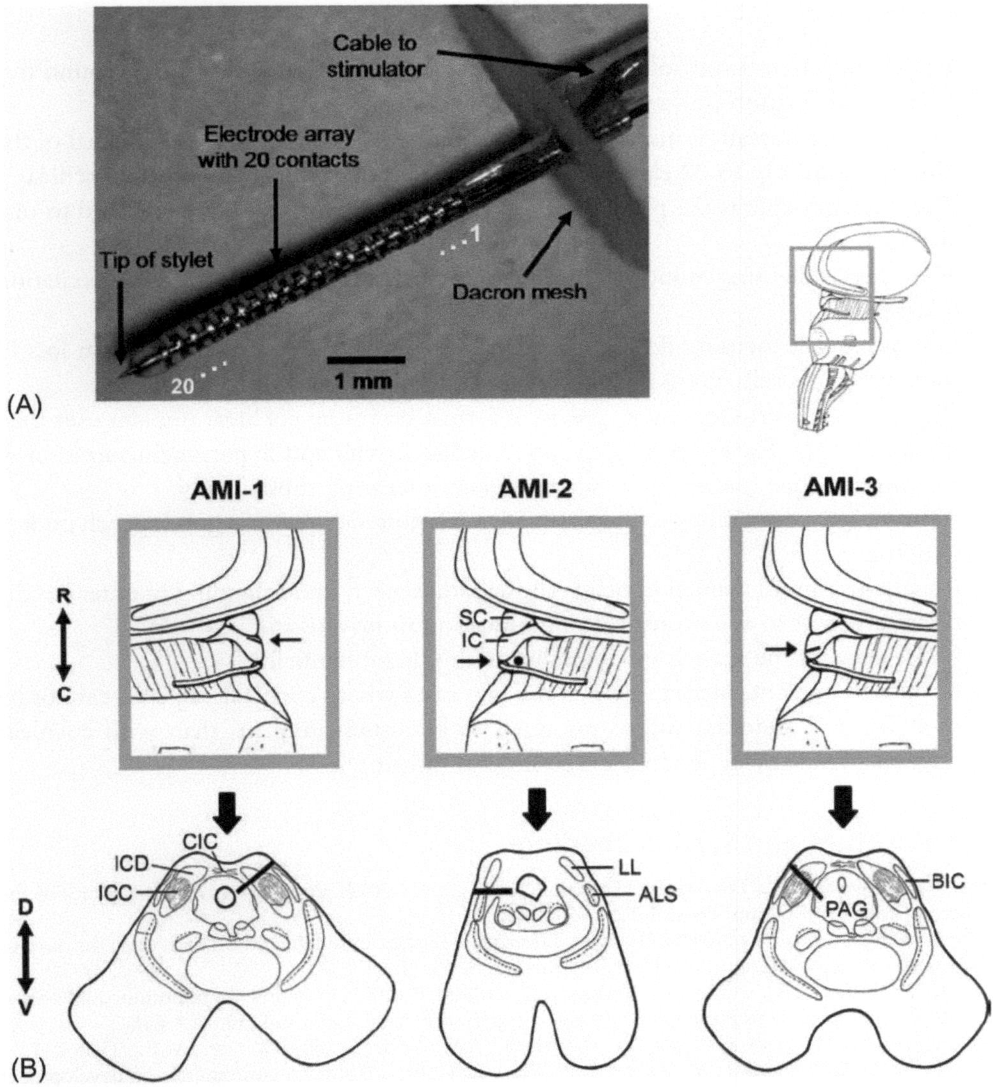

Fig. 11.21 Auditory midbrain from the first clinical study, device developed by Cochlear Ltd., Sydney, Australia, and used with a signal processor identical to the Nucleus Freedom cochlear implant. (A) Shape of the penetrating electrode carrier with 20 electrode contacts. The dacron mesh is used for stabilizing the array at the surface of the inferior colliculus. (B) Placement of the array in three subjects. AMI-1 is implanted in the dorsal cortex of the inferior colliculus, AMI-2 in the lateral lemniscus, and AMI-3 in the central nucleus of the inferior colliculus, the genuine target. AMI-3 also has the greatest benefit from the implant. *ALS*, anterolateral system; *BIC*, Brachium of the inferior colliculus; *C*, caudal; *CIC*, commissure of the inferior colliculus; *D*, dorsal; *ICC, inferior colliculus, central nucleus; ICD*, inferior colliculus, dorsal cortex; *LL*, lateral lemniscus; *PAG*, periaqueductal gray; *R*, rostral; *SC*, superior colliculus; *V*, ventral. *(Reproduced from Lim et al. (2007). Copyright 2007 Society for Neuroscience.)*

Brief summary

- The cochlea transforms sound into neuronal representation and separates sound frequency information into a place and a time code.
- The cochlear implant is inserted in a surgical intervention into the bony canal of the scala tympani. Up to 22 electrodes are arranged longitudinally along the cochlea.
- The implant exploits the place code by assigning an acoustic frequency band to one electrode.
- The place code using monopolar stimulation is inaccurate, as the spread of excitation is large.
- Use of current focusing does not provide benefit to subjects due to uneven loss of spiral ganglion cells along the cochlea and issues with perceived loudness.
- The time code provides more precise information to the cochlear implant user than the place code. However, lack of spontaneous activity and hypersynchronization of responses reduce the dynamic range of electric hearing substantially.
- At least eight to ten independent channels are required to provide good speech understanding in quiet.
- Present-day multichannel implants allow good speech understanding in quiet conditions sufficient to use acoustic communication in private and at work.
- Noise reduces the speech intelligibility with CIs substantially.
- Brainstem implants provide help in the rare cases where cochlear implants cannot be used. Speech understanding is poorer with brainstem implants than with cochlear implants, crucially depending on etiology of hearing loss.

Key literature and further reading

Avci, E., Nauwelaers, T., Lenarz, T., Hamacher, V., Kral, A., 2014. Variations in microanatomy of the human cochlea. J. Comp. Neurol. 522, 3245–3261.

Busby, P.A., Plant, K.L., Whitford, L.A., 2002. Electrode impedance in adults and children using the nucleus 24 cochlear implant system. Cochlear Implants Int. 3, 87–103.

Colletti, V., Shannon, R., Carner, M., Veronese, S., Colletti, L., 2009. Outcomes in nontumor adults fitted with the auditory brainstem implant: 10 years' experience. Otol. Neurotol. 30, 614–618.

Eisenberg, L.S., Hammes Ganguly, D., Martinez, A.S., Fisher, L.M., Winter, M.E., Glater, J.L., Schrader, D.K., Loggins, J., Wilkinson, E.P., Team LAPABI, 2018. Early communication development of children with auditory brainstem implants. J. Deaf. Stud. Deaf. Educ. 23, 249–260.

Fishman, K.E., Shannon, R.V., Slattery, W.H., 1997. Speech recognition as a function of the number of electrodes used in the SPEAK cochlear implant speech processor. J. Speech. Lang. Hear. Res. 40, 1201–1215.

Friesen, L.M., Shannon, R.V., Baskent, D., Wang, X., 2001. Speech recognition in noise as a function of the number of spectral channels: comparison of acoustic hearing and cochlear implants. J. Acoust. Soc. Am. 110, 1150–1163.

Fu, Q.J., Galvin, J.J., 2001. Recognition of spectrally asynchronous speech by normal-hearing listeners and Nucleus-22 cochlear implant users. J. Acoust. Soc. Am. 109, 1166–1172.

Fu, Q.J., Shannon, R.V., 1998. Effects of amplitude nonlinearity on phoneme recognition by cochlear implant users and normal-hearing listeners. J. Acoust. Soc. Am. 104, 2570–2577.

Fu, Q.J., Shannon, R.V., 2000. Effect of stimulation rate on phoneme recognition by nucleus-22 cochlear implant listeners. J. Acoust. Soc. Am. 107, 589–597.

George, S.S., Wise, A.K., Shivdasani, M.N., Shepherd, R.K., Fallon, J.B., 2014. Evaluation of focused multipolar stimulation for cochlear implants in acutely deafened cats. J. Neural Eng. 11, 065003.

Gourévitch, B., Edeline, J.-M., Occelli, F., Eggermont, J.J., 2014. Is the din really harmless? Long-term effects of non-traumatic noise on the adult auditory system. Nat. Rev. Neurosci. 15, 483–491.

Hartmann, R., Topp, G., Klinke, R., 1984. Discharge patterns of cat primary auditory fibers with electrical stimulation of the cochlea. Hear. Res. 13, 47–62.

Heid, S., Hartmann, R., Klinke, R., 1998. A model for prelingual deafness, the congenitally deaf white cat–population statistics and degenerative changes. Hear. Res. 115, 101–112.

Helms, J., Müller, J., Schön, F., Moser, L., Arnold, W., Janssen, T., Ramsden, R., von Ilberg, C., Kiefer, J., Pfennigdorf, T., Gstöttner, W., Baumgartner, W., Ehrenberger, K., Skarzynski, H., Ribari, O., Thumfart, W., Stephan, K., Mann, W., Heinemann, M., Zorowka, P., Lippert, K.L., et al., 1997. Evaluation of performance with the COMBI40 cochlear implant in adults: a multicentric clinical study. ORL J. Otorhinolaryngol. Relat. Spec. 59, 23–35.

Holden, L.K., Finley, C.C., Firszt, J.B., Holden, T.A., Brenner, C., Potts, L.G., Gotter, B.D., Vanderhoof, S.S., Mispagel, K., Heydebrand, G., Skinner, M.W., 2013. Factors affecting open-set word recognition in adults with cochlear implants. Ear Hear. 34, 342–360.

Komune, N., Yagmurlu, K., Matsuo, S., Miki, K., Abe, H., Rhoton, A.L., 2015. Auditory brainstem implantation: anatomy and approaches. Neurosurgery 11 (Suppl 2), 306–320 (discussion 320).

Kral, A., Kronenberger, W.G., Pisoni, D.B., O'Donoghue, G.M., 2016. Neurocognitive factors in sensory restoration of early deafness: a connectome model. Lancet Neurol. 15, 610–621.

Kral, A., Hartmann, R., Mortazavi, D., Klinke, R., 1998. Spatial resolution of cochlear implants: the electrical field and excitation of auditory afferents. Hear. Res. 121, 11–28.

Kral, A., O'Donoghue, G.M., 2010. Profound deafness in childhood. N. Engl. J. Med. 363, 1438–1450.

Kral, A., Tillein, J., 2021. Cochlear Implants. In: Fritzsch, B. (Ed.), Senses: A Comprehensive Reference. 2nd Elsevier Academic Press, pp. 923–944.

Laneau, J., Wouters, J., Moonen, M., 2004. Relative contributions of temporal and place pitch cues to fundamental frequency discrimination in cochlear implantees. J. Acoust. Soc. Am. 116, 3606–3619.

Lenarz, T., Lim, H.H., Reuter, G., Patrick, J.F., Lenarz, M., 2006. The auditory midbrain implant: a new auditory prosthesis for neural deafness-concept and device description. Otol. Neurotol. 27, 838–843.

Lim, H.H., Lenarz, T., Joseph, G., Battmer, R.-D., Samii, A., Samii, M., Patrick, J.F., Lenarz, M., 2007. Electrical stimulation of the midbrain for hearing restoration: insight into the functional organization of the human central auditory system. J. Neurosci. 27, 13541–13551.

McCreery, D.B., 2008. Cochlear nucleus auditory prostheses. Hear. Res. 242, 64–73.

Moon, A.K., Zwolan, T.A., Pfingst, B.E., 1993. Effects of phase duration on detection of electrical stimulation of the human cochlea. Hear. Res. 67, 166–178.

Moore, J.K., Osen, K.K., 1979. The cochlear nuclei in man. Am. J. Anat. 154, 393–418.

Nadol, J.B., Shiao, J.Y., Burgess, B.J., Ketten, D.R., Eddington, D.K., Gantz, B.J., Kos, I., Montandon, P., Coker, N.J., Roland, J.T., Shallop, J.K., 2001. Histopathology of cochlear implants in humans. Ann. Otol. Rhinol. Laryngol. 110, 883–891.

Osen, K.K., 1969. Cytoarchitecture of the cochlear nuclei in the cat. J. Comp. Neurol. 136, 453–484.

Pietsch, M., Aguirre Dávila, L., Erfurt, P., Avci, E., Lenarz, T., Kral, A., 2017. Spiral form of the human cochlea results from spatial constraints. Sci. Rep. 7, 7500.

Sato, M., Baumhoff, P., Tillein, J., Kral, A., 2017. Physiological mechanisms in combined electric-acoustic stimulation. Otol. Neurotol. 38, e215–e223.

Seyyedi, M., Eddington, D.K., Nadol, J.B., 2011. Interaural comparison of spiral ganglion cell counts in profound deafness. Hear. Res. 282, 56–62.

Shannon, R.V., Fu, Q.-J., Galvin, J., Friesen, L., 2004. Speech perception with cochlear implants. In: Zeng, F.-H., Popper, A.N., Fay, R.R. (Eds.), Cochlear Implants: Auditory Prostheses and Electric Hearing. Springer, pp. 334–376.

Shannon, R.V., Zeng, F.G., Kamath, V., Wygonski, J., Ekelid, M., 1995. Speech recognition with primarily temporal cues. Science 270, 303–304.

Shepherd, R.K., Hardie, N.A., Baxi, J.H., 2001. Electrical stimulation of the auditory nerve: single neuron strength-duration functions in deafened animals. Ann. Biomed. Eng. 29, 195–201.
Tillein, J., Hartmann, R., Kral, A., 2015. Electric-acoustic interactions in the hearing cochlea: single fiber recordings. Hear. Res. 322, 112–126.
van den Honert, C., Stypulkowski, P.H., 1984. Physiological properties of the electrically stimulated auditory nerve. II. Single fiber recordings. Hear. Res. 14, 225–243.
Wilson, B.S., Finley, C.C., Lawson, D.T., Wolford, R.D., Eddington, D.K., Rabinowitz, W.M., 1991. Better speech recognition with cochlear implants. Nature 352, 236–238.
Wilson, B.S., Dorman, M.F., 2008. Cochlear implants: a remarkable past and a brilliant future. Hear. Res. 242, 3–21.
Wrzeszcz, A., Steffens, M., Balster, S., Warnecke, A., Dittrich, B., Lenarz, T., Reuter, G., 2015. Hydrogel coated and dexamethasone releasing cochlear implants: quantification of fibrosis in guinea pigs and evaluation of insertion forces in a human cochlea model. J. Biomed. Mater. Res. B Appl. Biomater. 103, 169–178.
Zeng, F.G., 2002. Temporal pitch in electric hearing. Hear. Res. 174, 101–106.
Zeng, F.-G., Popper, A.N., Fay, R.R., 2004. Cochlear Implants: Auditory Prostheses and Electric Hearing. Springer Verlag, New York.
Zeng, F.-G., Rebscher, S., Harrison, W., Sun, X., Feng, H., 2008. Cochlear implants: system design, integration, and evaluation. IEEE Rev. Biomed. Eng. 1, 115–142.

CHAPTER 12

Visual neuroprostheses

The retina

The vertebrate retina is a layer of neural tissue located at the back of the eye responsible for the detection and early neural processing of visual information. Light, entering the eye through the lens at the pupil and projecting the visual scene onto the retina (Fig. 12.1), activates an electrochemical cascade starting at the photoreceptors located within the retina that culminates in a visual percept in the brain. A significant portion of information processing occurs within the retina. As such, the retina has a complex structure consisting of not only the photoreceptor sensory neurons, but also several other types of neural cells as well as non-neuronal cells that provide support and protection to the nervous tissue.

Photoreceptors are the light-sensitive cells of the retina. There are two primary types of photoreceptor within the vertebrate retina: **rods** and **cones**. Both transduce light into neural activity. In brief, in a compartmentalized portion of the photoreceptor known as the outer segment (Fig. 12.2), G-protein coupled receptors called *opsins* contain the chromophore 11-cis retinal. When struck by a photon, 11-cis retinal undergoes photo isomerization to all-trans retinal, which leads to a signal cascade culminating in the closure of cation channels and hyperpolarization of the photoreceptor cell. This is the opposite of most sensorineural pathways where the sensory cells depolarize upon sensory stimulation. The reason is energy efficiency: photoreceptors are some of the most metabolically active cells of the body. At night, the photoreceptor synthetizes glutamate, the neurotransmitter required for synaptic transmission in the depolarized condition, and during daylight it synthetizes the photopigment required for light sensitivity. This separation of the most metabolically active processes decreases the peak energetic demand.

Cone photoreceptors require more light than rods in order to hyperpolarize (have higher thresholds) but are less sensitive to over-stimulation, allowing them to function in bright-light conditions. Additionally, cone photoreceptors contain photopsins that are sensitive for particular wavelengths of light, providing color information from the visual scene. Rods, due to their lower thresholds, are more important for low-light vision.

The retina is arranged in a laminar structure with alternating synaptic and nuclear layers (Fig. 12.2). Light passes through the translucent inner neural layers before striking the photoreceptor inner and outer segments in the outer nuclear layer (ONL). Photoreceptors then influence *bipolar* and *horizontal cells* in the inner nuclear layer (INL) via synaptic transmission in the outer plexiform layer (OPL). Within the INL, horizontal cells provide *lateral feedback inhibition* to the photoreceptors and convey center-surround

Prostheses for the Brain
https://doi.org/10.1016/B978-0-12-818892-7.00011-0

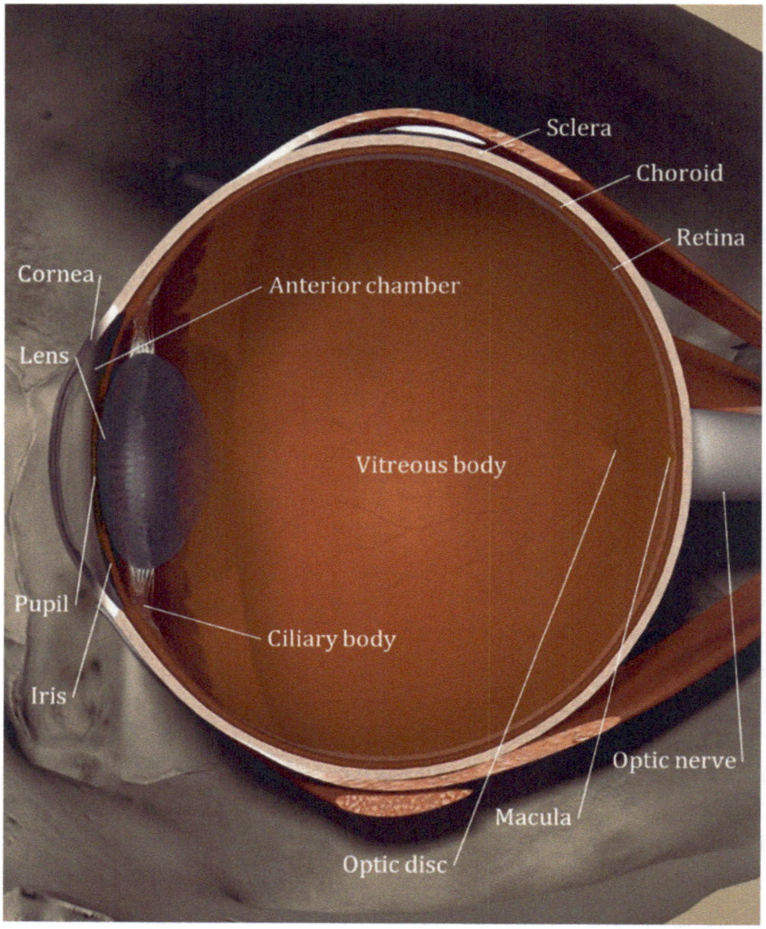

Fig. 12.1 Diagram of basic eye anatomy. Light passes through the pupil on the *left of the image* and is focused by the lens. It travels through the clear vitreous in the center and strikes the retina at the back of the eye. The area of the retina that is struck by the light receives a project of a flipped visual field: for example, light on the left side of the retina corresponds to the right visual field, and the whole picture is upside down. Photoreceptors in the retina convert light into neural signals via photo transduction. Neurons layered above the photoreceptors then process this signal before it leaves the eye via the optic nerve to be further analyzed in the brain.

relationships for receptive fields. The bipolar cells primarily perform simple spatial processing of the neural information before passing it to ganglion cells in the ganglion cell layer (GCL) and amacrine cells (ACs) in the INL via synaptic connections in the inner plexiform layer (IPL). ACs function to provide lateral feedback and feed forward for bipolar to ganglion cell input. *Retinal ganglion cells* (RGCs) function to summate and perform more complex signal processing on the visual information. RGC axons in the

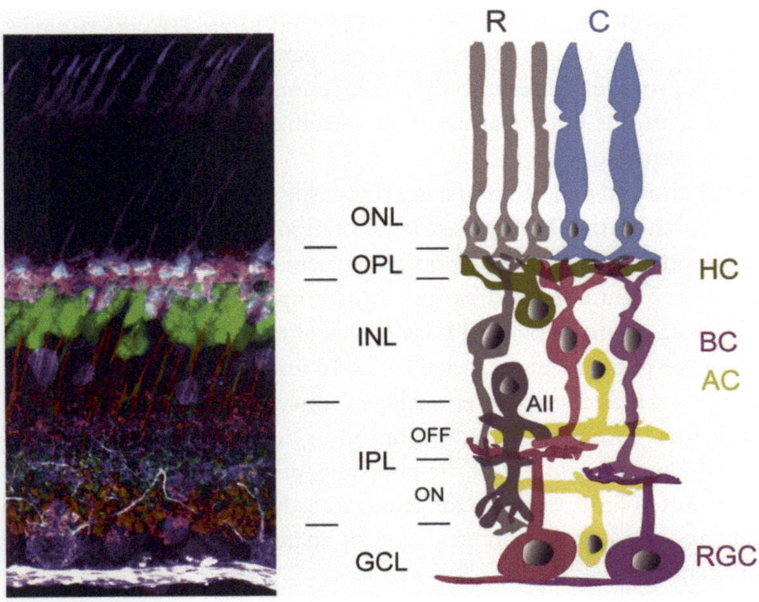

Fig. 12.2 Anatomical organization of neurons in a mouse retina, with drawn depictions of cell types and their connections on the right panel. The neural retina is organized into alternating nuclear and plexiform (synaptic) layers. Light enters the retina from the bottom of the image and passes through each layer before it is captured by the inner and outer segments of the rod (R) and cone (C) photoreceptors. The photoreceptors have their nuclei in the outer nuclear layer (ONL) and have synaptic connections to bipolar (BC) and horizontal (HC) cells in the outer plexiform layer (OPL). These cells in turn have their nuclei in the inner nuclear layer (INL). BCs have synapses in the inner plexiform layer (IPL) on retinal ganglion cells (RGCs) with nuclei in the ganglion cell layer (GCL). Amacrine cells (ACs) provide lateral feedback inhibition to IPL synapses. RGC axons forming the retinal nerve fiber layer (RNFL; *white strip* at image bottom) then project out of the retina via the optic nerve. The rod pathway *(in gray)* is distinct from the cone pathway *(colored)*, but a subset of ACs (AII ACs) convey information from the rod to the cone pathway. The IPL is further divided into sublamina depending on whether the cells respond (indirectly) to light with depolarization (ON) or hyperpolarization (OFF). *(From Hoon et al. (2014).)*

retinal nerve fiber layer (RNFL) project this information out to the brain via the optic nerve for continued processing and eventually the generation of a visual percept. This arrangement creates an opposing influence of the periphery of the receptive field (spatial sum of inputs) compared to its center. As an example, light in the center of receptive field leads to excitation of the neuron, but light in the periphery leads to inhibition of the neuron (**on-center receptive fields**). As will be discussed later, in some neurons the relationship is the inverse (**off-center receptive fields**).

The functions of the retina are influenced by both the **vasculature** within the retina and the neighboring tissues and cells, including the retinal pigment epithelium and the **choroid**, a separate vascular layer located at the external boundary of the retina (above the top of the image in Fig. 12.2). This layer provides nutrients for rod and cone photoreceptors in the outer retina. Blood vessels as part of the non-choroidal, intraretinal vascular network provide nutrients to the inner retina, including the GCL and INL. This intraretinal vasculature is not a feature of all vertebrate retinae, but is present in all primates including humans.

Between the choroid and the retina is a thin layer of epithelial cells known as the **retinal pigment epithelium (RPE)**. As a layer of pigmented cells, the RPE acts to absorb light that has passed the photoreceptor outer segments.[a] The RPE also acts as an epithelial transport layer and immunological barrier. Most importantly, RPE cells are involved in photo transduction, re-isomerizing 11-cis retinal after it has been converted to all-trans retinal as part of the photoreceptor visual cycle. In many nocturnal animals and predators there is an additional reflective pigmented layer between the RPE and choroid, called the **tapetum lucidum**. This layer is an adaptation to dim light conditions, reflecting light that has passed the outer segments of the photoreceptors back towards the outer retina to amplify the amount of light available for photo transduction. The tapetum lucidum is not present in humans but is an important tissue for anatomical consideration during animal model experiments.

There are important geographic landmarks in the vertebrate retina (Fig. 12.3). One is the **optic disc**, where axons of the ganglion cells exit the eye for the brain. Radiating out from the optic disc are the branches of the central retinal artery and vein. The area directly around the optic disc contains a greater percentage of axon fibers, and the optic disc itself does not contain any light-sensitive cells, making that portion of the retina effectively blind (the *blind spot*). As all ganglion cell axons must converge upon the optic nerve, it can be used to measure axonal health across the entire retina.

Furthermore, in many vertebrates there is an area of low vascular and high photoreceptor density called the **area centralis** (Fig. 12.3). It is the point where the lens generates a sharp (in focus) image and where greater acuity vision is achieved by a combination of greater photoreceptor density, a larger ratio of cones to rods, and a smaller number of photoreceptors per associated inner retinal neuron. In some vertebrates (particularly prey animals), this region is less defined and more spatially elongated, and is instead referred to as a **visual streak**. In primates, the area centralis has evolved into a specialized avascular form called the fovea. This area is comprised of cone photoreceptors, with ganglion cells and blood vessels displaced laterally to the foveal rim. There is a 1:1 association between photoreceptors, bipolar cells, and ganglion cells in the fovea. These adaptations create an area suited for detailed high-acuity vision in bright light. The fovea is essential for functional human vision and is important in many forms of human retinal disease, especially diseases of the photoreceptors.

[a] One is reminded of the black velvet curtain historically used to shield a camera from stray light that did not pass through the lens.

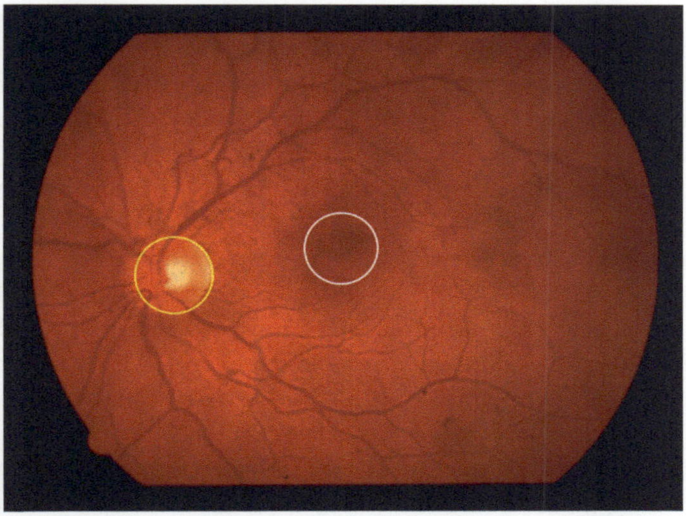

Fig. 12.3 Fundus camera image of a human retina. Fundus images are a clinical and experimental tool used to assess retinal health. Clearly visible are several important landmarks. The optic nerve *(yellow circle)* is the region where ganglion cell axons leave the retina and blood vessels enter (optic disc). This area has no photoreceptors and is effectively blind. The retinal vasculature can be seen throughout except at the area centralis *(white circle)*, which corresponds to an area of high-acuity central vision in humans called the fovea. The fovea contains a large density of cone photoreceptors. Many postsynaptic bipolar and ganglion cells are shifted laterally to the edges of the fovea to allow for an optimal, unobstructed light path.

Information processing in the visual system

Information processing within the initial visual pathways is primarily defined by the need to efficiently process the highly information-rich nature of a visual scene. Each synaptic connection in the primary visual pathway (from the photoreceptors to the visual cortex in the brain) can be thought of as an information consolidation step, where inputs from previous neurons are combined to define boundaries, initially of light and dark and then later of object borders, to generate increasingly complex models of visual space. The early visual pathway in particular achieves this using a set of general principles: **receptive fields**, **center-surround processing**, and **contrast sensitivity/edge detection**.

Receptive fields are a common feature of neural networks in the sensory systems. The receptive field of a neuron is the area of sensory space (e.g., sound frequency in hearing, or physical location in touch) that, when stimulated, will affect the activity of the neuron. In the visual system, receptive fields measure the size of the visual scene that a particular neuron will respond to. Individual photoreceptors only respond to light on a tiny segment of the retina. The collective responses of photoreceptors are then summed by the post-synaptic bipolar cells to create receptive fields that are a merge of many photoreceptors and sculpted by lateral input from the horizontal cells and ACs. Bipolar cells then synapse to ganglion cells, which consolidate the bipolar receptive fields into their own receptive fields. As a rule, receptive fields expand as visual information is consolidated at each synapse. Receptive fields remain smaller (and the consolidation is narrower) for areas of high-acuity vision such as the fovea in humans, where as mentioned earlier there is an almost 1:1 relationship between photoreceptor and bipolar and ganglion cell inputs.

Downstream neurons with significant convergent input can compare information between periphery and center of their fields to detect transition zones between light and dark. This property is called **center-surround processing.** Typically, the center of a cell's receptive field is sensitive (will fire in response) to either light or dark, while the surrounding area has the opposite relationship (initially conveyed by the retinal *horizonal cells*). For example, an *on-center bipolar cell* is excited by the presence of light in the center of its receptive field but will be inhibited if there is light in the surround. As such, this cell will only respond well if there is a bright spot in the center surrounded by darkness. In a fully bright field, the "off" surround will cancel out the "on" center. Likewise, an *off-center bipolar cell* will only respond if there is a dark spot surrounded by light. A visual representation of center-surround receptive fields is shown in Fig. 12.4. Specialized cells and systems further extract complex information from their receptive fields. For example, motion-selective neurons in the visual pathway may only respond if stimuli move through their receptive field in a particular direction. As the visual information continues down the primary visual pathway, simple center-surround receptive fields are combined to detect specific information about the properties of the visual scene, which are then used to detect further properties, and so on.

A primary processing goal of the early visual system is to generate **contrast sensitivity**. Because the visual scene is so information rich, it is necessary for the visual system to define regions of interest that should be the focus of further discrimination and attention. It does this by identifying, via the center-surround processing system discussed previously, areas of greatest contrast or complexity, which represent the edges of objects and other regions of spatial interest. **Edge detection** is a vital step in early visual processing and, as a result, the human visual system is much more sensitive to changes in contrast than it is to the total luminance of a visual scene. This is of particular importance for prosthetic stimulation since this is the key feature that has to be conveyed to the brain to allow appropriate visual perception.

The advantage of the information processing strategies discussed in this section is that they enable **high spatial sensitivity** for the human visual system. Minor details in a visual scene can be efficiently extracted by the visual system and allocated appropriately to higher-order neural pathways. However, the need for so many consolidation steps (each with one or more synapses associated with them) means that vision has relatively **low temporal sensitivity**. A good example of the relative importance of these two factors for vision is TV or computer monitor technology. We easily detect poor spatial

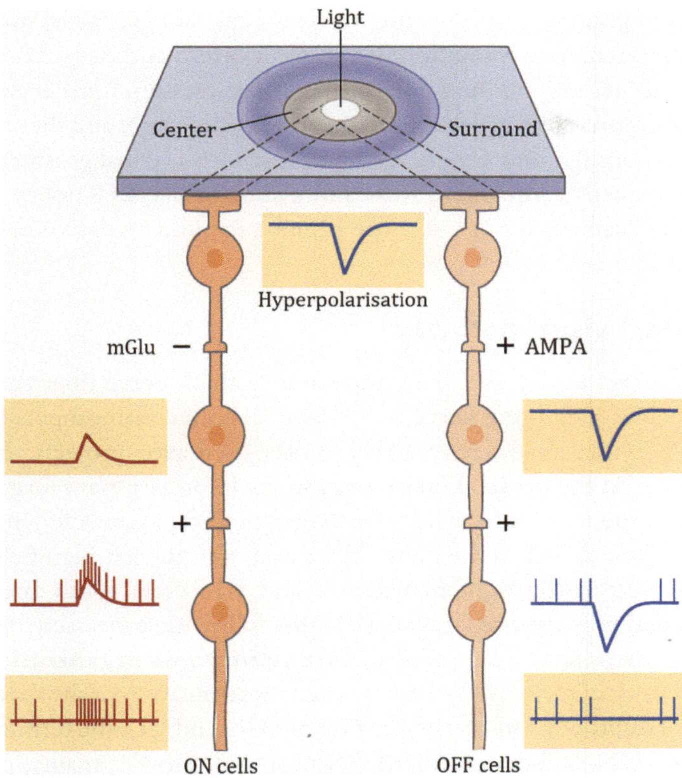

Fig. 12.4 A simplified example of on-center and off-center receptive fields in retinal processing. When ganglion cells receive input corresponding to light in the center of the field, they respond with either excitation (on-center cells) or inhibition (off-center cells). This is a function of inhibitory or excitatory bipolar cell synaptic inputs. The opposite is true of the periphery of the field, where on-center cells will be inhibited, and off-center cells are excited. Center vs. surround input is further gated by GABAergic horizontal interneurons (not shown). By combining the input of many such fields, it is possible to precisely map the edges of light and dark areas in the visual scene.

resolution in computers or TVs: movie or computer graphics quality from even 10 years ago are noticeably worse and a great deal of technological effort is directed towards improving spatial detail. The temporal resolution of computer monitors and TVs ("refresh rate"), however, has undergone few changes for nearly a century, as the human eye can barely perceive differences greater than 30–60 Hz. Visual reflexes that rely on good temporal responsiveness and accuracy, such as the pupillary light reflex (constriction of the pupil in response to light), use secondary pathways that bypass the slow primary visual pathway.

These factors are important to consider for the development of electrical stimulation of the visual system. Compared to the cochlear implants discussed in **Chapter 11**, an ideal visual implant requires much greater spatial resolution, but the temporal resolution is less important. This is potentially challenging for prosthesis design, as electrical stimulation tends to have high temporal resolution, but current spread at the electrode-tissue interface can impose limitations on the achievable spatial resolution. Furthermore, the neural population in the retina consists of cells that respond both to light and the absence of light. It is important to consider how electrical stimulation with a retinal prosthesis might affect these cell populations as a whole; the broad stimulation of all cells is not an ideal outcome if it results in the "canceling out" of many center-surround receptive fields.

The post-retinal visual pathway

Neural activity leaves the eye via the optic nerve, a thick nerve fiber consisting of the axons of the RGCs. The optic nerve has a loose anatomic retinotopy: RGCs spatially co-located in the retina are also more likely to have their axon projects physically closer in the optic nerve. At the **optic chiasm**, retinotopic information is reorganized according to visual field: the right visual field in both eyes projects to the left hemisphere of the brain and the left visual field to the right. This means that the left hemifield of the visual space is represented in the right hemisphere and vice versa. Both lateral geniculate nucleus (LGN) and primary visual cortex (V1), the following processing centers of visual information, are characterized by a well-defined **retinotopic organization**. While distorted by the density of the retinal receptors (i.e., representation of the foveal parts of the retina occupies a disproportionally large region of LGN and V1), the terminal projections of RGCs to the LGN, and then further LGN projections to V1, maintain a spatial relationship that projects a physical "map" of visual field location onto the neural surface. This makes them an attractive target for prosthetic stimulation.

Three main segregated pathways have been described in the central visual system, denominated by the form of ganglion neurons in the retina that initiate them: (1) the **parvocellular system** is initiated by ganglion cells with small dendritic fields, has neurons with small receptive fields, is sensitive to red-green contrasts, and processes visual form; (2) the **magnocellular system** is initiated by ganglion cells with large dendritic fields, has correspondingly large receptive fields, and processes visual motion and visual depth perception; (3) the **koniocellular system** is characterized by small ganglion cells and sensitivity to blue light.

Lateral geniculate nucleus

The lateral geniculate nucleus is a compact structure that serves as an intermediate between the retina and the visual cortex. Each side of the LGN receives input from both eyes, organized according to visual field (the left LGN receives input from the right visual field, and vice versa). LGN neurons project to the primary visual cortex (V1). The LGN is organized into six distinct layers (see Fig. 12.5). Each layer contains its own retinotopic

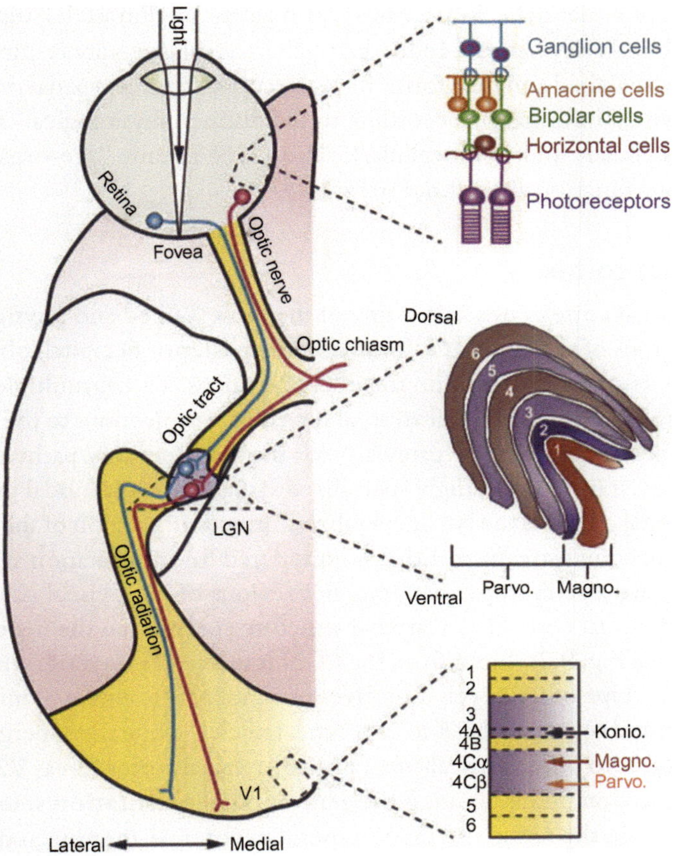

Fig. 12.5 Diagram showing the primary visual pathway in a macaque monkey, including the basic physiological organizations at each step. The retina *(top of the image)* is organized into laminar layers that take the neural signal generated by the photoreceptors in response to light and convert it into (primarily) contrast information via center-surround receptive fields. Ganglion cell axons leave the eye via the optic nerve where they are split at the optic chiasm into contralateral and ipsilateral visual fields. The ipsilateral visual field then passes through the optic tract to each lateral geniculate nucleus (LGN), a thalamic structure organized into discreet layers each of which processes and organizes receptive field properties according to their origin (ipsilateral or contralateral eye) and different functional aspects of the visual information such as motion and color. Each layer of the LGN then projects through via the optic radiation to the primary visual cortex (V1) where visual information from the LGN is received in the intermediate layers according to function, with a processing focus on even more complex aspects of the image such as orientation and edge detection. V1 then further projects on to either higher cortical regions (e.g., V2-6) via the superficial layers of V1, or to subcortical regions via the deeper layers. *(From Jeffries et al. (2014).)*

map of (half) the visual field. In primates this map has an almost 1:1 input relationship from RGC to LGN relay neuron. Individual cells in LGN layers are responsive to specific regions of the visual field and map forms of visual contrast, either spatial or temporal. The layers process visual information according to the distinct physiological circuits (magnocellular, parvocellular, and koniocellular). The LGN is thus "pre-organizing" retinal information into functionally distinct streams.

Primary visual cortex

The primary visual cortex (area V1) is one of the most studied and physiologically well-understood regions of the brain. It is located in the posterior occipital lobe with approximately 67% of its surface area within the calcarine sulcus. V1 has multiple projections to downstream visual areas, non-visual areas, and feedback projections to the LGN. As such, it can be considered the cortical "gateway" for the visual sensory pathway, which continues on to branch into increasingly specialized visual and multimodal processing areas. The primary visual cortex is the last "generalized" processing region of the visual pathway and thus the most downstream area that is considered for implantation with visual prostheses. It maintains a retinotopy that amplifies regions of high visual acuity.

The primary visual cortex has a laminar structure common to the neocortex, with six defined layers (see Fig. 9.2). Input from the LGN is received in layer 4, where it is further segregated by the type of LGN cell it receives (magno/parvocellular/koniocellular). The deeper layers (5 and 6) project back to subcortical nuclei, while the supergranular (superficial) layers project to other cortical areas, primarily visual cortex (areas V2-6). A primary (but not sole) function of this circuit is the generation of **orientation selectivity**. While upstream neurons in the retina and LGN respond to contrast, motion, and relative intensity, the output response of V1 responds to the orientation, direction of motion, and size of shapes in the visual scene, as well as more complex properties such as binocular disparity required for visual depth perception. This increasing complexity of stimulus responses as information moves downstream in the visual pathway is characteristic of sensory processing. Output from V1 is thought to inform the higher visual and associative areas about what regions of the visual scene are of high saliency (that require further analysis), as well as generating "saliency maps" that are used to direct gaze and attention towards interesting parts of the visual scene. In other words, V1 helps the visual system identify what regions of a visual scene are important for the discrimination of objects, such as borders and corners (**edge detection**).

Vision loss

Visual prostheses are designed to restore vision in patients with a loss of visual function. Blindness is a common disability, with nearly 250 million people suffering from impaired vision worldwide. However, many patients with visual impairment have easily treatable conditions such as cataracts or uncorrected vision that go untreated due to poverty and a lack of adequate medical care. Electrical stimulation of the visual system instead addresses a specific subset of visual impairments that arise from otherwise untreatable forms of degeneration or injury. For retinal implants in particular to be an effective treatment option, *the presence of surviving and functional ganglion cells in the retina is a necessity*. In the Western world, the most common conditions that still leave ganglion cells intact are inherited photoreceptor degenerations (retinitis pigmentosa in particular) and age-related macular degeneration. Other common forms of retinal degenerations also destroy the RGCs and so are not suitable for treatment with a retinal implant. These instead are only eligible for visual prostheses that are implanted in the LGN or primary visual cortex. Of these, the most common are diabetic retinopathy (DR) and glaucoma.

Photoreceptor degenerations

The rod and cone photoreceptors within the retina are a specialized cell type with a high metabolic load, which makes them particularly susceptible to degeneration or malfunction in response to stress. In particular, mutations in genes responsible for photoreceptor development or function can lead to the dysfunction of the photoreceptor and subsequent loss of the cell. There are more than 100 individual genes implicated in these degenerative conditions. The complex interaction of genes and environment creates a family of conditions with diverse phenotypes, but the late-stage progression of many of these diseases remains similar due to secondary pathological changes within the inner retina as a result of the initial photoreceptor loss (discussed in more detail in the next section). Photoreceptor degenerations are typically divided into three main categories: **rod-cone dystrophies**, **cone-rod dystrophies**, and **macular degeneration/dystrophy**. Each category is broadly defined by the initial location and progression of the disease process.

Rod-cone dystrophies

Rod-cone dystrophies are a family of photoreceptor degenerations characterized by a primary dysfunction of the rod photoreceptors. The most common form of rod-cone dystrophy is **retinitis pigmentosa (RP)**, which has an incidence rate of approximately 1 in 5000 in western countries. RP is a group of diseases classified by an initial loss of rod photoreceptors or the RPE, followed by secondary loss of cone photoreceptors and pathological changes in inner retinal neurons. As the outer retina in humans contains a greater percentage of rod to cone photoreceptors, the symptomatic progression of RP typically begins with a loss of peripheral vision; the fovea remains relatively intact until late-stage disease progression. Secondary signs as the disease progresses can include constriction of the retinal vasculature, pallor of the optic nerve, and a characteristic RPE bone spicule pigmentation, as is evident in Fig. 12.6. RP onset typically occurs in early adulthood,

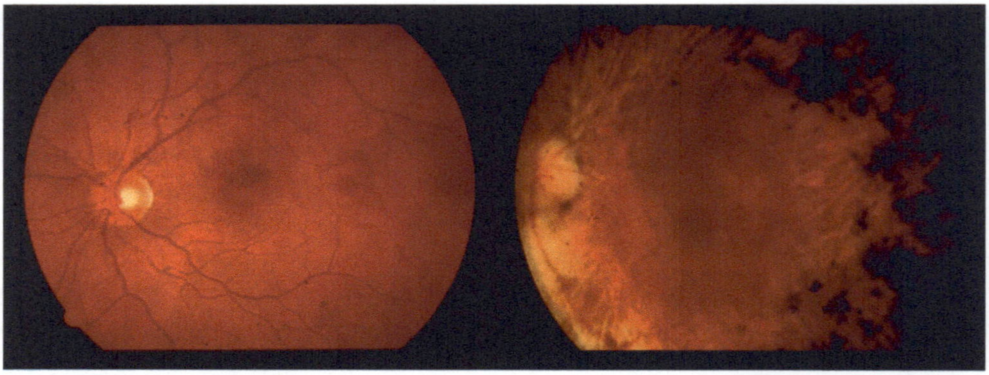

Fig. 12.6 Fundus photography images of a healthy and degenerated human retina. *On the left image,* we can clearly see the healthy fovea in the center with the optic nerve and vasculature. *On the right image,* we see a patient with late-stage retinitis pigmentosa. The retina is clearly degenerated, particularly in the periphery where we see characteristic bone-spicule pigmentation of the retinal pigment epithelium *(dark areas on the right).* The retinal vasculature is thinner (constricted), with only the central retina near the fovea showing roughly normal anatomical appearance.

with visual impairment occurring over the course of several decades. However, rate of onset and disease progression is highly variable between patients, defined in part by the interaction between the many individual genetic factors involved in RP.

Cone-rod dystrophies

Cone-rod dystrophies differ from rod-cone dystrophies in that the primary cause of degeneration lies in a malfunction of the cone photoreceptor pathway. Cone-rod dystrophies are not as common as rod-cone dystrophies, with an incidence rate of 1 in 40,000 in the developed world. The initial disease progression in cone-rod dystrophies is the opposite of rod-cone dystrophies such as RP. Typically, in these conditions the cone photoreceptors degenerate first, affecting visual acuity, color vision, and the central retina over the periphery. Cone-rod dystrophies tend to be more severe due to the relative importance of cone photoreceptors in functional vision; most sufferers are diagnosed during childhood and are legally blind by adulthood. Over time, rod photoreceptors also begin to degenerate, and the end stage of degeneration is similar to rod-cone dystrophies. Like rod-cone dystrophies, cone-rod dystrophies are genetically and phenotypically heterogeneous with many of the same gene loci implicated in the two conditions.

Diseases of the macula

The macula is the central foveal area of the retina that provides our high-acuity vision. Loss of macular function is rapidly debilitating as we rely so heavily on precise visual discrimination tasks for much of social living (reading, driving, facial recognition, etc.). The two main diseases of the macula are **macular dystrophies** and **age-related macular degeneration (AMD)**. Macular dystrophies are a cluster of conditions with a primarily genetic trigger that are relatively rare. While the precise etiologies vary between individual conditions, they share a similar disease progression (loss of macular vision). By far the more common form of macular degeneration is AMD, with high prevalence in the developed world (~170 million worldwide). The disease is expressed in two forms: "wet" and "dry" AMD, distinguished by the presence of abnormal angiogenesis (blood vessel formation) and a much more severe disease progression in wet AMD. Dry AMD is characterized by atrophy of the RPE and the presence of characteristic spots in the macular region called "drusen." Like the other conditions mentioned previously, disease progression varies between patients and, while no cause has been definitively identified, it is likely that a multitude of genetic and environmental factors combine to determine the nature and progression of this disease cluster. AMD is complex and attempts to characterize the etiology and variation within AMD comprises an entire sub-field of ophthalmology.

While there is no cure, AMD has several treatment options already available (particularly for the more aggressive wet form of the disease) that can slow the disease progression. Laser treatment aims to inhibit the growth of new blood vessels in the macular. Anti-vascular drugs have also shown considerable success in slowing angiogenesis and thus the rate of vision loss. However, even with these treatment options irreversible vision loss occurs over time, and many patients still go on to lose functional central vision. At this point, there is potential for the restoration of vision using a retinal prosthesis.

Glaucoma

Glaucoma is an umbrella of conditions characterized by degeneration of RGCs resulting in progressive and irreversible vision loss. Glaucoma is responsible for visual impairment in ~70 million people worldwide, with ~7 million sufferers being legally blind, making it the second greatest cause of vision loss after cataracts (and the greatest cause of irreversible vision loss). Glaucoma has such a high rate of blindness in part because the progressive loss of vision is slow and originally asymptomatic.

The etiology of glaucoma is not well understood, but is related to circulation of fluids in the eye. There are two main drainage pathways for the aqueous humor: the trabecular meshwork and the uveoscleral outflow pathway. In **open-angle glaucoma**, there is reduced outflow through the trabecular meshwork, while in **angle-closure glaucoma** there is reduced outflow through the uveoscleral outflow pathway. Glaucoma can also occur as a secondary condition resulting from damage to the retina from trauma, tumor, or inflammation. Increased intraocular pressure results from an imbalanced rate of inflow vs. outflow of aqueous humor in the eye. Increased intraocular pressure causes mechanical stress on the retina and its supporting structures. In particular, the optic disc and nerve is particularly susceptible to changes in pressure as it is the weakest part of the external wall of the eye. Damage to the optic disc initially disrupts normal function, causes loss of RGC axons and, subsequently, a loss of both RGC cell bodies and LGN terminal synapses. Although initially photoreceptors are functional, without a functional optic nerve or RGC layer there is no way to transmit the sensory information to the brain and the patient becomes blind.

If glaucoma is diagnosed early enough, treatment can slow the progression of the disease. However, there is no cure and the condition will eventually progress to complete blindness in the affected eye/s. As glaucoma destroys RGCs, visual prostheses that rely on surviving RGC populations as stimulation targets cannot be used for patients blinded by glaucoma progression. This includes all retinal and optic nerve implants. Moreover, late-stage glaucoma causes some progressive degeneration at the LGN, although whether this affects perceptual outcomes with an LGN-implanted prosthesis is not currently known. Cortical prostheses are an option for these subjects.

Diabetic retinopathy

Diabetic retinopathy (DR) is a microvascular complication secondary to diabetes mellitus, which also causes progressive retinal damage. Diabetes mellitus affects ~400 million people globally, with roughly a quarter of those suffering from DR as a consequence. The early stages of DR are called **non-proliferative diabetic retinopathy (NPDR)**, with mild retinal pathology. The later stage is **proliferative diabetic retinopathy (PDR)**, characterized by the formation of new, intrusive blood vessels in the retina (neovascularization), which can hemorrhage profusely, clouding vision and destroying the local retina. This creates a "patchy" blindness where regions of edema and hemorrhage can have total vision loss while other areas are relatively well preserved. Hyperglycemia (high blood sugar) is a risk factor for both the initiation and progression of DR. If the condition is diagnosed early and managed well, it is often possible to maintain good visual acuity for many years.

Vascular endothelial growth factor (VEGF) plays a role in the neovascularization. Some treatments to slow the progression of the disease therefore include intraocular injections of substances that bind to VEGF and inhibit it. Another option is laser ablation or surgery. However, if the disease progresses to blindness, there are no current treatment options available to restore the lost vision. Due to a complete degeneration of ganglion cells, retinal prostheses are an unviable option. LGN or cortical visual prostheses have been proposed as potential vision rescue strategies after the main-line therapies have been unsuccessful in slowing the disease progression.

Retinal remodeling

The loss of photoreceptors has extensive consequences for the remaining tissues in the retina. The retina undergoes a series of atrophic and pathological changes following loss of the photoreceptors, which are independent of the initial disease. These changes are collectively referred to as "**retinal remodeling**" and involve widespread gliosis, the formation of aberrant synaptic connections and ultimately inner retinal death and degeneration. In rod-cone photoreceptor degenerations, three general phases of retinal remodeling commonly occur, each corresponding to widespread anatomical, neurochemical, and physiological changes in one or more retinal layers. **Phase I** corresponds to a progressive loss of rod photoreceptors, cone photoreceptor stress, and a thinning of the outer retina as the ONL degenerates. A change in glia (Müller cells) activity in response to the stressed retina has been described. At this stage, inner nuclear layers remain relatively intact, although aberrant photoreceptor neurites begin to sprout and bipolar cell dendrites retract. **Phase II** remodeling begins when the majority of rod outer segments are lost. This stage is typified by widespread cone loss with horizontal and bipolar cells undergoing dendritic retraction and aberrant neurite growth into the inner plexiform and ganglion cell layers, leading to significant functional changes. Glial cells migrate into the sensory retina en masse, presumably in order to remove photoreceptor debris, forming a fibrotic seal in the distal retina. Finally, the onset of **phase III** remodeling corresponds to near complete loss of all photoreceptors and leads to a thickening of the fibrotic seal in a dense gliotic scar, the appearance of Müller cell "columns" that extend throughout all layers of the retina, neuronal and glial migration, microneuroma formation and, ultimately, progressive death of inner retinal neurons.

A histological example of retinal remodeling (Fig. 12.7) is documented on a 12-μm section from a cat area centralis. The contralateral retina (right image) has a chronic, pharmacologically induced photoreceptor degeneration. Both images have been stained with the nuclear stain DAPI in blue, vesicular glutamate (VGLUT) in red, indicating the presence of synapses, and calretinin (CALRET) in green, indicating the presence of some amacrine and ganglion cell soma and synaptic processes. The normal, healthy retina (left image) has a typical strong laminar structure. In the contralateral retina the photoreceptor layer (ONL) is obviously highly degenerated, with far fewer cell bodies. Numerous other effects are also visible. For example, processes and even cell bodies that would normally be contained with the OPL and INL have infiltrated deeply into the ONL (white arrowheads). Furthermore, the IPL synapses (red) have almost completely degenerated even though the cell nuclei remain. Clearly, following retinal remodeling electrical stimulation will not be as straightforward as in the laminar and well-organized healthy tissue.

Retinal remodeling in late-stage photoreceptor degenerations poses both a challenge and opportunity for visual rescue strategies. Many such strategies rely on surviving and

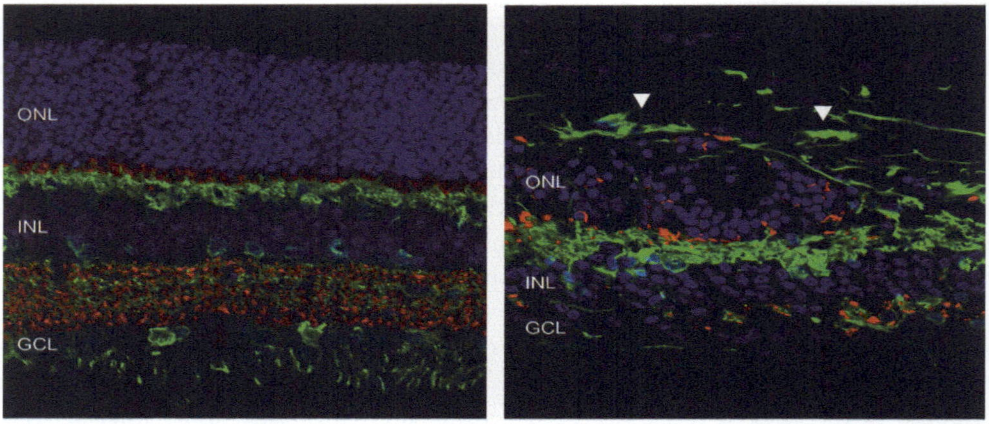

Fig. 12.7 Histological sections of healthy *(left)* and degenerated *(right)* retina from a cat model of retinal degeneration. Cell nuclei are shown in *blue* (DAPI), glutamatergic synapses in *red* (VGLUT), and amacrine/ganglion cell bodies and processes in *green* (VGLUT). In the healthy retina we can see the neat, laminar tissue consisting of an outer nuclear layer (ONL), inner nuclear layer (INL), ganglion cell layer (GCL), and alternating nuclear/synaptic layers. In the degenerated retina, the primary insult (loss of photoreceptors in the ONL) can be seen, but also a thinning of the other layers, a loss of synaptic inputs, and aberrant connectivity resulting from a loss of the laminar architecture *(white arrowheads). (Adapted from Aplin et al. (2016).)*

functional inner retinal neurons in order to successfully restore vision. In any photoreceptor degeneration where vision loss is severe enough to warrant an invasive treatment, the surviving retina will likely exhibit changes associated with phase II or III remodeling as discussed above, and thus have aberrant inner retinal function as well some inner retinal cell death and gliosis. This may interfere with or even prevent successful treatment in some cases. The heterogeneous, haphazard nature of remodeling events in degenerate retina may also combine with the similarly complex disease progression in many photoreceptor degenerations to create a difficult predictive environment for optimal patient selection.

Although individual remodeling events are hard to predict, retinal remodeling as a whole follows a general pattern of progression that appears to remain consistent across many models of photoreceptor degeneration. Thus, the end-stage progression of many photoreceptor diseases is similar, even though the initial pathogenesis might be very different. The consequence of this is that visual restoration strategies that attempt to treat late-stage disease for one form of photoreceptor degeneration have the opportunity to be broadly transferable for the treatment of other photoreceptor degenerations. However, how changes in the inner retina may negatively or positively affect the functional restoration of vision continues to be an open question.

Animal models of blindness

Testing and optimization of retinal prostheses rely on the use of animal models to make predictive judgments on device function in the human retina. Human trials (see **Chapter 3**) are necessary to confirm the viability and safety of a device designed for clinical practice; however, human trials are often limited to a small number of patients and the precise degenerative state of any given human retina cannot be tightly controlled. The effect of late-stage retinal remodeling events on device function is extremely difficult to determine in human trials because one cannot implant healthy human retinae. Animal models enable researchers to test device safety, form, biocompatibility, stimulation limitations, and functional response without putting human patients at risk.

The majority of animal models used to investigate photoreceptor degenerations are transgenic small mammal rod-cone photoreceptor dystrophies; typically mouse (rd1/rd10) or rat (P23H, RCS). Mice and rats are ideal animals for use as models of disease because they are widely available, well documented, have very short generational turnover, and are easy to manipulate genetically. However, their dissimilarity to humans, particularly anatomically, means that larger-eyed animal models of retinal disease are also used in visual prosthesis development. Unlike in the auditory system, where the cat dominates as a model of profound hearing loss (as described in **Chapters 9** and **11**), there is no unified large-eyed animal model of blindness. Rather, different groups across the world have developed blind models across several species and with several different techniques. Table 12.1 outlines some of the more widely used animal models of blindness and their differentiating features. The axial length is a good measure of the relative size of the eye, with a similar size enabling a better surgical comparison to the human eye. The presence of a central cone-dense retinal area for high-acuity vision is useful to compare the functional outcome of centrally vs. peripherally implanted devices, especially as human implantations typically aim to restore central vision.

Pharmacological models of photoreceptor degeneration

Pharmacological models of photoreceptor degenerations initiate photoreceptor death via the application of a phototoxic compound. These models do not mimic the initial pathogenesis of a disease but instead rely on the shared end-stage progression of retinal remodeling seen in most photoreceptor degenerations to create a pathology with broad applicability. The primary advantage of toxic models is pragmatic rather than academic: they reduce the cost and time associated with the development and maintenance of a model of blindness. Pharmacological models can be recreated in any lab that has access to the normal-sighted animal and the relevant compound, allowing them to achieve greater penetrance in the research community. Some models also offer the possibility for the development of a unilateral blindness, which can offset ethical and housing concerns for bilaterally blind animals. These models have the potential for translation

Table 12.1 Features of common animal models used in visual prosthesis research, compared to humans.

Animal model	Axial length (mm)	Central retina	Common dystrophies	Notable advantages	Notable disadvantages
Mouse	3	None	RD1/ RD10	Easy genetic manipulation	Eye too small for in vivo implantation
Rat	6.3	None	P23H, RCS	Low cost and high sample size	Poor surgical comparison to human
Rabbit	7	Visual streak	TgP347L	Low cost relative to size	Lacking internal retinal vasculature
Cat	21.3	Area centralis	CEP290, CRX	Well understood visual pathway	Poor access to genetic models
Dog	21.7	Area centralis	RCD1, RPE65	Common inherited dystrophies	Expensive housing, slow vision loss
Pig	24	Visual streak	TgP347L, ELOVL4	Comparable eye size/immune response	Afoveate, poorly understood visual pathway
Macaque	14.5	Fovea	R565Q	Visual cortex most similar to human	Expensive, greater ethical considerations
Human	24	Fovea	RP, AMD, LCA	Most direct comparison	Very low sample size, high subject variation

between species, meaning that initial development of the model can occur in smaller animals such as rats before they transition to a larger animal. The most well-documented and suitable models of retinal degeneration are **N-methyl-N-nitrosourea (MNU)**, **sodium iodate (NaIO3)**, **iodoacetic acid (IAA)**, and **adenosine triphosphate (ATP)**. Each has specific advantages and disadvantages, mostly centered on the specificity of the degeneration, general toxicity of the substance (and thus risk to researchers/animals), and the rate of disease progression. The use of pharmacological models should be considered whenever the development or procurement of a genetic model of retinal disease is too prohibitive for practical use.

Retinal implants: Basic principles

The push towards a successful retinal implant design has been driven by the success of cochlear implants and advancing materials technology that enabled higher-density electrode arrays (and thus higher spatial resolution inherent in visual information). There was and still remains a substantial population of otherwise untreatable patients who have photoreceptor loss but at least partially intact RGCs and/or bipolar cells. These patients stand to benefit substantially from the development of retinal implants and provide an active potential market for such devices. However, the retinal tissue is more complex than the cochlea and the approach is less obvious, leading to many challenges and pitfalls that have in turn been addressed very differently by the varied retinal implant research groups. This means that, unlike the auditory implants discussed in **Chapter 11** that follow very similar surgical placements and device designs, there is considerable variation in retinal implant design and function. Regardless, there remain basic principles of operation that are shared between most retinal implants.

The objective of all retinal implants is to generate a visual percept by electronically stimulating the surviving neural tissue of the retina. The most common operational flow is as follows (Fig. 12.8):

1. A camera, typically attached to a pair of glasses, captures the visual scene and transmits it to an external processing unit.
2. The visual scene is pre-processed by the unit and converted into a set of stimulation instructions for the retinal implant. The data, along with power, is then transmitted (via wire or wirelessly via radiofrequency coil, see Chapter 3) to a subcutaneous implanted receiver and digital-to-analog converter.
3. The receiver then transmits this signal to the implanted pulse generator and electrode array in the retina, where the electrodes produce current pulses to stimulate retinal neurons.
4. Action potentials from RGCs either directly or indirectly stimulated by the implant travel via the optic nerve to the brain, where their combined activity is interpreted by the brain as visual percepts.

This basic operational flow holds for most retinal implant designs, with differences stemming from specifics in electrode design, pre-processing strategies, and implantation location. Most retinal implant designs are originally based on cochlear implants and much of the discussion in **Chapter 11** about general design principles applies here. The vision acquisition system and physical electronics associated with the external unit are unremarkable from a biomedical perspective and will not be discussed in detail here, except to mention that they, like all biomedical devices worn on the body, are optimized for low power consumption and small/ergonomic size/shape. The power transmission and lead designs are overall similar to the cochlear implant. A substantial difference and the reason for many issues is that the eye is a moving structure, with constant high-velocity rotations exceeding many hundreds of thousands per day. Therefore the connection to the retinal electrode must be resistant to the stress of this movement. This is important since most resistant multi-strain wires will break when repeatedly bended at the same position. Spiral-shaped lead wires can reduce stress on the electrode (**Chapter 3**).

Retinal implants are typically flat (slightly curved) paddles with a grid of implanted electrodes, to maximize available surface area on the axis normal to the stimulation

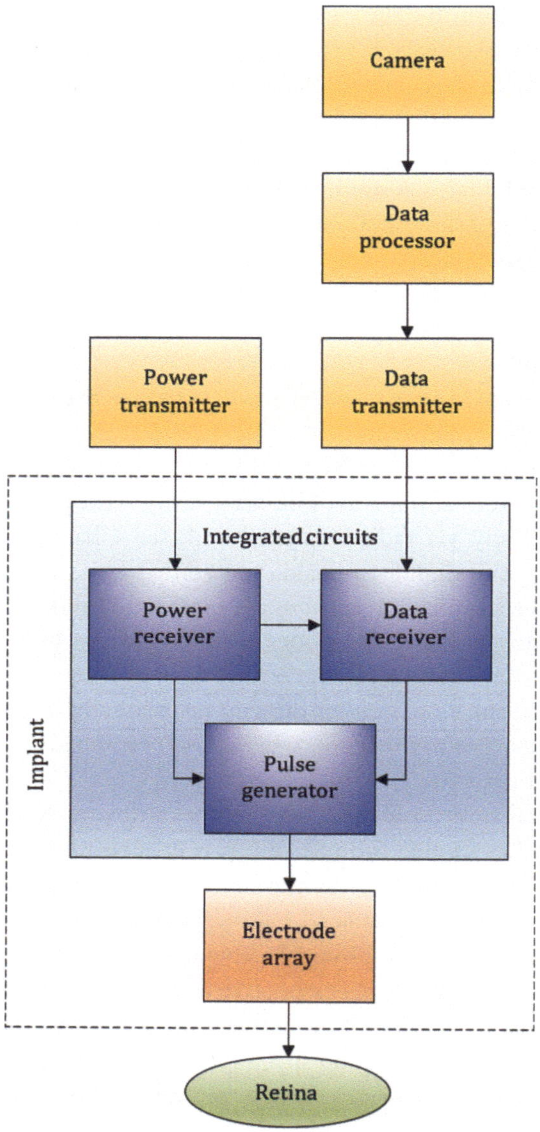

Fig. 12.8 Operational flow for a retinal implant. A camera usually located on a set of glasses captures the visual scene and transmits it to an external processor. This processor transforms the data into a set of stimulation commands for the implanted device and then transmits them (along with power) via an implanted receiver. Finally, the commands are transmitted to the implanted pulse generator that drives a retinal electrode array, stimulating the surviving retinal neurons.

surface. They are implanted as close to the fovea as possible due to the higher density of ganglion cells available and relative importance of this region for functional vision. A thin and flexible material is of greater importance for retinal implants when compared to cochlear implants, due to the limited space for implantation and vulnerable tissue on either side of the implant. A greater electrode density is also more important due to the need for greater spatial resolution and the theoretically closer contact to reduce current spread.

Electrical stimulation of the retina results in gross activation of surviving tissue, which cannot encode information as precisely as the center-surround receptive field processing that begins as early as the bipolar cells in a healthy retina. Electrical stimulation will activate both on-center and off-center cells, which limits the ability for implants to encode physiological information associated with edge-detection. Instead, electrical stimulation evokes a generalized percept in the higher visual system associated with an area of the retina. This percept is called a **phosphene** and is commonly described by patients as an irregular smear, smudge, or blot of light. Phosphenes range from simple "flashes" of light to complex percepts with both a spatial and temporal component. Phosphenes are usually described as achromatic but do sometimes vary in color, although this is not normally a directly controllable property.

Phosphenes can be perceived from a single biphasic charge-balanced pulse, with the intensity and shape of the phosphene as a function of the amplitude and pulse width of the stimulus. It is also possible to integrate pulses over time to control phosphene intensity and duration (**temporal integration**). However, this is not widely used, as it is not as effective as amplitude or pulse width modulation (also called pulse duration modulation) for intensity control. There is a perceptual desensitization that occurs when repetitive stimulation occurs at rates greater than 60 Hz called **fading**, that limits the ability of prostheses to generate stable percepts via the integration of repetitive stimulation. As such, most stimulation paradigms focus on fixed stimulation rates between 5 Hz and 60 Hz, with some exceptions such as the high frequency stimulation discussed in the stimulation strategies section of this chapter. Phosphenes co-located in perceptual space can also spatially integrate ("**fuse**") to produce single, larger, percepts. Phosphene fusing can be a linear summation of the two discrete phosphenes but is more commonly a complex amalgamation that may even contain perceptual space not present when the percepts are presented individually. For example, by stimulating electrode pairs simultaneously it is sometimes possible to produce a color perception that was not present for individual electrode stimulation. The precise characteristics of phosphene shape are currently unpredictable between electrodes and between patients, although they are generally well conserved across time. This can be compensated for by psychophysically mapping the relative position and shape of phosphenes generated by the electrodes of an implant. This information can then be fed back to the processing unit to allow for the generation of individualized maps of the electrode-to-phosphene spatial relationship.

While phosphene percepts may not be a physiological sensory stimulus, it is expected that, like auditory implant input, over time the brain will adapt and associate spatially discrete phosphene patterns with objects in a visual scene. It seems logical to generate this "non-physiological input" as upstream in the primary visual pathway as possible to enable multiple, potentially plastic processing steps before the visual percept is generated. However, it is not well understood how phosphenes generated via retinal vs LGN or cortical stimulation might differ in their level of plastic adaptation. There has not yet been any conclusive experimental evidence to suggest that stimulation further upstream in the visual pathway produces "better" functional outcomes.

Common materials and stimulation parameters

Retinal implants have largely used similar design principles to cochlear implants, except that the devices are a flat sheet rather than long cylinders (Fig. 12.9). The most common electrode material for retinal implants is platinum or iridium-oxide for reasons discussed in **Chapter 6** (biocompatibility, high charge injection capacity). Photodiode arrays have also used titanium nitride or gold as alternative electrode materials. The electrode array encapsulation is a soft silicone or polyimide with an emphasis on mechanical softness to avoid damage to the fragile retina. The device in Fig. 12.9 is a 23-electrode (21 stimulating, 2 return) design for use in pre-clinical studies. The design emphases a large, flat surface area for the electrode contacts with soft implantable edges. The housing of

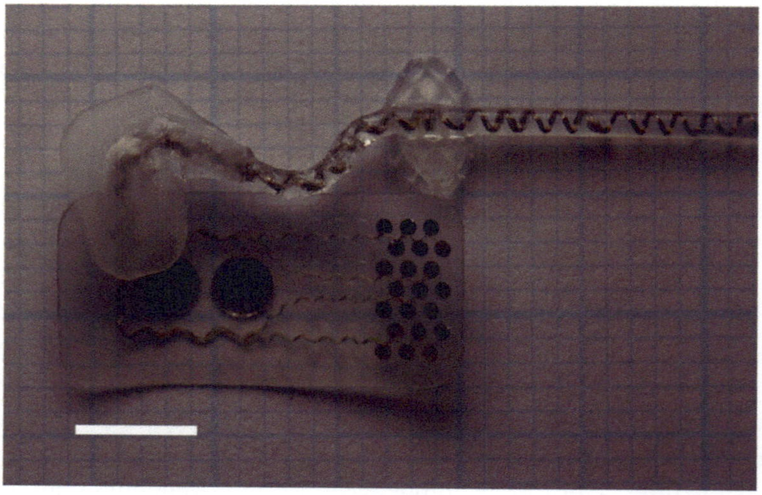

Fig. 12.9 Example electrode array for a suprachoroidal retinal implant (placed between the sclera and the choroid). 21 platinum stimulating electrodes can be seen on the right of the array, with 2 large platinum returns on the left. The electrodes and lead wire (above the array) have been encased in soft silicone and designed to be flexible and easy to insert/position surgically. Scale bar is 1 cm.

electronic components is either made from silicone, with a focus on softness and flexibility, or a more traditional titanium shell, with a focus on chronic electrochemical stability. While a soft silicone encapsulation may seem the obvious choice, there have been problems with encapsulation failure over long periods (years) as the soft material is worn down over time, making the choice of electronic housing material less straightforward.

Similar to cochlear implants, retinal prostheses use **charge-balanced**, **biphasic pulses** to deliver their charge. Biphasic pulses can excite neural tissue without generating toxic irreversible reactions that would corrode the electrodes and damage neurons, as discussed in **Chapters 6 and 7**. Pulses with a cathodic leading phase typically produce better thresholds than anodic-leading pulses and are the standard stimulation paradigm. The considerable variation between patients, implant locations, and electrode designs means that pulse duration and amplitude ranges used clinically vary. Perceptual thresholds vary within the order of 10–1000 μA and pulse durations between 100 and 1000 μs. As electrode contact diameters in current clinically implanted devices range between 40 and 600 μm, perceptual thresholds in some designs can result in charge delivery above the 400 $\mu C/cm^2$/phase safety limit for platinum contacts, necessitating the use of materials with higher safety limits such as iridium-oxide (1 mC/cm^2/phase) or surface-etched platinum (platinum-gray, ~0.9 mC/cm^2/phase).

Several groups have experimented with alternative electrode materials, particularly for implant designs that seek to optimize the spatial resolution of the visual percept. New materials have been used in an attempt to reduce the individual electrode size and thus increase the density of the implanted array. The simplest approach has been to surface-etch platinum to increase the available surface area and thus the charge injection capacity of the material. Other alternatives that have been used are nitrogen or boron-doped nanocrystalline diamond, carbon nanotubes, and conductive polymers such as PEDOT, which can result in electrode safety limits above ~2.5 mC/cm^2/phase depending on the material and fabrication technique. While these materials have been promising in vitro, their translation into clinical devices has been slow due to issues associated with biological stability and safety. Further innovation and translation of these novel materials is a vital step to overcome the material limitations of clinically approved devices.

The electrode array used for stimulating the neural tissue in a retinal prosthesis is commonly implanted into one of three main locations within the retina: **epiretinal**, **subretinal**, and **suprachoroidal**[b] (Fig. 12.10).

[b] To date only one company, Second Sight Medical Products Inc., has received full regulatory approval and is active commercially in the United States. Second Sight devices currently use an epiretinal surgical approach.

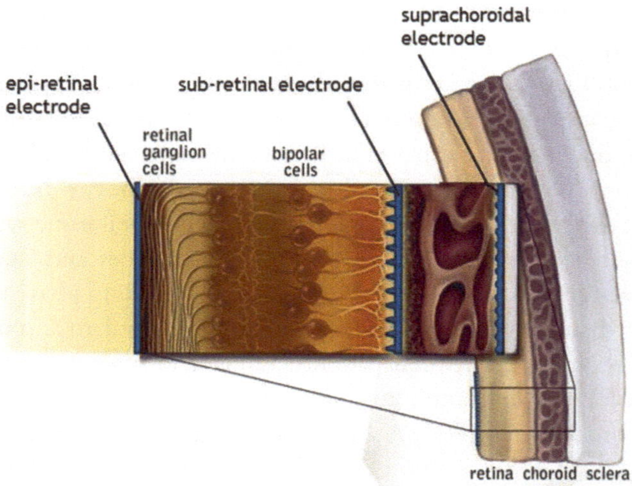

Fig. 12.10 Location of various retinal implant surgical approaches in a degenerated retina. Epiretinal electrodes are positioned on top of the retina closest to the surviving ganglion cells and their axons. Subretinal electrodes are positioned underneath the retina where the photoreceptors were located before their degeneration and death. Suprachoroidal electrodes are positioned on the other side of the blood supply of the outer retina (the choroid). *(Adapted from Ayton et al. (2019).)*

Epiretinal prostheses

Epiretinal prostheses place an electrode array either in contact with or directly adjacent to the GCL within the inner retina (Fig. 12.11). Epiretinal prostheses aim to stimulate surviving RGCs and their axonal projections in the closest possible proximity. By placing the stimulating electrode so close to the target tissue, epiretinal prostheses should have the lowest thresholds for activation of RGCs and thus the smallest amount of current spread within the retina, increasing the potential spatial resolution of the device. However, close proximity to the neural tissue means any immune encapsulation and/or mechanical or thermal stress generated by the implant runs the risk of directly damaging the target tissue. The internal position of epiretinal devices means more invasive surgery involving a full removal of the inner content of the eye (corpus vitreum, the procedure is called vitrectomy) and, if wires to an external controller are required, a possible avenue of infection directly into the eye. Devices are also in the least physically stable position, as they are not constrained by two tissue substrates, and thus need to be secured to the retina in order to avoid the risk of mechanical stress or device detachment as a result of natural eye movements.

Subretinal prostheses

Subretinal prostheses are positioned between the RPE and surviving inner and outer retina, in the potential space previously occupied by the photoreceptors. Subretinal prostheses aim to stimulate surviving inner retinal neurons from the bipolar cells onward

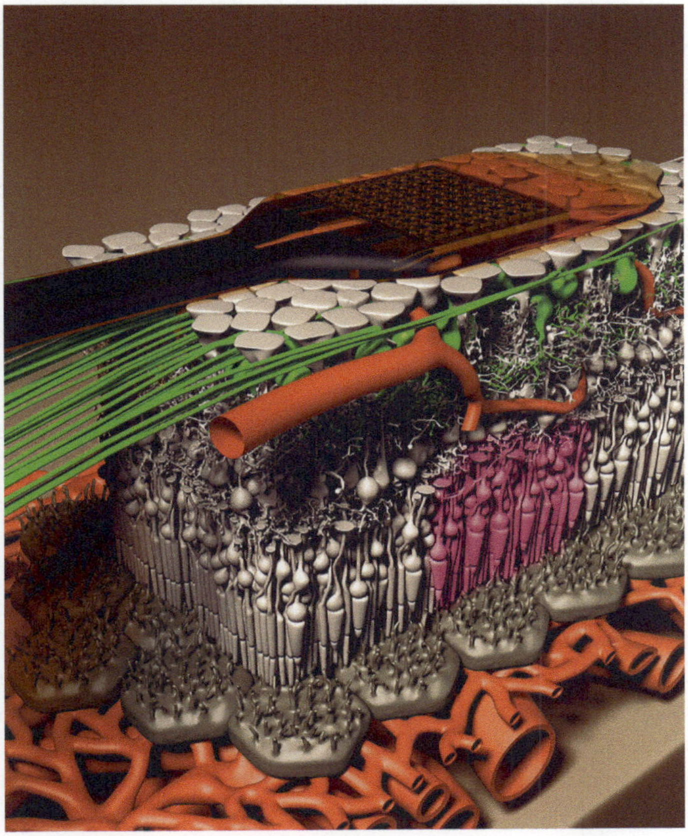

Fig. 12.11 Position of an epiretinal electrode relative to the retina. The array *(orange)* is implanted above the retina and sits on a network of Müller cells and retinal ganglion cell axons in the nerve fiber layer. The primary stimulation target of the device is the ganglion cell axons and, more ideally, the ganglion cell bodies *(green)*. In doing so it attempts to replace the input of the photoreceptors *(purple)* and subsequent retinal processing, much of which has been lost in patients with severe photoreceptor degenerations. However, the epiretinal position can be unstable, and the immediately adjacent tissue is vascularized *(red)*, which can pose issues with chronic surgical stability. This is often addressed with a "retinal tack" that penetrates the tissue and provides an anchor point for the electrode array.

by emulating the output of photoreceptor cells. By physically positioning the array at the very beginning of the visual pathway, subretinal prostheses include as much physiological neural processing as possible, and thus create a more natural (in theory) percept. Given that the ganglion cell population is already processing somewhat complex center-surround information from bipolar input, this is an intuitively logical stimulation approach. However, it is debatable to what extent bipolar cell inputs to ganglion cells remain functional following late-stage retinal remodeling in patients.

Subretinal arrays have the advantage of being located between two tissue layers, making their position more stable than an epiretinal device. However, this comes at the cost of an even more delicate surgical operation and more restrictive device specifications to prevent mechanical tissue damage. If supply of data or power to the array is required, this must be achieved by either penetrating the retina or choroid, both of which are delicate tissues. The array is interposed between the choroid and inner retina, which may reduce the nutrient supply from the choroid to the surviving retina. Thus, the implant is potentially unsuitable for patients with residual photoreceptor survival as a loss of choroidal nutrient supply may exacerbate further degeneration.

Suprachoroidal prostheses

Suprachoroidal prostheses are positioned behind the retina in the suprachoroidal space between the choroid and sclera. Suprachoroidal prostheses aim to stimulate any surviving inner retinal neurons (ganglion cell or bipolar cell). As the suprachoroidal space is not in direct contact with the retina there are fewer constraints on device design, allowing for a bulkier device and thus the possibility for a larger stimulated surface area. The suprachoroidal space can be accessed from the sclera and is in a mechanically stable position, allowing for a relatively safe, simple, and fast surgery when compared to other device placements, including the possibility of explantation in the case of device malfunction. Given how delicate retinal structures are, this is a major advantage over subretinal and epiretinal approaches.

The greater distance from electrode to retina in suprachoroidal implants results in higher thresholds and less spatial resolution than other surgical positions, which is a major disadvantage. Thus, suprachoroidal prostheses are better positioned to enable low spatial density electrode configurations that provide a larger visual field at lower spatial resolution, compared to epiretinal and subretinal prostheses that are more suited to high-density stimulation but in a much smaller area of retina. A larger visual field may enable suprachoroidal prostheses to maintain a separate clinical niche as an effective mobility aid, even if the devices cannot provide the same level of high-acuity central vision as other device positions.

Photodiode arrays

The prosthesis designs discussed above all function via electrical current generated from an external current source, much like a cochlear implant. However, there is another form of prosthesis that takes advantage of the natural access to light at the retina. Rather than powering the retinal implant externally, an alternative is to provide power intrinsically via photodiode arrays that generate an electrical current when exposed to photons (light). Photodiode arrays are implanted in the subretinal or (occasionally) epiretinal position and consist of typically circular or square arrays 1–3 mm in diameter, where each photodiode is 50–250 μm.

Initial photodiode designs relied on ambient light passing through the pupil to activate passive photovoltaic circuits that were linked directly to stimulation electrodes. While this idea is attractive on paper, it fails in practice because the ambient light in the eye is much too low to enable the generation of currents sufficient for neural stimulation. Photoreceptors are orders of magnitude more efficient than current photodiode technology! The initial failure of these devices led to an adaptation of a concept wherein the necessary light would be provided directly using pulsed light in the infrared or near-infrared spectrum to avoid direct stimulation of surviving photoreceptors. The function of passive photodiode arrays has also been extended via the inclusion of an active element where the signal is further amplified by an external current. While this may seem an unintuitive design direction, it is an attractive alternative because the external power requirement for active photodiode arrays is still small compared to a standard retinal implant.

The basic principles of photodiode arrays are substantially different to other retinal implant designs. Rather than visual information being converted to analog electrical signals, it is instead converted from visible light into infrared (IR) pulses that are directed through the lens towards specific photodiode-implanted retinal areas. This requires a unique external unit design including IR light sources that must be mounted over the eyes, as well as associated power/processing units. The externalization of these sources is advantageous as it reduces the need for surgically implanted electronics. However, this unique approach is also a disadvantage. Traditional implant designs benefit from similarities to the cochlear implant, which enables the transfer of technologies and solutions for a faster development and regulatory cycle. The technical complexity of photodiode-based retinal implants means that more effort (time, money) must be put into solving the technical challenges and obtaining regulatory approval.

Optic nerve implants

Optic nerve prostheses are located around the optic nerve and target surviving ganglion cell axons as they project to the LGN. An optic nerve prosthesis involves the implantation of a spiral cuff or circular array of penetrating electrodes in the optic nerve behind the eye. Optic nerve prostheses benefit from an easily accessible location for surgical placement and a well-contained target population. Stimulation at the optic nerve allows for close contact with neural tissue while avoiding proximity to the fragile and potentially heterogeneously degenerated retina. In contrast to flat retinal prostheses, optic nerve prostheses use a cuff design to envelop the cylindrical nerve. Penetrating electrodes with multiple contacts per shank can also be used in conjunction with a cuff design to better stimulate surface vs deep fiber bundles; the trade-off is that penetrating the epineurium of the optic nerve will increase the tissue reaction and thus make the device less chronically stable.

Although they are not positioned within the eye, optic nerve prostheses still rely on the survival of RGCs in the retina (the axons of which they stimulate) for the generation of a functional percept and thus have been grouped with retinal implants here. Perhaps the most challenging aspect of optic nerve stimulation is that the target ganglion cell axon fibers are densely packed. Stimulation of a subset of ganglion cell axons is difficult given current technology. Additionally, while the retinotopic map is somewhat conserved in the optic nerve, it is not as consistent as in the retina or brain structures. This means that stimulation of nearby ganglion cell axons is not guaranteed to produce spatially confined visual percepts. Although it has been shown that the generation of a consistent spatial map of elicited phosphenes is possible, the shape of this map is irregular and varies between patients. There has been recent research in animal models suggesting that paired retina and optic nerve stimulation may improve the specificity of this stimulation.

Cortical and lateral geniculate nucleus visual implants

The retina and optic nerve are attractive locations for visual prosthesis implantation due to their surgical accessibility. However, both of these locations rely on the stimulation of surviving retinal tissue (particularly RGCs) and their axon projections to convey information to the brain. Many common diseases of blindness such as glaucoma and DR also kill ganglion cells and are thus untreatable with a retinal implant. To address these conditions with electrical stimulation it is necessary to look for stimulation targets further into the visual pathway: either in the LGN or cortex. This is possible because a retinotopic organization is well maintained in the visual pathway.

The challenges associated with cortical and LGN implant development are very different to the retina. Firstly, brain regions have distinct anatomic and physiological structures as discussed in **Chapter 9**. They are also downstream in the visual pathway, meaning that neural activation encodes more complex information features. Finally, the brain requires a very different surgical approach. Further discussion on the challenges brain implants face in general can be found in **Chapters 13 and 15**. There are also numerous advantages to implanting a prosthesis further up the visual pathway, if these challenges can be overcome. Access to a larger patient population is a significant clinical and business advantage. In addition, brain implants avoid the problems associated with retinal remodeling and the general fragility of the diseased retina. Importantly, visual brain regions may allow for better spatial resolution in areas corresponding to the retinal fovea (central vision), for reasons that will be discussed below. These advantages combine to make visual prostheses in either LGN or cortical visual areas an attractive alternative to retinal implants.

Lateral geniculate nucleus prostheses

The lateral geniculate nucleus has several properties that make it a potential target for electrical stimulation. It is compact and anatomically well defined, it maintains a strong retinotopy, it is organized in such a way that the encoding of different visual functions (notably, color and motion) are anatomically distinct, and it has a larger spatial region dedicated to foveal processing (the high acuity region of vision and an ideal stimulation location). The LGN is disadvantaged by an anatomic location that complicates surgery; however, the recent popularity and advances in deep brain stimulation (see **Chapter 13**) have allowed for the rapid development of safe and reproducible surgical access methodologies for the midbrain, mitigating what was previously a chief drawback. There is some LGN remodeling that occurs as a result of retinal loss, but the impact of this on the efficacy of a chronically implanted device is not well understood.

The development of LGN visual prostheses is relatively recent compared to retinal or cortical approaches, meaning that the field is only now entering pre-clinical and early clinical phases of development. Device operational principles are not too dissimilar to other visual prostheses (Fig. 12.12), with the main differences being the surgical approach and position of the electrode array at the end of a thin penetrating shaft. Electrodes are spaced within and across LGN layers so that different spatial and functional regions can be stimulated. One distinct physiological difference from the retina is that spatial information in the LGN is organized according to left or right visual field rather than left or right eye, meaning that a single unilateral implant can only at best represent half of the visual scene. As such, LGN prostheses are expected to require bilateral implantation. There are currently no studies assessing stimulation parameters in human patients for LGN prostheses. However, an animal model study has demonstrated behavioral thresholds using biphasic sinusoidal pulses in the range of 50–500 μA, with a pulse duration of 1000 μs and pulse frequency of 100–200 Hz. Further research is necessary to determine whether this approach can chronically and reliably produce visual percepts at high spatial resolution in humans.

Primary visual cortex (V1) prostheses

The primary visual cortex, or V1, is an area of the visual cortex that acts as the endpoint for the majority of LGN projections. Functionally, V1 creates a map of orientation and salient visual regions constructed from the edge and contrast-sensitive receptive field inputs from the LGN. V1 has long been considered an attractive stimulation location for a visual prosthesis as it is an accessible cortical region with a large surface area and a strong retinotopy that amplifies high acuity regions of the retina (i.e., the fovea). In theory, this would allow for V1 stimulation to produce much greater spatial resolution than upstream in the visual pathway. Studies in the 1960s and 1970s established that spatially discreet phosphenes could be generated in response to V1 surface stimulation

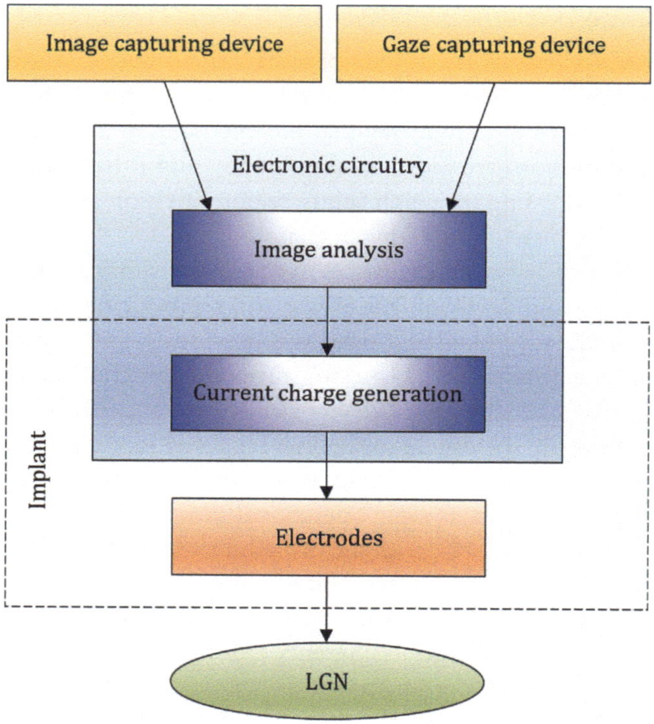

Fig. 12.12 Example design schematic for an LGN prosthesis. The individual components are very similar to other visual prostheses, including an external capture device and image processing suite. The implant uses identical principles (biphasic pulse stimulation via a current source and platinum electrode contacts) except that the electrodes are positioned at the end of a long shaft that is inserted through the brain to the LGN. *(Redrawn and adapted from Tangutooru et al. (2014).)*

(see also **Chapter 2**). However, research progressed slowly due to serious surgical and long-term stability concerns. Early cortical electrodes provoked a strong tissue reaction, with high charge densities required to overcome the subsequent high impedances and thresholds. Only recently with the expanding development of chronically implantable microelectrode arrays has the prospect of low-threshold chronically safe V1 prostheses reopened as a viable or potentially preferable alternative to retinal implantation.

Much like the LGN prosthesis, the external components of a cortical visual prosthesis remain similar to other visual prostheses, with a camera for image acquisition and a processor for image analysis (Fig. 12.13). The electrode array instead resembles other intracortical microstimulation (ICMS) arrays with either a surface electrode grid or a "bed" of penetrating shank electrodes that can stimulate different cortical layers and/or compensate for the uneven topography of the cortex (**Chapter 9**). The materials used for these arrays are typical of other ICMS devices (generally platinum or iridium oxide).

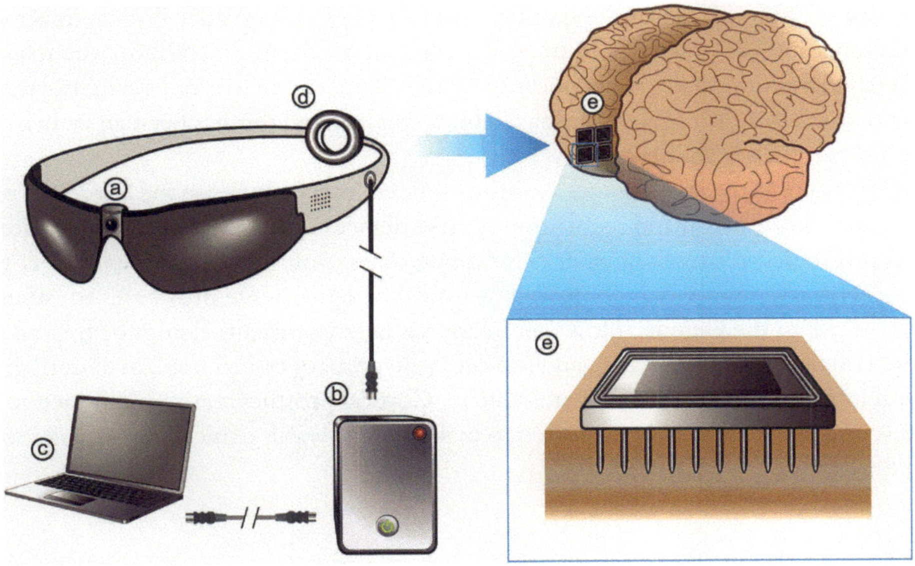

Fig. 12.13 Representation of a cortical prosthesis system. The initial components (A)–(D) are similar in function to those of a retinal prosthesis as shown in Fig. 12.8. The primary difference is the cortically implanted ICMS electrode array (E), which is designed to stimulate cortical, rather than retinal, physiology. A primary difference is the inclusion of penetrating "shanks" on many cortical prosthesis designs that can be used to stimulate different cortical layers. *(From Lewis et al. (2015).)*

Substantial variation exists in the specific designs of prototype human-implanted devices. Electrodes are typically larger than retinal prosthesis electrodes (~500–3500 μm in diameter) due to the larger available surface area. Stimulation is delivered via biphasic pulses, with the lowest thresholds consistently reported using a 100–1000 μs pulse duration and a 100–200 Hz pulse rate. Stimulation amplitudes vary considerably between studies and patients, from ~10 to 7500 μA, owing to a wide range of stimulation parameters, electrode sizes and surgical positions. This makes it difficult to report "average" perceptual thresholds. Generally, penetrating stimulation has lower perceptual thresholds in the range of tens of μAs, with lower thresholds in deeper cortical layers. Surface stimulation has higher perceptual thresholds in the range of hundreds or thousands of μAs. As in retinal implants, phosphene perception suffers from **fading** (loss of intensity with repetitive stimulation). The use of dynamic stimulation to "trace" shapes rather than display them statically appears to produce better perceptual thresholds in patients.

The challenges faced in cortical visual prosthesis development are similar to those of other cortical implants. Chiefly, there is inherent risk associated with brain surgery when compared to peripheral nerve surgery, which is coupled with a systemic risk of chronic tissue responses to electrode implantation and stimulation. An additional problem is the possibility of inducing a seizure response,[c] which has been observed in both animal model experiments and previous human trials of a cortical prosthesis. In addition, the mapping of electrode position to perceived location within the visual field is not straightforward as it is with pitch in a deaf subject with a cochlear implant and this has been an issue in previous human trials (**Chapter 3**).

While none of these challenges are insurmountable, they increase the burden of proof for the safe introduction and regulation of these devices in a clinical setting compared to retinal prostheses: relatively greater clinical outcomes must be demonstrated for cortical (and LGN) prostheses when compared to retinal or optic nerve prostheses to offset the increased risk to the patients. However, many visual impairments cannot be treated with a retinal implant due to a loss of ganglion cells (the primary retinal implant target), giving cortical implants their own therapeutic niche. Cortical prostheses are a highly active area of pre-clinical research that is expected to make steps towards clinical implementation in the near future.

Data processing and stimulation strategies

The visual system operates at very high spatial fidelity. For visual prostheses to be successful the devices must produce high spatial resolution (i.e., a large number of perceptually distinguishable phosphenes). This can be addressed by increasing the number of individual stimulating electrodes present on the device. In reality, a higher electrode density has not always resulted in a greater spatial fidelity. This is because there are several major physiological confounds that limit the distinguishability of the resulting visual percept. Often electrodes that are co-located produce phosphenes that are identical or at least so similar that patients cannot meaningfully distinguish between them. The most significant limiting confounds are:

- The retina contains many cell types and structures and the pattern of degeneration is heterogeneous. Current spreads between electrodes due to stimulated axon fibers, retinal remodeling, and the presence of the foreign body reaction increasing the electrode impedance.
- Indiscriminate stimulation of RGC populations activates the off- and on-center pathways of the retina indiscriminately. This may lead to higher stimulation thresholds and less distinct percepts.
- Likely due to the above reasons, phosphene shape and size is not consistent across electrodes, patients, and sometimes time. It is not possible to map 1:1 a visual scene from the capture device to the electrode grid.

[c] Often the seizure was preceded by phosphenes that persisted after the stimulation had been switched off.

It is necessary to develop data processing and stimulation strategies that overcome or minimize the impact of the above effects. Several popular strategies are commonly employed or under active development across multiple labs.

Pre-implant data processing

Most visual implants, including many photodiode arrays, use an external camera to capture the visual scene. The input from the external camera has many orders of magnitude more information than can be faithfully encoded into the stimulation array (millions of pixels vs. dozens, hundreds, or at best thousands of individual electrodes, and that assumes a 1:1 electrode to phosphene ratio). Therefore, it is first necessary to downsample (reduce) the high-resolution visual image into a low-resolution format that can be delivered to the stimulation array. This image processing must be done online (i.e., in real time) without introducing a significant delay in timing between capture and stimulation, and must also be tailored ("fitted") to individual patients as the map of phosphene position, size, and shape will be unique for each subject.

Initial data processing strategies have focused on down-sampling methods that preserve as many salient features in the visual scene as is possible. These strategies are relatively straightforward to develop as they can first be tested on normal sighted patients (with a simulated output) and have shown subsequent, if modest, success in implanted patients. The most common initial processing methods have been regional averaging (summing the output of pixels that are similar spatially and/or in luminance) and the application of Gaussian filtering algorithms (the transformation of an image via a Gaussian function, to create a low-pass filter of the visual information). Subsequent processing has focused primarily around contrast enhancement and highlighting edges. Improved contrast sensitivity and edge detection are particularly important parameters given that they are core functions of the physiological visual pathway.

Many patients state that the ability to see faces and the ability to easily navigate their environment are the functions they desire most. Reading is also a concern but this can often be sufficiently compensated via text-to-speech or other "low-vision aids." Face-detection algorithms can increase the stimulation output in areas where a face has been detected, although no visual implant yet has the resolution to resolve facial features. Many algorithms seek to separate and amplify the differences between the ground plane of motion and obstacles that pose a collision or fall risk. These have shown moderate success in trials, although their usefulness in natural environment is still unclear.

Finally, the connection of two cameras to enable depth-processing strategies, and thermal cameras to highlight living or potentially dangerous objects in the environment, have been suggested. It is exciting to consider that prosthetic vision does not necessarily need to be limited to the standard visual spectrum of light.

Although image processing has shown great success in the lab, the usefulness of these algorithms for daily prosthesis use is still unknown. Image processing algorithms are helpful to better optimize the stimulation output, but they alone cannot overcome the bottleneck of perception caused by the low phosphene resolution generated by current generation implants. Similarly, improved perceptual resolution without the development of innovative processing strategies will also likely not be enough to overcome the acuity gap between physiological and prosthetic vision in the near future. Thus, a combined approach is necessary for prosthesis development.

Current steering

While increasing the number of electrodes in an array is the most straightforward way to increase the perceptual resolution of resulting stimulation, often physically co-located electrodes can produce indistinguishable percepts. Rather than adding more electrodes or repositioning them physically, it is instead possible to stimulate electrodes in concert to direct the resulting electric field creatively. The combined overlapping electric fields created via stimulation across two or more "real" electrodes results in a summed "virtual electrode," which allows for additional stimulation options and potentially more perceptual differentiation. This method is called **current steering** in the field of neural engineering, related to but distinct from the identically named concept in pure electrical engineering. Current steering has been experimentally used in cochlear implants to focus the stimulated area in an attempt to increase frequency specificity (Fig. 11.10), and in the retina is used with the intention to direct fields spatially towards new targets.

Fig. 12.14 provides a simplified example of how simultaneous stimulation on two or more electrodes can shift the resulting electric field. When identical amplitudes of current are used, the peak of the electric field sum is precisely between the two electrodes. However, when one electrode has a higher amplitude current applied, the field is shifted towards that electrode. In this way, the peak of the stimulation (and thus the area of greatest neural activation) can be "steered" over a continuous space between electrodes. Unlike a cochlear implant, retinal implant electrodes are spaced across a roughly two-dimensional plane (e.g., Fig. 12.9) meaning that the addition of a third or fourth stimulated electrode can result in further steering to any point on the retina, which lies between the outermost electrodes of the implant array. Current steering holds promise to improve the range of spatial locations available for retinal stimulation and so increase the number of discreet percepts available to the patient. However, in the visual system, the technique still remains relatively unproven outside of pre-clinical studies.

Cell-selective stimulation

Retinal implants use biphasic pulses to excite the retina. This stimulation excites both on-center and off-center pathways, as well as non-target tissues such as ganglion cell

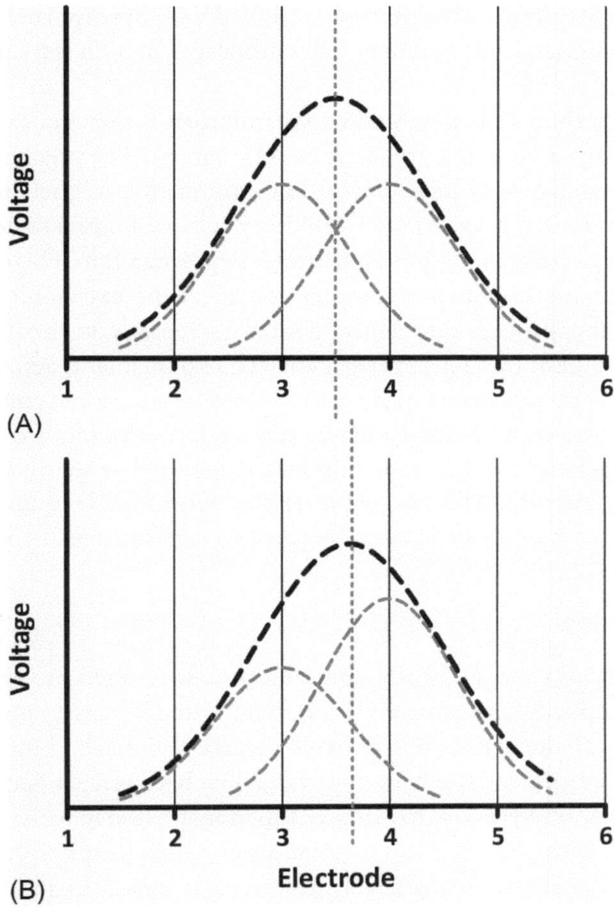

Fig. 12.14 Schematic demonstrating the concept of current steering in retinal prostheses. (A) shows the summed "virtual electrode" electric field *(dashed black line)* resulting from the fields generated by stimulating simultaneously on electrode 3 and 4 *(dashed gray lines)*. (B) shows the resulting electric field when stimulation is uneven between the two electrodes (30% on electrode 3 vs 70% on electrode 4). By varying the relative amplitude of stimulation between the physical electrodes it is possible to shift the peak of the virtual electrode relative to its initial position (*gray dotted line*, for comparison) and so reach different populations in the excitable tissue.

axons that may be passing across the retina from more distant areas. This is likely why phosphene shapes are often described as highly irregular or as elongated streaks. Regions within the same cell, or cell types with differing morphologies, can have different electrical properties. This means that it may be possible to selectively excite specific cell types or regions of cells by tailoring the stimulation waveform to best match the properties of the targeted region or cell morphology. For example, very short, anodic-first pulses (non-standard, as discussed in **Chapter 6**) combined with hyperpolarizing pre-pulses (to act as a "priming" stimulus) may preferentially stimulate ganglion cell soma over ganglion cell axon processes.

A promising method of **cell-selective stimulation** is the application of sinusoidal stimulus, particularly at very high frequencies (kHz range). The precise mechanisms that drive differential excitation or inhibition at high stimulation frequencies are both complex and poorly understood, yet cortical inhibitory cells are known to be able to generate action potentials at a particularly high rate under depolarization. The experimental evidence suggests that high frequency stimulus can affect the excitability of on- and off-center pathway ganglion cells differently, with a discrepancy in the optimal amplitude for stimulation of inhibition. This property may be exploitable to generate percepts that are driven primarily by one or the other pathway, rather than some combination of both as is currently the case with standard pulsatile stimulation. This requires testing in human subjects. Current generation clinical prostheses are not rated or approved for the delivery of high-frequency stimulus. Thus, some pre-clinical work is still required to demonstrate the potential efficacy and safety of high-frequency waveforms in the retina.

Clinical outcomes

Several retinal implants saw successful clinical trials but resulted in very limited market success. Retinal implants have struggled with stability and longevity problems associated with the fragility of the retina and difficult surgical approach. Functional outcomes remain low in all devices, with high levels of variability between patients. The high spatial resolution requirements necessary to produce functional vision in patients was never consistently met, even with high-density electrode arrays (often the phosphenes produced by co-located electrodes are not recognizably different). It is clear that the achievements of the cochlear implant cannot be so easily replicated in the retina without further innovation and engineering. In an attempt to overcome the continued challenges associated with visual prosthesis design, competition between research groups has resulted in considerable variation in surgical approaches, electrodes, and housing materials for retinal implants. In order to improve the functional outcomes of patients implanted with these devices, it is necessary to develop more advanced technologies, but also to better understand how these technologies can be optimized to compensate for individual particular disease pathologies.

After implantation with a visual prosthesis, it is important to assess the visual outcomes of the intervention in a manner that can be compared between patients, clinics, and devices. There is a broad set of tests in ophthalmology to determine visual function, encompassing central visual acuity, size of the visual field, performance in light vs. dark areas, motion detection, color discrimination, and so on. There are also qualitative tests for functional tasks that assess a patient's ability to perform activities associated with unassisted daily living. Functional tasks are arguably as or more important to assess as they give a better understanding of how a medical intervention has improved quality of life in a patient. Unfortunately, no tests have been universally adopted to compare the outcomes of different devices, and because the visual percepts in patients are not similar to natural vision, an objective comparison to standardized outcomes is also difficult. There have at least been some common assessments shared between all clinical trials.

Visual acuity is used to assess the spatial resolution of the perception. Visual acuity tests are straightforward to perform using a forced-choice paradigm on a computer screen, typically where the patient must determine differences in grating stimuli. However, it is important to remember that the identification of gratings is not necessarily an indication of the minimum acuity needed to perform functional tasks such as reading. There are many units used to describe visual acuity across the world. The most common clinical measure in the United States is the Snellen ratio, defined as the distance of the test over the distance at which the smallest correctly identified optotype (normally a letter) subtends an angle of five arcminutes. "Standard" vision is 20/20 in the imperial system (feet) or 6/6 in the metric system (meters), and "legally blind" is commonly defined as 20/200 or 6/60. The unit most often used scientifically is the log of the minimal angle of resolution (MAR) in arc minutes, where a logMAR of 0 is normal vision and logMAR of 1 is legal blindness. The best visual acuity reported for retinal implants so far is 20/546 (logMAR 1.43), but most patients perform well under this bar, meaning that even in the best case patients with a retinal prosthesis are currently still considered legally blind. Legal blindness does not mean patients do not have any restoration of visual perception at all, but rather that they legally remain blind for the purposes of disability.

Perimetry is the assessment of the size of the visual field, and is often tested alongside **motion detection** as a quantitative measure of the ability of a patient to navigate an environment that includes moving objects in the periphery (e.g., many external environments that contain traffic, people, animals, etc.). These tests are difficult to perform or even properly define on retinal implant patients because the "size" of the visual field is a complex function of the input (how much area the camera is sampling) and the perception of the patient (how much of their subjective visual field contains a percept, and in what locations). At best, motion detection assessments have reported a discrimination threshold of 35 degrees/s, which is still well below normal vision ($\sim<0.5$ to 2 degrees/s depending how peripherally the stimuli is presented).

Functional vision tests such as the **orientation and mobility** and **daily living** tests attempt to quantify the ability of patients to navigate and function in their daily lives and environments. These tests have not always been applied consistently leading to difficulties in comparing results from different device manufacturers. However, a standard tool called the **Functional Low-Vision Observer Rated Assessment (FLORA)** that improves the comparative ability has been recently developed. Patients are capable of some basic daily tasks such as navigating simple environments, avoiding obstacles, and locating sources of light such as lightbulbs or windows. As the goal of visual prostheses is to restore quality of life to patients, the inclusion of more qualitative assessments, including patient-reported outcomes, is important because it helps identify the "real" benefit of the clinical intervention outside of a carefully controlled laboratory setting.

Current retinal prostheses reached the regulatory threshold for safety and efficacy, but have so far failed to reach a market "threshold" of vision restoration that would enable widespread adoption and translation beyond severe visual impairments. Visual prostheses (~150,000 USD) are marketed only as a complementary, not replacement, device for a cane (a simple mobility aid, ~20 USD). It is clear that the field of visual prosthetics requires significant further innovation and iteration if it seeks to achieve the same level of success as the cochlear or brainstem implants discussed in **Chapter 11**. This innovation must be driven by the integration of multiple upcoming technologies as briefly discussed throughout this chapter, including new material interfaces, higher density arrays, better stimulus encoding, and novel stimulation parameters. The clinical translation of cortical prostheses may also provide a new niche for visual prosthesis therapies. In addition, a robust system to measure and compare the clinical outcomes of new devices is an overlooked but vital component in retinal prosthesis research to ensure real progress is being made.

Brief summary

- The retina is a complex neural tissue consisting of photoreceptors and sensory neurons.
- The post-photoreceptor visual system focuses on the consolidation of high spatial resolution information using center-surround receptive fields, edge detection, and contrast sensitivity.
- Receptive fields are conserved through the visual pathway and into the cortex, but become increasingly more complex in the types of information they encode.
- Blindness can occur due to dysfunction at any point along this pathway. Many common forms of blindness primarily affect the photoreceptors, but leave other retinal neurons alive as a potential stimulation target.
- Retinal remodeling occurs in response to a loss of photoreceptor input. It corrupts the surviving retinal physiology and influences the outcomes of prosthetic therapies.
- Most visual implants are similar in design to cochlear implants, with components that capture the sensory input, process and convert them to stimulation patterns, relay these patterns and power to the implant, and finally, stimulate the neurons electrically.
- Many different surgical positions are available for visual prostheses near or in the retina, with different advantages and disadvantages. The most common are epiretinal, subretinal, suprachoroidal, and optic nerve.

- Photodiode retinal arrays are different to other retinal implants. They convert light (typically infrared) into a potential difference that can be used to electrically stimulate the retina.
- Another viable visual prosthesis strategy is to bypass the retina and instead stimulate the LGN visual cortex. This has a greater associated risk but may enable treatment in a larger patient population.
- Electrical stimulation does not produce "natural" visual percepts. Data processing and stimulation strategies are essential to convert the captured visual scene into patterns of electrical stimulation that can be understood by the patient.
- Understanding how patient outcomes are assessed is necessary to judge treatment success and compare device performance. Current generation devices have had limited patient outcomes.

Key literature and further reading

Aplin, F.P., et al., 2016. Retinal changes in an ATP-induced model of retinal degeneration. Front. Neuroanat. 10, 46. https://doi.org/10.3389/fnana.2016.00046.

Ayton, L.N., Blamey, P.J., Guymer, R.H., 2014. First-in-human trial of a novel suprachoroidal retinal prosthesis. PLoS One. 9(12), e115239. https://doi.org/10.1371/journal.pone.0115239.

Barriga-Rivera, A., et al., 2017. Visual prosthesis: interfacing stimulating electrodes with retinal neurons to restore vision. Front. Neurosci. 11, 620.

Chen, D.L., Greenberg, P.B., Borton, D.A., 2017. Advances in retinal prosthetic research: a systematic review of engineering and clinical characteristics of current prosthetic initiatives. Curr. Eye Res. 42, 334–347.

Foroushani, A.N., Pack, C.C., Sawan, M., 2018. Cortical visual prostheses: from microstimulation to functional percept. J. Neural Eng. 15, 021005.

Hoon, M., Okawa, H., Della Santina, L., Wong, R.O., 2014. Functional architecture of the retina: development and disease. Prog. Retin. Eye Res. 42, 44–84.

Jeffries, A.M., Killian, N.J., Pezaris, J.S., 2014. Mapping the primate lateral geniculate nucleus: a review of experiments and methods. J. Physiol. Paris 108, 3–10.

Lewis, P.M., Ackland, H.M., Lowery, A.J., Rosenfeld, J.V., 2015. Restoration of vision in blind individuals using bionic devices: a review with a focus on cortical visual prostheses. Brain Res. 1595, 51–73. https://doi.org/10.1016/j.brainres.2014.11.020.

Marc, R.E., Jones, B.W., Watt, C.B., Strettoi, E., 2003. Neural remodeling in retinal degeneration. Prog. Retin. Eye Res. 22, 607–655.

Masland, R.H., 2001. The fundamental plan of the retina. Nat. Neurosci. 4, 877–886.

Nguyen, H.T., et al., 2016. Thalamic visual prosthesis. IEEE Trans. Biomed. Eng. 63 (8), 1573–1580.

Palanker, D., et al., 2020. Photovoltaic restoration of central vision in atrophic age-related macular degeneration. Am. Acad. Ophthalmol. 127 (8), 1097–1104.

Priebe, N.J., 2016. Mechanisms of orientation selectivity in the primary visual cortex. Annu. Rev. Vis. Sci. 2, 85–107.

Tangutooru, S.M., Yoon, W.J., Troy, J.B., 2014. Early design considerations for a thalamic visual prosthesis to treat blindness resulting from glaucoma. 2nd Middle East Conference on Biomedical Engineering, Doha, 249–252.

Tong, W., Meffin, H., Garret, D.J., Ibbotson, M.R., 2020. Stimulation strategies for improving the resolution of retinal prostheses. Front. Neurosci. 14, 262.

CHAPTER 13

Pacemaker for the brain: Deep brain stimulation

We actively interface with the world through the motor system. The motor system allows us not only to influence the material world around us, but is also required for vocalizations and for speech. The motor system is responsible for breathing, walking, and standing upright.

Every motor act is complex and involves machinery that uses energy stored in the muscle (in adenosine triphosphate (ATP) and in creatine phosphate) and transforms it to a change in length of the muscle. Muscle contraction and relaxation require calcium for coupling excitation of the muscle membrane to contraction of the muscle. Furthermore, the muscle has sensors in the muscle fibers and in tendons that ensure that muscle length is a precisely controlled entity in the body. Finally, muscles have agonists (other muscles that act in a similar way) and antagonists (that oppose the action of the muscle). Simultaneous contractions of agonists and antagonists may lead to stiffening of the corresponding joint in the given position. Every healthy muscle receives a certain level of activity from the innervating axons of the spinal cord even at rest so that it has a certain tension ("tone"). There are sensors for this muscle tone so that the information comes back to the spine to regulate it actively. Only a muscle in absence of any innervation is completely flaccid.

Muscle contraction regulation is a distributed neuromuscular phenomenon, with certain tasks performed autonomously. An early part takes place in the spine. The spine ensures muscle tone and regulates a constant length of the muscle, but also includes pattern generator circuits. For example, there are pattern-generating circuits responsible for the alternating contraction of muscles during walking. These are inborn motor programs. The brain itself sends signals that modulate this pattern (e.g., increase the walking speed). By such outsourcing of automatic movement patterns to the spine, more central parts of the nervous system can take care of the more variable, less automatic motor acts.

The central structure responsible for voluntary motor action is the cerebral cortex (Fig. 13.1). Layer V of the *primary motor cortex* (M1) contains particularly large pyramidal cells that send out signals to the spine and control the spinal circuits. The neurons do not represent individual muscles but rather movements of a given part of the body in a certain direction (Chapter 15). Thus, whenever we perform a voluntary movement, the primary motor cortex must be active. However, when a motor pattern is planned, further areas are required that organize the individual movements into the pattern. This is performed by

Prostheses for the Brain
https://doi.org/10.1016/B978-0-12-818892-7.00012-2

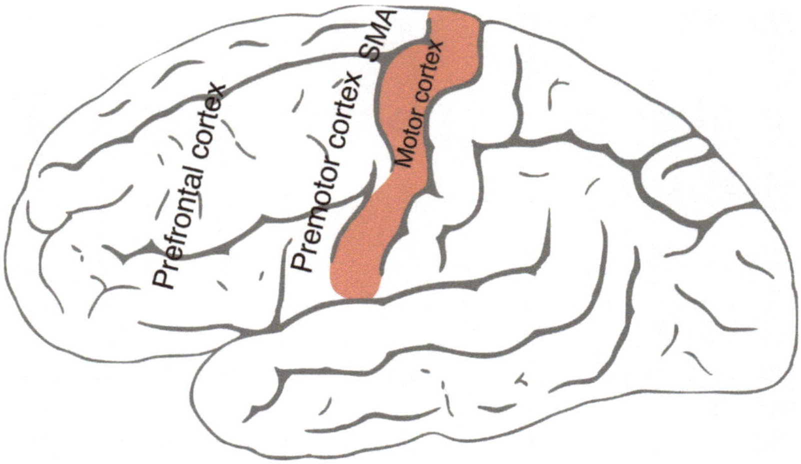

Fig. 13.1 Location of the motor cortex (field M1) and the planning regions, supplementary motor area (SMA), and premotor cortex, on the lateral view of the brain.

the areas rostral (in front) of the primary motor cortex, and particularly by the *supplementary motor area* (SMA) and *premotor cortex*.

Not all complex movement patterns can be performed under complete voluntary control. Particularly when fast and complex reactions are required, a coordinated pattern of movements must be first learned, become automatic, to be fast and efficient. This is how we learn to play tennis, to ride a bike, or to ski. The motor patterns are initially a slow sequence under (nearly) full voluntary control, and with repetition they become more efficient, more automatic, and by that also faster. Interestingly, the more efficient we become the less voluntary control we have and the less we are capable of describing how we do what we do; the exact motor program thus escapes voluntary control and becomes involuntary.

Even complex movements are not programmed from scratch, but often take advantage of reflex patterns stored, for example, in the spinal cord. For an ice hockey goalie, many of the moves when catching the puck are similar to simple neck and spine reflexes that can be already observed in a very young infant a few months after birth. These innate "fixed action patterns" can be released by appropriate stimulation and may be chained into new more complex patterns. Thus the motor system behaves like a complex program that chains existing subroutines in a new order and adds new subroutines to it.

The innate action patterns are, as a rule, stored in the spinal cord and subcortical centers of the CNS (like the red nucleus in the brainstem). New coordinated patterns also require a structure that can handle them and store them by reorganizing the existing circuitry. This thus requires a neuronal structure that is sufficiently plastic and complex enough so that it can handle temporal patterns of activity over a long time scale. This circuitry includes the basal ganglia, motor part of the thalamus, and the cerebellum. The cerebellum is required for fine motor coordination and is involved in the integration of movement and balance (**Chapter 15**). We will not discuss this further here but will focus more on the basal ganglia. The basal ganglia consist of the caudate nucleus, the putamen (together called the striatum), the pale globe, substantia nigra, and subthalamic nucleus. Their connections are well known and include excitatory and inhibitory synapses and a large number of neurotransmitters (Fig. 13.2).

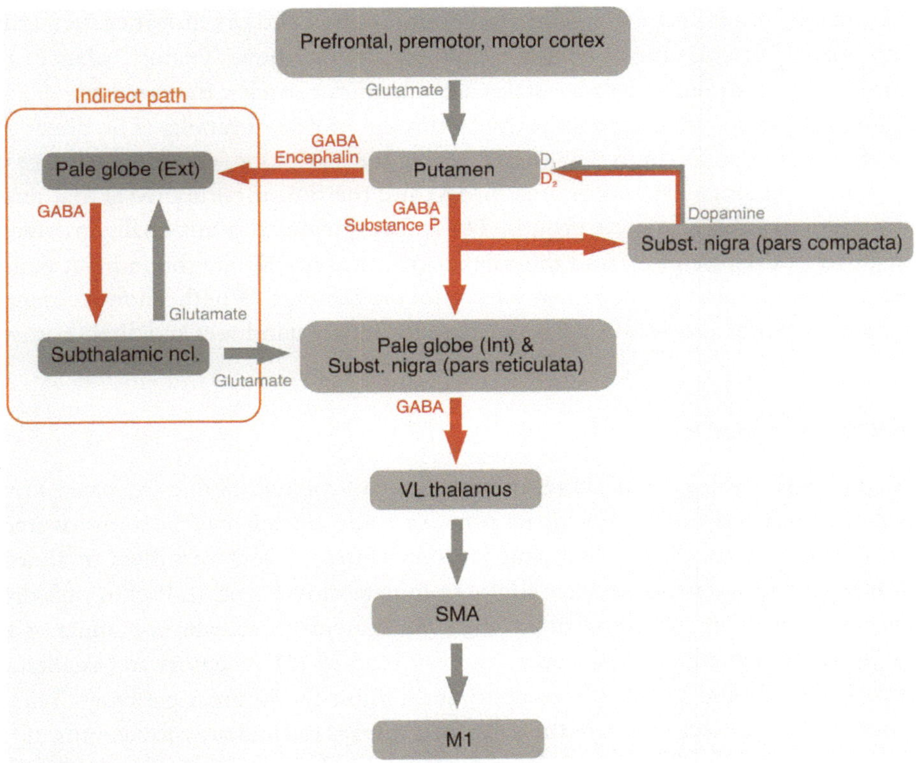

Fig. 13.2 Circuitry in the basal ganglia. Excitatory connections (with glutamate as transmitter) are shown in *gray*, inhibitory in *red*, with transmitters shown at the structure of origin of the projection (remember that the transmitter is synthetized in the soma of the neuron, thus in the structure of origin, but acts at the target synapse). The path to the primary motor cortex (M1) and supplementary motor area (SMA) is divided into the direct path (from putamen to the internal segment of the pale globe to the ventrolateral (VL) thalamus) and the indirect path (from putamen to the external segment of the pale globe, subthalamic nucleus and finally to the internal part of the pale globe). The indirect path inhibits movement, while the direct path facilitates movement. The circuit through substantia nigra (pars compacta) to putamen is dopaminergic, but the receptors in the putamen are different: D_1 receptors have a facilitating effect on the direct pathway, while activation of D_2 receptors inhibits the indirect pathway.

This dedicated circuitry receives input from the premotor and motor cortex and outputs the additional stored elements of complex movement as required; in other words, the basal ganglia store the subroutines for complex movement. The basal ganglia also act on the motor system at rest. They contain neurons that are spontaneously very active. It has been suggested that the individual nuclei with excitatory and inhibitory connections are in a dynamic balance that is precisely controlled. Thus, the oscillatory activity between the nuclei is in resonance both at rest and during movement. During planning, the motor and premotor cortex send information to the basal ganglia, which process it and directly influences the cortical neurons that are responsible for the movement preparation and execution in the supplementary motor cortex and the motor cortex. During execution of a particular movement the circuitry attains a new dynamic balance, and a transition through different balance states accompanies complex movements.

There is a direct and an indirect pathway through the basal ganglia. The direct pathway leads from the putamen to the internal part of the pale globe, ventrolateral (VL) thalamus to the supplementary motor area (SMA) and the motor cortex (M1) that directly initiates the activation of muscle groups. The indirect pathway additionally involves the external part of the pale globe and the subthalamic nucleus. While the indirect pathway inhibits movements, the direct pathway activates movements. Whether a movement will be executed depends also on the balance of activity between indirect and direct pathways.

Parkinson's disease

This complex physiology may sometimes become a problem. While the exact mechanisms are not understood in detail, neurons in some nuclei may become overactive and bring the concert of the basal ganglia "out of tune." This manifests in abnormal and unintended movements or the inability to initiate movement. In Parkinson's disease *dopaminergic neurons* in substantia nigra[a] die. These neurons release dopamine at their synapse in the putamen, and the dopamine may bind to D1 receptors and facilitate the direct pathway or bind to the D2 receptor and inhibit the indirect pathway. Thus the net action of the connections from the substantia nigra is to facilitate movements. If these neurons are lost in significant number, a functional imbalance in the circuitry of basal ganglia shows up, starting from the putamen. The activity in the indirect pathway is increased, with synchronized activity throughout many structures, particularly the subthalamic nucleus, and prominent pathological *oscillatory activity in the beta band* (Fig. 13.3). In this condition, initiation of a movement, critically dependent on the balance between the direct and the indirect path, is thus compromised. The consequence is a clinical picture characterized by *rigidity* or stiffness (there is no increase in muscle tone, but a particular

[a] Substantia nigra is Latin for "black substance," named for the higher levels of neuromelanin in the dopaminergic neurons found in this brain region.

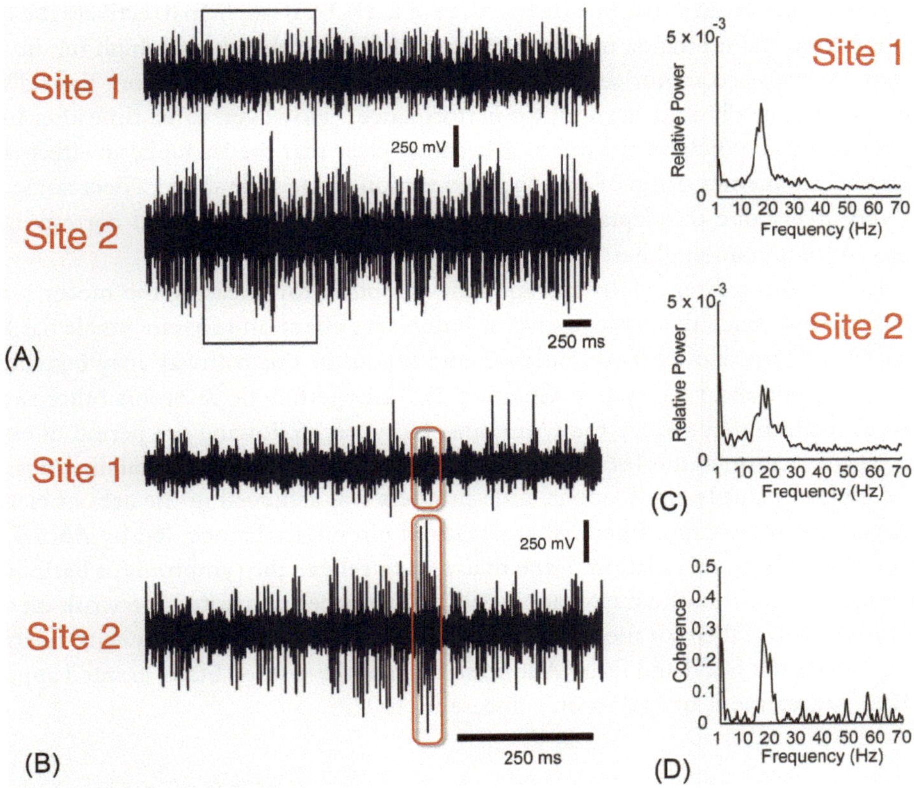

Fig. 13.3 Extracellular recording of spiking activity in the subthalamic nucleus of a Parkinson's patient. (A) Original traces of simultaneous recording from two electrodes. (B) Same recording, timescale expanded for the part delineated by the black rectangle in A. Note the repeating bursts of activity *(highlighted by the red rectangles)* are synchronized between sites. (C) Frequency analysis of the power showing a peak in the beta range for both sites. (D) Coherence analysis demonstrating that the oscillatory activity in both recorded neurons is synchronized in the beta range. *(Reproduced from Moshel et al. (2013).)*

step-like increase in resistance when the limbs are moved passively, known as the cogwheel phenomenon), inability to initiate movements, typical parkinsonian stance, shuffling gait, and tremor of the hands. The tremor occurs at rest and may appear as counting of invisible coins. It can also be so extensive that the subject cannot drink water out of a glass. The tremor may thus impair daily life substantially. Abnormal beta oscillations in neurons of the basal ganglia are synchronized with the frequency of the tremor. However, the clinical picture can vary substantially. Some subjects have a stronger rigor (akinetic form) and some have a stronger tremor. Therefore, the intervention must consider the subject's complete clinical picture.

Supplementation of dopamine (in the form of L-DOPA) can help to activate the feedback loop from the substantia nigra to the striatum. Even subjects with high rigidity and substantially impaired motor reactions may miraculously "wake up" from their disease and show substantially improved motor performance.[b] However, some time after introduction of this very helpful treatment it becames clear that the therapeutic effect is not permanent. Supplementation of dopamine over a long time scale shows a decreasing efficacy, very likely due to adaptation of the receptors for dopamine and corresponding changes in the putamen. Therefore, other solutions are needed.

Lesions in the indirect pathway represent an option for releasing the motor system from its rigidity, since this pathway has an inhibiting effect on movements. It has been historically known that electrostimulation and lesions in this pathway may beneficially modulate tremor and rigidity (see **Chapter 2**). In hyperkinetic disorders other sites of electrostimulation may reduce the symptoms. However, following the period of extensive experimentation in the 1960s, and beyond the extensive experimental investigations by Jose Delgado and Irving Cooper, little progress was achieved in the area of electrostimulation for some time. Eventually, a team in Grenoble, France, led by Alim-Louis Benabid, used electrostimulation in the thalamus to relieve the symptoms of Parkinson's disease and reported on the outcomes in 1991. This paper reinitiated the work on deep brain stimulation (DBS) for motor diseases. Due to its efficacy and safety with relatively few side effects the Food and Drug Administration of the United States granted approval for DBS for treatment of Parkinson's disease in 2002.

Mechanism of deep brain stimulation

The first attempts at DBS were aimed at thalamic stimulation since it appears plausible that these drive the tremor. Soon it became clear that for treating tremor and rigidity, the subthalamic nucleus is the best (most effective) target of DBS. Of course, the small size of the nucleus makes it a more difficult target. However, oscillations in the subthalamic nucleus are synchronous with the tremor and can be used for detecting the desired stimulation targets. The stereotactic path through the basal ganglia allows for monitoring of the trajectory of the electrode, especially when combining the stimulation electrode with recording (either through the stimulation electrode to record local field potentials or using additional microelectrodes, advanced before the stimulating electrode). Such an

[b] The book of Oliver W. Sachs *Awakenings* (Sachs O, 1976, Harmondsworth: Pelican Books) and the movie *Awakenings* with Robert de Niro and Robin Williams based on the book describe patients that suffered from a disease called encephalitis lethargica (that includes parkinsonian symptoms) and after introduction of L-DOPA awakened from their state of heavily reduced motor activity. Sachs (1933–2015) was a professor of neurology who wrote many very valuable books about different neurological conditions providing insights to the functioning of the brain. Oliver Sachs had an exceptional empathy for patients trapped in severe neurological conditions.

approach provides feedback on the actual trajectory (the penetration is not blind) and thus a good orientation. However, use of recording electrodes increases the risk of bleeding during the intervention.

The stimulation itself is aimed at suppression of the neuronal activity in the beta range that is associated with tremor. Therefore, the stimulus is a high-frequency pulse train (>100 Hz). It has been well documented that such stimulation alleviates the tremor and rigidity. This suppression has been further documented in animals using invasive recordings in different structures of basal ganglia. One mechanism might be a depolarization block, as discussed in **Chapter 4**. On the one hand, as also outlined in **Chapter 11**, neurons can normally follow a pulse train at 100 Hz well and can synchronize to this frequency in the auditory nerve and most other structures in the brain. It could be that it is the specific composition of ionic channels of the neuronal membranes in basal ganglia that is more susceptible to a strong adaptation of firing as a result of high-frequency stimulation. On the other hand, even if the neurons show an entrainment to the stimulation, such high-frequency stimulation will override the low-frequency oscillations in the beta range that are coupled to the tremor. This override effect may be effective since muscles cannot contract at rates above the beta range. Alternatively, more likely is that the oscillatory network in the basal ganglia cannot appropriately relay this information and thus the stimulation has the effect of an "information lesion" (jamming). Another possibility is that such filtering of the high-frequency information is performed at the synaptic level ("synaptic filtering") subsequent to the axons, and thus while the neurons entrain to the stimulus, the synapses and thus the subsequent stages of processing cannot follow such fast rhythms. This is obviously different from, for example, the auditory system that uses such high-frequency information. We need to consider that neurons in the brain differ in their electrical properties, even in one (the same) structure, and thus it appears plausible that downstream neurons may not be capable of transferring such high firing rates in the basal ganglia as observed in the auditory system. Interestingly, the therapeutic effect of the stimulation saturates some weeks after stimulation onset, indicating that long-term adaptation of the stimulated region and its downstream target are indeed involved in the therapeutic effect. A modulatory influence of the glia (astrocytes) has also been discussed in this long-term effect, among others. The situation is complex, and how the stimulation is related to changes of symptoms is a focus of ongoing research. Fortunately, it is possible to imitate Parkinson's disease using a pharmacological destruction of dopaminergic synapses using 1-methyl-4-phenyl-1,2,3,6-tetrahydropyridine (MPTP) in animals. This allows for a better investigation of the neuronal mechanisms of Parkinson's disease and the effects of electrostimulation. The mechanisms of the beneficial effect of DBS in motor diseases are still subject to research and in this sense is a "work in progress."

Alternatively to the subthalamic nucleus, the internal part of the pale globe remains another potential target of stimulation. In some constellations of Parkinson symptoms, neurologists may decide for this target instead of subthalamic nucleus.

Design of the stimulator

The design of the system consists of an implantable pulse generator (IPG) that is placed on the chest under the skin (Fig. 13.4), a lead wire connecting the pulse generator to the electrode, and finally the implant itself that is inserted deeply into the brain. While the structure of this device is similar to the one discussed in previous chapters, it differs by its simplicity and smaller energy requirements. Therefore, both the electronics and the batteries can be completely placed under the skin (without an extracorporal part as exists in cochlear implants). This provides a major advantage, for example, for the contact with water: taking a shower does not require unplugging of the stimulator. The disadvantage is that over time (1–4 years) replacement of the batteries is required and thus so is a cut into the skin. This procedure is, however, well tested in cardiac pacemakers and very safe. Modern DBS systems also offer rechargeable batteries that require recharging in regular intervals. Programming of the device is performed transcutaneously through a radio frequency link. Since the stimulation setting is, compared to cochlear implants for example, restricted to few parameters, this programming has to be performed only very rarely during the regular clinical check-ups.

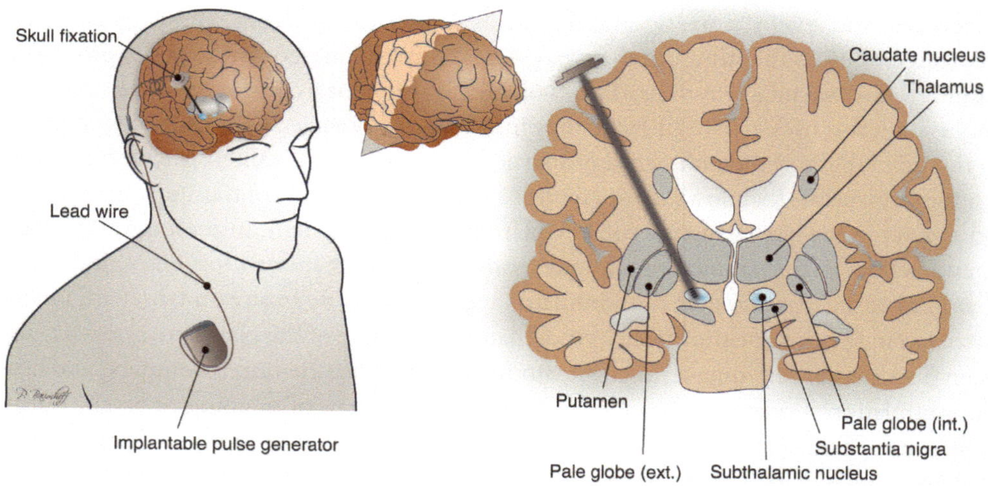

Fig. 13.4 Deep brain stimulation for Parkinson's disease. *Left*: Position in the subject. The implantable pulse generator (IPG) is placed subcutaneously, the lead wire leads to the fixation point in the skull. The electrode penetrates deeply into the brain. *Right*: Section through the brain (inset) showing the placement of the electrode in the subthalamic nucleus. Unilateral placement is sufficient to alleviate motor symptoms. Potential stimulation targets are the subthalamic nucleus, pale globe, and motor thalamus.

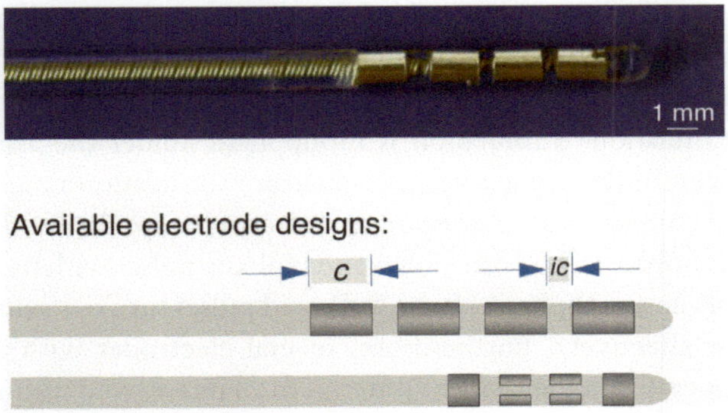

Fig. 13.5 Example of a deep brain stimulation electrode. Topmost is a photograph of an electrode (Medtronic Comp., MN, USA). Below are designs currently available, with contact length (designated c) of 1.5 or 3.0 mm, and inter-contact spacing (designated ic) of 0.5–4.0 mm, with 4 or 8 electrode contacts in total. In some designs, the electrode is not a ring, but rather has the contact segmented into three segments (shown are only two) to allow current steering (electrodes produced by Boston Scientific and St. Jude). *(Top: Figure courtesy of Dr. Roger Calixto, Calixto (2004).)*

The electrode

The stimulation electrode is substantially larger than in cochlear or retinal implants. It is not supposed to deliver structured information by anatomic location. Rather the goal is to limit the spread of the electric stimulation to the size of the target. Therefore the optimal size of the electrode is of approximate similarity to the target structure. Over the years, different designs of the electrodes have been developed (Fig. 13.5). Principally, however, there are four to eight electrodes with longitude of 1.5 mm with an interelectrode spacing of 0.5–1.5 mm in the majority of devices. Some electrodes have the ring broken into three subparts so that the current can be steered into the radial direction. The contacts are made of platinum-iridium, and the isolation is by polyurethane.

Stimulation configuration

The original Medtronic stimulator was a voltage source, and many systems are still voltage sources or can be operated in the voltage mode. Only in recent years have current sources become available for DBS. Although the true charge delivery cannot be controlled in voltage sources (for reasons, see **Chapters 5 and 6**), these systems were mainly designed for suppression of abnormal activity and not for delivery of detailed information structured in amplitude and time. This imprecision was thus in DBS of lesser consequence compared to systems where stimulus amplitude is key and thus charge delivery must be carefully controlled (like in sensory implants). Recently, current sources are preferred by providing over time more stable clinical outcomes.

Stimulation is in most cases monopolar (with the case of the system as a return electrode), however bipolar and multipolar stimulation modes are possible, too. The systems allow for the operating of each electrode separately as a cathode, anode, or off. Most effective is cathodic stimulation. Stimulation is monophasic under the assumption that the stimulators are driven in the capacitive (non-faradaic) stimulation range. This is possible because of the large contacts with corresponding electrode capacitance. Recently, charge-balanced pseudomonophasic, biphasic pulses and biphasic pulses with interphase gaps have become the state of the art. Biphasic charge balanced pulses suppress symptoms of Parkinson's diseases most effectively. Furthermore, several electrodes with different stimulus amplitude can be operated in the modern systems, in an interleaved stimulation mode similar to cochlear implants (see **Chapter 11**).

The usual effective setting in clinical environment is monopolar, with the working electrode as cathode and return electrode as anode. The electrode surface area is large ($\sim 0.06\,cm^2$ in most applications). Pulse widths range between 10 and 507 μs, and voltage between 1 and 3 V (charge $<1\,\mu C$/phase). The stimulation rates can be set from 2 to 255 Hz, depending on the system in use. However, stimulation at low frequencies tend to increase the tremor, whereas stimulation of 120–185 Hz is typically more effective in suppressing the tremor. This corresponds to the physiology of the basal ganglia as described previously.

Clinical approaches

It has been estimated that 160,000 subjects worldwide have undergone DBS surgery. The clinical use of DBS aims mainly at motor diseases, as already mentioned in **Chapter 2**. Here, tremor and rigidity are the main targets in Parkinson's disease. In Parkinson's disease, the first attempt is usually pharmacological treatment, and only later is electrostimulation indicated to alleviate remaining motor symptoms. However, the progression of cognitive symptoms, speech deficits, and gait pathology is unaffected by DBS. Therefore, this approach has introduced a new clinical picture with less rigidity and tremor, but that still presents other symptoms. From the medical point of view, DBS is thus only a part of the neurological therapy of Parkinson's disease.

In some centers, microelectrode recordings are performed to guide the stimulating electrode towards the target. Here, recording of ongoing activity in the structures on the penetration track can identify the exact position of the electrode. However, microelectrode recording is connected with a greater risk of bleedings, which are a serious complication in 2%–3% of the subjects treated with DBS. The risk-benefit ratio of such microelectrode recordings has not been established yet. Seizures and infections are the next most frequent complications. Wire breakage or IPG malfunction may occur in 8%–19% of the devices. If other functional contacts can be used for achieving the desired therapeutic effects, stimulation can be switched to the other electrodes.

Other motor disorders treated with DBS are dystonias (pathological changes of muscle tone, often limited to one part of the body). Here the usual target is the internal part of the pale globe. The beneficial mechanisms of DBS are even more obscure in dystonia than in Parkinson's disease and the therapeutic effect is delayed (months) and progressive. Interestingly, in some cases after a long stimulation time, the beneficial effects persist even days after the stimulation has been switched off. In essential tremor, stimulation of the subthalamic nucleus has been a successful treatment. Both essential tremor and dystonia treatment with DBS are approved by the FDA.

Animal models suggested that DBS might be an effective treatment of epilepsy, with targets in the mammilothalamic tract, anterior nucleus of the thalamus, and hippocampus. These are components of one important brain circuit called the circuit of Papez (involved in memory). Lesioning of these targets increases the threshold for induction of epileptic seizures. This has led to a clinical trial on this therapy using DBS, with promising outcomes. However, subjects rarely become seizure-free.

With respect to modulation of mood (as originally suggested by Jose Delgado), potential targets investigated are the nucleus accumbens and lateral habenula as well as the ventromedial prefrontal cortex.

Other diseases where DBS could potentially ameliorate the symptoms (at least in a subset of subjects) are Tourette syndrome, major depression, bipolar disorder, obsessive-compulsive disorder, and anorexia nervosa. In these diseases, clinical trials are still needed to prove the effectiveness of electrostimulation.

Concluding remarks

It is interesting that such simple design of a stimulator is sufficient to cause clinically relevant effects. The effect of DBS is not a transmission of information to the brain, but rather a functional lesion (i.e., inactivation of the structure). This effect does not require an understanding of the neuronal representations at the stimulated structure, and the beneficial clinical outcome is sufficient for its usefulness.

Readers at this point may be surprised that voltage sources have been clinically used in this area despite what has been written in **Chapters 5 and 6**. However, since the amplitude of the electric stimulus in DBS is only of importance with respect to functional suppression threshold, the changes in applied charge over time as a consequence of the voltage-controlled power source may be of limited importance. Nonetheless, in more recent devices current sources are replacing voltage sources also in this domain due to better stability of the clinical outcomes over time.

It may be surprising to read that clinically, monophasic (thus not charge-balanced) pulses have been used for decades in this area. However, as mentioned above, the large size of the contact expands the range where charge is delivered via capacitive effects. Small lesions around the electrode, an effect observed in DBS and partly attributed to stimulation, may not be a problem in an application that is aimed at suppressing activity in the target region. Lesion and functional suppression lead to the same effects. Charge-balanced biphasic pulse stimulation is more effective in alleviating the symptoms, and therefore recent technology supports such modes.

Functional inactivation, compared to anatomical lesions, has the advantage of reversibility. This is of key importance. The basal ganglia are also involved in cognitive and linguistic tasks. Repeating the experience with frontal lobotomy, where initially the outcome appeared so beneficial and only later did the devastating cognitive consequence of the intervention become apparent, has led us to use caution when lesioning the brain, even when it is small in size or scope.

Finally, it remains to be emphasized that as we learn more about the exact functional characteristics of the nuclei that are the target of DBS, we will very likely come also to more refined stimulation strategies that will help to provide a more focused therapy. Closed-loop approaches, where the stimulation is delivered on demand (similar to cardiac pacemakers), may be a first step in this direction.

Brief summary

- Deep brain stimulation (DBS) uses pulse trains to functionally inactivate regions in the brain.
- DBS is clinically helpful in motor diseases that rely on a dynamic functional balance in the basal ganglia. Pathology causes an imbalance and leads to tremor and rigidity.
- Parkinson's disease, caused by loss of dopaminergic neurons in substantia nigra, causes such an imbalance.
- Inactivation of the subthalamic nucleus or part of the pale globe alleviates the symptoms of Parkinson's disease.
- DBS may also prove effective in other diseases that lead to a functional imbalance in the brain.

Key literature and further reading

Amon, A., Alesch, F., 2017. Systems for deep brain stimulation: review of technical features. J. Neural Transm. 124, 1083–1091.

Bain, P., Aziz, T., Liu, X., Nandi, D., 2009. Deep Brain Stimulation. Oxford University Press, Oxford.

Benabid, A.L., Pollak, P., Hoffmann, D., Gervason, C., Hommel, M., Perret, J.E., De Rougemont, J., Gao, D.M., 1991. Long-term suppression of tremor by chronic stimulation of the ventral intermediate thalamic nucleus. Lancet 337, 403–406.

Calixto, R., 2011. Investigation of Novel Auditory Implants of the Inferior Colliculus. PhD Thesis. Medizinische Hochschule Hannover.

Engel, A.K., Moll, C.K.E., Fried, I., Ojemann, G.A., 2005. Invasive recordings from the human brain: clinical insights and beyond. Nat. Rev. Neurosci. 6, 35–47.

Grill, W.M., 2005. Safety considerations for deep brain stimulation: review and analysis. Expert Rev. Med. Devices 2, 409–420.

Krauss, J.K., Lipsman, N., Aziz, T., Boutet, A., Brown, P., Chang, J.W., Davidson, B., Grill, W.M., Hariz, M.I., Horn, A., Schulder, M., Mammis, A., Tass, P.A., Volkmann, J., Lozano, A.M., 2020. Technology of deep brain stimulation: current status and future directions. Nat. Rev. Neurol. In press.

Lozano, A.M., Lipsman, N., Bergman, H., Brown, P., Chabardes, S., Chang, J.W., Matthews, K., McIntyre, C.C., Schlaepfer, T.E., Schulder, M., Temel, Y., Volkmann, J., Krauss, J.K., 2019. Deep brain stimulation: current challenges and future directions. Nat. Rev. Neurol. 15, 148–160.

Moshel, S., Shamir, R.R., Raz, A., de Noriega, F.R., Eitan, R., Bergman, H., Israel, Z., 2013. Subthalamic nucleus long-range synchronization-an independent hallmark of human Parkinson's disease. Front. Syst. Neurosci. 7, 79.

Okun, M.S., 2012. Deep-brain stimulation for Parkinson's disease. N. Engl. J. Med. 367, 1529–1538.

Sharott, A., Gulberti, A., Zittel, S., Tudor Jones, A.A., Fickel, U., Munchau, A., Koppen, J.A., Gerloff, C., Westphal, M., Buhmann, C., Hamel, W., Engel, A.K., Moll, C.K.E., 2014. Activity parameters of subthalamic nucleus neurons selectively predict motor symptom severity in Parkinson's disease. J. Neurosci. 34, 6273–6285.

CHAPTER 14

Peripheral nerve and spinal stimulation

Physiology of the nociceptive and somatosensory periphery

Animals are dependent on sensory information to navigate and interact with their environment. Our peripheral nervous systems use a complex network of sensory neurons that detect the position of the body (proprioception), the presence of other objects in physical contact with the body (somatosensation), and potentially body-damaging stimuli (nociception). These systems are closely interwoven as they provide complementary information about our internal and external environment, primarily with the goal of monitoring our body, its position in space, and its integrity.

The most common sensory receptors of these sensory pathways are **mechanoreceptors**. Mechanoreceptors convert mechanical information (pressure, stretch/strain, deformation) into neural signals, a process called **mechanotransduction.** The mechanotransductive elements within these cells have an ancient evolutionary history that can be traced across many diverse vertebrate and invertebrate animal groups. Typically, they use a specialized mechanosensitive apparatus connected to **mechanotransducer channels** on sensory nerve endings that depolarize neuronal membrane potential in response to mechanical forces and thus initiate an action potential. In mammals, there are many different types of mechanoreceptors, each with a specialized sensory apparatus that activates these channels in response to different stimuli properties (Fig. 14.1). Working in concert with mechanoreceptors are **thermoreceptors** and **pH-sensitive chemoreceptors** that give information about heat and acidity at the receptor site. **Polymodal** receptors respond to more than one type of stimuli, often in complex relationships that are dependent on priming or sensitization. Information from different receptor types can convey complex information about internal and external mechanical forces, including whether these forces are innocuous or represent a risk of tissue damage.

Somatosensory and nociceptive information is conveyed to the central nervous system (CNS) via afferent nerve fibers (conveying information from the periphery to the brain) that, in mammals, have their cell bodies located in the dorsal root ganglia (DRG) of the spinal cord or trigeminal ganglia in the head. Peripheral nerves have a complex anatomy consisting of a protective fatty nerve sheath called the **epineurium** that contains blood vessels and nerves bundled in an additional protective sheath called the **perineurium** (Fig. 14.2). Fibers within these bundles are classified according to their myelination and axonal diameter, originally for efferent fibers (from the brain to the muscle or effector organ) with letters (A, B, C), and for afferent fibers by Roman

Prostheses for the Brain
https://doi.org/10.1016/B978-0-12-818892-7.00013-4

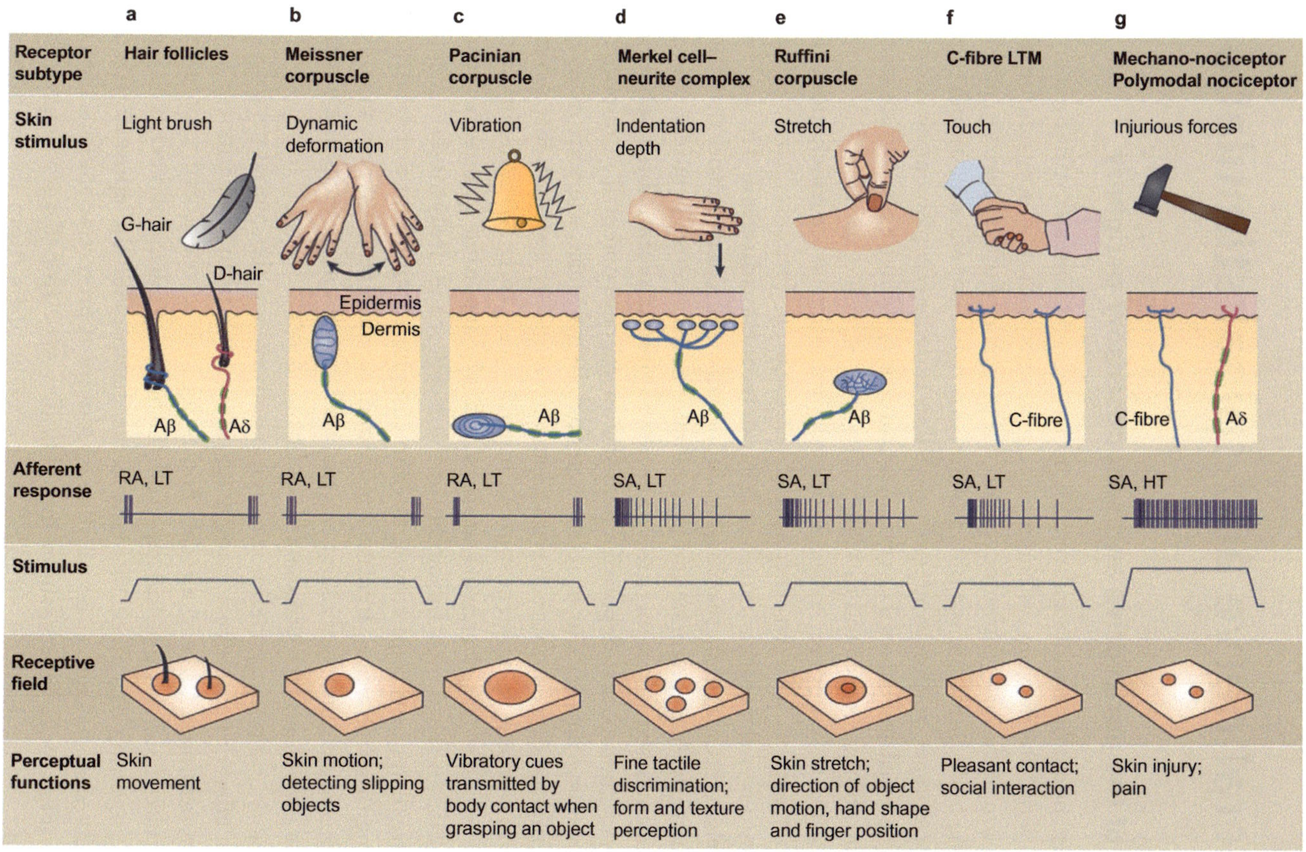

Fig. 14.1 Diagram of receptors in the human peripheral nervous system. The peripheral somatosensory and nociceptive system is comprised of receptors, primarily mechanoreceptive but also multimodal, with distinct sensory endings. The physical differences between the sensory apparatus, along with firing properties of the accompanying fibers (Aβ, Aδ, and C), allow for the detection and encoding of different forms of skin stimulus. *LTM*, low-threshold mechanoreceptor; *RA*, rapid adapting; *SA*, slow adapting; *HT*, high threshold; *LT*, low threshold. *(Figure from Delmas et al. (2011).)*

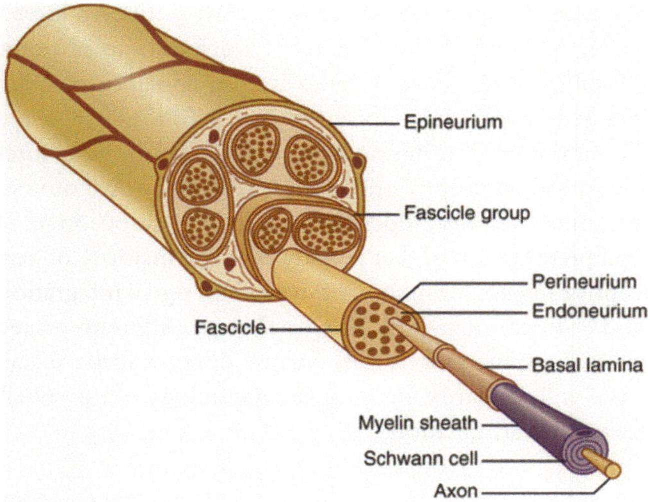

Fig. 14.2 Cross-sectional representation of a peripheral nerve. Peripheral nerves contain afferent and efferent axons that are bundled into fascicles, between which lies connective tissue and blood vessels. The entire nerve is encased in a protective sheathe called the epineurium. A surface electrode on a nerve is not in direct contact with neurons; it must still penetrate multiple layers of non-neural tissue across and within the epineurium and individual fascicles. Nerves in fascicles close to the electrode are likely to have lower thresholds. *(Figure from Neligan et al. (2013).)*

numerals (I–IV). However, the alphabet classification is today also used for afferents. **A-fibers** are myelinated fibers with either a large (**Aβ**) or medium (**Aδ**) axonal diameter and a higher conduction velocity.[a] Aβ fibers receive input from low-threshold mechanoreceptor nerve endings, while Aδ fibers receive a mix of input. **C-fibers** are unmyelinated, small diameter afferents with a slow conduction velocity. C-fibers convey vegetative information, but are also used for classification of afferent input from both low- and high-threshold mechanoreceptor and polymodal receptor nerve endings. In the afferent fibers, **group I/II fibers** have the thickest and most heavily myelinated axons and exclusively convey proprioceptive information about muscle/tendon position and tension. **Group III and IV fibers** are unmyelinated afferent fibers that convey thermoreception, pain, nociception, and information from chemical receptors.

As a rule of thumb, the Aβ input transmits somatosensory "touch" information, while the Aδ and C-fiber input transmit nociceptive "painful" information. Low-threshold C-fiber endings can also transmit the sensation of pleasant touch, and sensory priming (the expectation of a potentially painful stimulus) or sensitization/desensitization (via injury or inflammation, or receptor adaptation via repeated stimuli) can influence the resultant classification of the percept as "painful" or "innocuous." It is important to

[a] Aα fibers are the largest type and convey information to the skeletal muscles. They will not be considered here.

understand that nociception and the sensation of pain are distinct, if interdependent, concepts. Nociception is the purely physical detection of injurious or potentially injurious forces that can be used to either generate reflexes at the spinal cord or further relay them to the brain for the generation of a painful percept. Pain is the sensory experience and subsequent behavioral response to injurious or potentially injurious forces. Nociceptive sensory nerve endings and nociceptive fibers are essential for the conveyance of the percept of pain, but somatosensory, nociceptive, and proprioceptive elements are all involved in the final presentation of that percept. For the majority of peripheral somatosensory and nociceptive information, the first step of this signal integration and processing occurs at the A- and C-fiber synapses in the **spinal cord**. Afferents projecting from facial nerve endings bypass the spine and instead synapse directly at the thalamus via the **trigeminal nerve**. We will primarily focus on the physiology of the spinal cord as a more common site for electrical stimulation.

Neurophysiology of the spinal cord and dorsal horn

The spinal cord is a component of the CNS that extends from the medulla at the base of the brain down to the conus medullaris in the lower back. The primary role of the spinal cord is to process and convey both "**ascending**" sensory information to the brain, and "**descending**" motor commands from the brain (or via internally generated spinal reflexes) to the peripheral muscles. As part of the CNS, the spinal cord is surrounded by meningeal layers (dura, arachnoid, and pia mater) and bathed in the same cerebrospinal fluid (CSF) that surrounds the brain (Fig. 14.3). This is an important consideration for surgical implantation within the spinal cord; penetrating these protective layers is analogous to and carries similar risks to surgery on the brain itself.

The spinal cord itself is divided into regions defined by a combination of location, cellular anatomy, and function. Along the spine are longitudinal segments where paired motor and somatosensory nerve bundles (corresponding to physical regions of the body) leave or are integrated into the spinal cord, respectively. In essence, spinal segments are the semi-exposed entry/exit points for neural axons between the protective plates of the vertebrae. In the human, from the head downwards, these consist of the eight cervical, twelve thoracic, five lumbar, five sacral, and one coccygeal segments (thirty-one in total). At the spinal cord, combined somatosensory/motor nerve bundles are separated into **dorsal** (afferent) and **ventral** (efferent) nerve roots. The cell bodies of the ascending peripheral afferents for each segment are contained within the **dorsal root ganglia (DRG)** directly external to the **dorsal root entry zone (DREZ)**.

In cross-section, the spinal cord itself has three gross anatomical layers, which are further subdivided into regions. The outermost layer of the spinal cord contains the myelinated axonal tracts of the ascending and descending pathways, giving it a pale coloration. Further within is a gray region that contains neural cell bodies and synaptic connections, again separated into dorsal (ascending, afferent) and ventral (descending, efferent) regions or

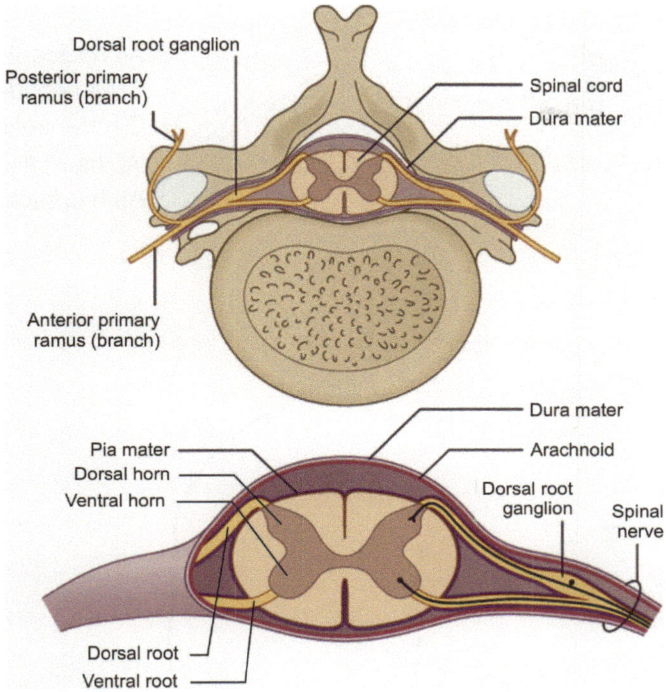

Fig. 14.3 Diagram showing gross spinal neuroanatomy. Like the brain, the spinal cord is encased in meningeal layers and bathed in CSF. The outer layer of the spinal cord contains white matter (ascending and descending nerve axons), while the inner layer contains gray matter (cell bodies and synapses). The most central part of the spinal cord is the CSF-containing central canal (not shown here). Peripheral nerves enter or leave the spine at each spinal segment and synapse at the dorsal horn (forked terminal in the lower image). The dorsal root ganglion contains the soma of the peripheral sensory neurons. *(Figure modified from Neligan et al. (2013).)*

"**horns**." The dorsal and ventral horns contain distinct layers with their own interneurons and complex synaptic connections that process information and generate spinal reflexes. Finally, the innermost chamber of the spinal cord is the central canal, which contains CSF and is directly connected to the ventricles within the brain. The spinal cord is heavily integrated with the structures of the brain and is more than a simple "tract" or pathway. For example, it contains the pattern generator circuit that controls walking gait. For the purposes of this chapter, we focus on a brief description of the dorsal horn, and in particular the superficial layers of the dorsal horn that are involved in the processing of nociceptive inputs, as this is the primary site of neuromodulation using implanted neuroprostheses.

Nociception at the dorsal horn

The **dorsal horn**, or posterior gray column, is a gray-matter region within the spinal cord that contains synapses between first-order ascending peripheral nerves and

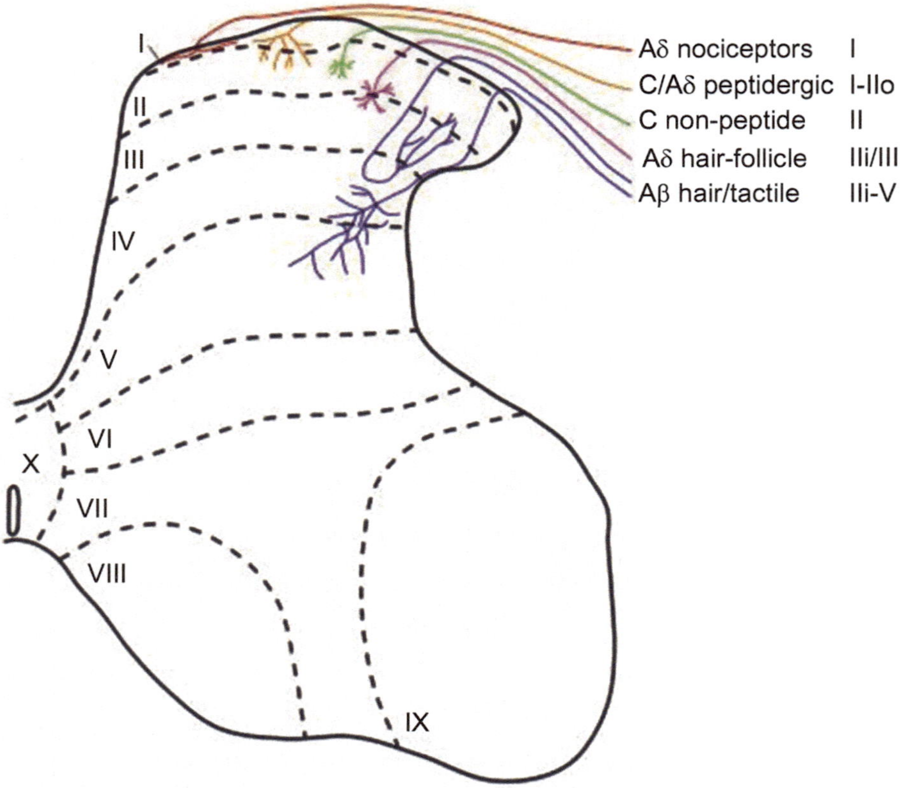

Fig. 14.4 Schematic showing the laminae of the dorsal horn and associated peripheral inputs relevant for the processing of pain. Nociceptive and somatosensory afferent terminations in the dorsal horn are organized into distinct laminae. Peripheral nociceptive information is received in lamina I, lamina II, and lamina V. Lamina II (substantia gelatinosa) is further divided into sublamina IIo (outer), IIid (inner dorsal), and IIiv (inner ventral). Interneurons with processes that span between these layers create a web of modulatory inhibition and excitation that shapes ascending input to the brain. *(Figure adapted from Todd (2011).)*

second-order neurons as well as the cell bodies of these second-order neurons. The dorsal and ventral horns are further separated into **laminar regions** I through X (Fig. 14.4). These laminae are not always anatomically discrete and their precise shape and location can vary from segment to segment. Instead, the laminae are better defined as functional regions that contain specific cell types and receive input from distinctive groups of A- and C-fibers. Synaptic transmission in the dorsal horn is primarily via glutamate release, mediated by secondary neuropeptides and GABAergic inhibitory interneurons.

Peripheral nociceptive information is received in three regions: lamina I, lamina II, and lamina V. **Lamina I**, or the *Marginal zone*, contains synaptic input from Aδ and

C-fibers, interneurons, and the synapses for ascending projections to the brain. Lamina I receives substantial input from both inhibitory and excitatory cells located in lamina II. **Lamina II**, or the *Substantia Gelatinosa*, is a complex layer that receives inputs from lamina I, C-fibers, and somatosensory Aβ/Aδ fibers from lamina III. It is further divided into sublamina II_o (*outer*), II_{id} (*inner dorsal*), and II_{iv} (*inner ventral*). Each sublaminae is defined by its discrete cellular and synaptic composition. Importantly, lamina II neurons do not project beyond the dorsal horn and are instead involved in processing of combined nociceptive/somatosensory information and subsequent modulation of lamina I ascending projections. Finally, **lamina V** contains input from Aβ and polysynaptic secondary inputs from the other nociceptive laminae. Laminae IV, V, and VI are involved in the multimodal processing of somatosensory input to convey more complex information such as texture and direction of movement as well as noxious percepts such as itch. The primary outputs of these laminae are wide dynamic range neurons (WDR neurons) that project to somatosensory regions in the brain.

There is no single brain "region" associated with the processing and sensation of pain as there is with visual or auditory sensory input. Instead, there is a "**pain matrix**" of areas that integrate and process aspects of the pain percept. Nociceptive information first reaches the brain at the brainstem, where it is relayed to higher brain areas such as the somatosensory cortex, the cingulate gyrus/insula, the prefrontal cortex, and the hypothalamus. Cortical processing of painful stimuli will not be further discussed in this chapter; along with spinal and dorsal horn physiology, it is a complex topic and, while this section provides a limited introduction, more detailed descriptions have been recommended in the further reading section at the end of the chapter.

Information processing principles in peripheral/spinal nociception

Information processing in the somatosensory and nociceptive systems must compensate for several discreet properties of the somato-nociceptive periphery. These systems carry a wide range of responses that are all behaviorally relevant and context dependent, ranging from soft touch/itch through to injurious forces. Somatosensory and nociceptive responses are integrated across a large spatial range and between many different cell types with unique or multimodal receptor properties and afferent fiber characteristics. Fast identification and reaction are vital for potentially injurious forces, but "false positive" responses must be avoided. Reflexive responses, where the sensory-motor loop is resolved in the spinal cord, are used to reduce response time for clear-cut injurious stimuli (e.g., rapid temperature changes), but often it is non-trivial for the system to quickly discriminate between various injurious and non-injurious stimuli.

Here we summarize several general principles that are particularly important for understanding how the nociceptive and somatosensory systems differentiate and encode information.

Gate control theory

The wide range of responses that can be elicited by closely associated sensory neurons in the nociceptive and somatosensory periphery creates a "gray area" between injurious and harmless forces, particularly when the system is deliberately under strain (e.g., when lifting a heavy object). Given that nociceptive stimuli carry a large energetic burden for the animal (in the form of escape responses, or stress/suffering), the normal-functioning system must have a mechanism to limit nociceptive "false positive" pain sensations arising from deliberate somatosensory interactions. The **gate control theory of pain** outlines one of the mechanisms by which somatosensory interactions can override pain sensations. Increased somatosensory activity in a peripheral region may block or "gate" the transmission of nociceptive activity in the same region. This is thought to occur at the dorsal horn where projection cells receive synaptic input from inhibitory interneurons, C-fibers and Aβ fibers (Fig. 14.5). The inhibitory "gate" shuts down the projection cell when activated. Excitatory inputs onto the inhibitory gate from the Aβ fiber enhance this inhibition ("gating" the nociceptive pathway), while inhibitory inputs from the C-fiber will reduce this inhibition ("opening" the nociceptive pathway). This allows for a discrimination between painful and somatosensory stimuli based on the dominant sensory input. A common behavioral example used to describe gate theory is the human tendency to "rub" or apply pressure on injured areas to relieve the associated painful sensation.

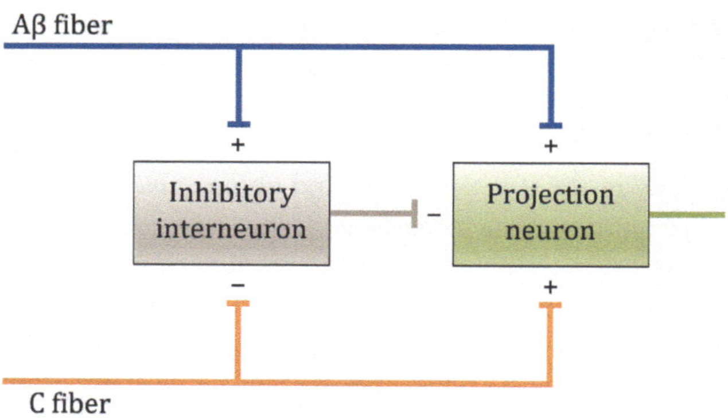

Fig. 14.5 The gate theory of pain control, as originally proposed by Melzack and Wall. Both somatosensory Aβ fibers and nociceptive C-fibers synapse on to projection neurons, which send output to the brain. Projection neurons received inhibitory modulation by inhibitory interneurons, which are in turn modulated by Aβ and C-fiber activity. The presence of somatosensory input excites the inhibitory interneuron, which in turn inhibits the projection neuron, "closing the gate" for nociceptive input. Nociceptive input at high enough intensities instead downregulates interneuron activity and so keeps the gate "open" for signal transmission to the brain. While the concept of gated nociceptive output is widely considered valid, the specifics of the circuit and molecular mechanisms remain controversial.

The significance of gate control and the physiology of gate control circuits is controversial. Gate theory has been a historically dominant explanation for pain control in the dorsal horn, and there is evidence to suggest that it does exist as one of several spinal control mechanisms to discriminate nociceptive and somatosensory stimuli. However, as the field of nociception and pain has matured, there has been continued recognition that teaching gate control theory as the *only* or even *primary* function of dorsal horn regulation of somatosensory/nociceptive input is overly reductionistic. Regardless, gate control theory plays an important role in the development and mechanistic explanation of many traditional spinal/peripheral neural implants used as therapies for the alleviation of pain. We discuss this further in the implant design and principles section of this chapter.

Short-term and long-term plasticity in the spinal cord

Another way the peripheral somatosensory/nociceptive systems can prioritize information, to both save energy and correctly identify the importance of the nociceptive component, is to either **sensitize** or **desensitize** peripheral input depending on the multimodal and temporal context of the stimuli. For example, inflammation due to bodily injury (e.g., bleeding) or infection sensitizes C-fibers, reducing their activation thresholds and changing their action potential characteristics. This ensures that detection of nociceptive input can be prioritized over somatosensory input when there is pre-existing evidence of injury or vulnerability. Conversely, repeated activation of some peripheral fibers leads to their **adaptation**, reducing their firing rate and desensitizing them to further input. In combination, this lets the peripheral neurons respond optimally when there is multi-modal evidence of injury, or when there is a sudden change in sensory input, without overburdening the system during normal behavior. At the dorsal horn, information can be prioritized via **short-term potentiation (STP)** (as in the above processes of sensitization), **long-term potentiation (LTP)**, and other cellular memory processes. While these processes were described in more detail in **Chapter 9**, in short, the relative timing of synaptic inputs can bias the responsiveness of a neuron to further input. For STP this can occur for short periods <30 min, whereas for LTP, this can last many hours or days and lead to epigenetic changes that are potentially lifelong. This allows for spinal nociceptive processing to further prioritize repeated stimuli when the pattern of repetition may indicate continued injury (and de-prioritize irrelevant stimuli). Moreover, stimuli with a strong temporal cohesion (i.e., that arrive in synchrony or with well-defined timing) are more likely to represent detection of a "real" stimulus and thus can be prioritized over random, desynchronized activity. Together with peripheral mechanisms, spinal horn sensitization/desensitization is another mechanism by which stimuli can be classified according to their relative behavioral importance. In addition, sensitization mechanisms act as a form of "gain control" that allow for a larger dynamic range of responses to be encoded for each sensory input.

Sensitization and desensitization mechanisms have direct application both as an explanation for the failure of some neuroprosthestic devices to provide chronic relief and as a potential therapeutic mechanism for others.

Central control in the peripheral and spinal nociceptive pathway

There is a level of subjective context involved in whether stimuli from the nociceptive periphery are interpreted as painful. Multi-sensory cues such as additional visual information can give context to nociceptive stimulus, to better identify the location and extent of physical damage. Similarly, the expectation of a painful stimulus can enhance the sensitivity of the painful percept, while thermal stimuli can even become pleasurable rather than painful depending on the environmental context (e.g., a cold shower when you are hot and vice versa). Brain areas involved in reward can gate activity in the spinal ascending pathways associated with the sensation of painful stimuli. This is thought to be part of a **feed-forward** system that can be biased depending on the *expectation* of a painful or pleasurable stimulus.

Context-dependent classification is performed by central cognitive processes to create a **central representation of pain**. These processes use descending serotonergic and noradrenergic **feedback control** mechanisms to further regulate the balance between spinal nociceptive and somatosensory processing. For this, a dedicated circuit exists. The serotoninergic and noradrenergic neurons synapse on opioid neurons in the spinal cord and opioid synapses effectively reduce the excitability within the pain neurons of the spinal cord. This descending pain pathway originates in a nucleus in the brainstem called periaqueductal gray and the application of opioids to relieve from pain acts primarily (but not exclusively) on this circuit. Thus, central processes are inextricably linked with peripheral processes in the classification of nociceptive stimuli as painful or innocuous. This is an important consideration for the interpretation of patient outcomes in peripherally implanted devices: the patient's *perception* of possible therapeutic outcomes and stimulation percepts can influence not only subjective patient reports but also peripheral measures of the response.

Chronic neuropathic pain

The sensation of pain is the most common reason that people seek medical attention. However, for many cases, this pain plays a vital protective role, signaling the presence of bodily harm or damage. While it may be unpleasant to experience, by causing sufferers to seek aid, the sensation of pain is helping them receive treatment for their underlying condition, preventing further injury and potentially saving their lives. This is fundamentally distinct from chronic pathological pain, which no longer serves a useful physiological purpose and can occur separate from the presence of injury, or else persist for months or years after the initial injury has been repaired. When this occurs, the sensation of pain itself becomes a pathology that needs to be treated. Chronic pain is one of the world's most common healthcare conditions, affecting >20% of the world population and severely impairing quality of life. Plastic adaptation to pain that occurs as a consequence of brain plasticity may represent a maladaptive consequence of the ability of pain circuits to undergo LTP on their synapses (as described previously). Chronic pain is a varied and complex phenomenon that can be broadly classified into two main forms: **nociceptive pain** and **neuropathic pain**. There are other forms of pathologic pain that do not fit neatly into these categories, although they will not be discussed in further detail here.

Nociceptive pain occurs when non-neural tissue has sustained injury or inflammation that results in the perception of pain even after the original tissue has healed. For the most part, current pharmacologic analgesic treatments (including non-steroidal analgesics and opioids) that are used to treat acute pain are also effective at treating nociceptive pain, although these may come with associated risks of serious negative side effects including toxicity, in the case of opioid addiction and abuse. Electrical stimulation is usually only indicated for nociceptive pain as a second-line treatment for the subset of patients where analgesic drugs are ineffective or contraindicated.

It is also possible for an injury or disease process to cause direct damage or otherwise interfere with the function of the somatosensory and nociceptive tissues themselves. This creates a malfunction in the processing or perception of pain that leads to the sensation of a chronic painful stimulus even when there is no tissue damage. This form of pain is called **neuropathic pain** and it is strikingly common, affecting between 1.5% and 8% of the world population. Neuropathic pain is much more difficult to diagnose and treat. This has created an opportunity for the therapeutic use of electrical neurostimulation as a first-line treatment for patients with neuropathic pain.

There are multiple underlying etiologies that can lead to the formation of neuropathic pain, including peripheral nerve or spinal injury, brain injury or stroke, diabetes, pathogens such as HIV/AIDS, cancer, or even as a side effect of other pharmaceutical therapies (particularly chemotherapies). Symptoms can vary considerably depending on the etiology and include **hyperalgesia** (increased pain response) and **allodynia** (pain in response to an innocuous stimulus) (Fig. 14.6). **Spontaneous** ("shock"-like) and **continuous** ("burning") pain without any accompanying physical stimulation can also occur. These sensations are not only intrinsically unpleasant but can also interfere with normal somatosensory and nociceptive function in the affected area, which can lead to further injury or dysfunction. They can also interfere with normal motor function, as pain increases muscle tone to immobilize the affected body region. A comprehensive treatment of neuropathic pain has proven difficult. Opioids are particularly ineffective at treating neuropathic pain. Other first-line pharmaceutical treatments have been developed that are more effective (e.g., gabapentinoids); however, these treatments are typically only efficacious for a subset of neuropathic pain patients. It is also difficult to predict patient

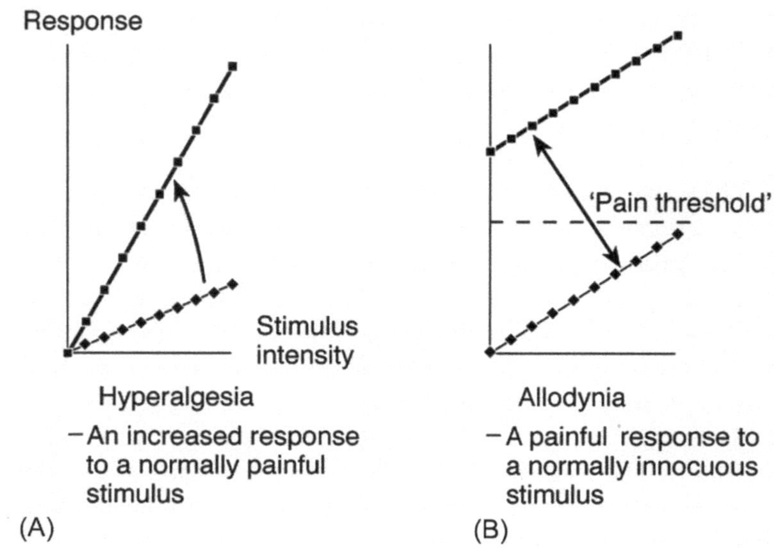

Fig. 14.6 Graphical representation of stimulus intensity vs system response in the somatosensory/nociceptive systems. During hyperalgesia (A), as stimulus intensity increases, the sensitized nociceptive system has an inappropriately amplified output. This leads to mildly painful stimuli becoming severely painful. During Allodynia (B), the nociceptive system interprets all output as painful regardless of the intensity of the stimulus, but does not further amplify this output as the intensity increases. This leads to normally painless mechanical stimulus (i.e., somatosensory stimulus) becoming painful. *(Figure from Campbell et al. (2006).)*

outcomes from their underlying etiologies or presenting symptoms. The reason why treatment success has been so variable should be clear if one considers the complexity of pain signal control discussed in the previous section. Neuropathic pain can create a fundamental reorganization of the classification of pain that occurs not only at the initial site but also up and downstream in the nociceptive and somatosensory periphery, the spinal cord, and in the brain (both the thalamus and cortex). This reorganization occurs slowly over the course of weeks to years and can lead to permanent alterations in synaptic weights, connectivity, epigenetic expression, and eventually entire cortical and spinal anatomies. **Acute and neuropathic pain have fundamentally different mechanisms.** This explains why acute and chronic neuropathic pain respond so differently to pharmacologic treatments. While acute pain occurs due to a stimulus response to injury, neuropathic pain occurs due to a fundamental "re-classification" of what constitutes a painful stimulus, potentially at all levels of the nociceptive and somatosensory pathway.

Neuropathic pain is so heterogeneous in its presentation and treatment because the precise *form* of reorganization leading to the chronic painful percept is also heterogeneous. For example, following nerve injury, excitatory synaptic processes in the dorsal horn are enhanced (sensitized), while inhibitory processes are attenuated. This can occur due to changes in the expression of voltage-gated sodium or calcium channels within the nociceptive periphery (Aδ and C-fibers). Alternatively, changes in genomic expression in glial "support" cells in lamina II can create hyperexcitability or influence the susceptibility of lamina II neurons to LTP, enhancing responses to previously innocuous stimuli. Continuing along the same line of thought, central changes in cortical and subcortical areas of pain processing can increase responses of the spinal cord to nociceptive stimuli (in effect, creating a physiological unconscious increase in the *expectation* of pain, which in turn sensitizes spinal responses).

These are just several of many mechanisms by which reorganization of pain pathways in neuropathic pain can produce a single outcome. The overall conclusion of this intricate web of pain signal reorganization is a disease with a complex molecular underpinning, making it difficult to treat pharmacologically. The persistent and debilitating effect of neuropathic pain on behavior and quality of life can persist or progress even after the original initiating cause of the pain has long since been treated. Given our current level of understanding of neuropathic pain and its systemic complexity, it is a condition that will likely only be managed by therapeutic treatments rather than comprehensively cured, at least in the near future.

Pain neuromodulation

Electrical neuromodulation in neuropathic pain provides an avenue for pain management that holds several advantages over traditional pharmaceutical approaches and helps to improve the quality of life of those where other therapeutic options are not sufficiently helpful. The use of implantable electrical stimulation for the treatment of neuropathic and other chronic pain disorders has historically been an area of clinical interest, owing to the large patient population, high disease burden, relative accessibility of the spinal and peripheral nociceptive/somatosensory systems compared to the brain, and the lack of efficacious pharmacological treatment options. The first commercially available semi-implantable stimulators used for the treatment of chronic pain were developed in 1968, but difficult surgery, a bulky external power source, and poor patient outcomes meant that the field remained nascent until advances in technology led by the success of the cochlear implant (CI) and deep brain stimulation (DBS) created a resurgence of interest in fully implantable pain control devices. Pain control is distinct from many other forms of electrical stimulation of the nervous system in that it is focused on the elimination or modulation of a gained sensory dysfunction, while most other applications seek to restore a lost sensory function (e.g., cochlear or retinal prostheses). This is why electrical stimulation for the control of pain is more commonly called **neuromodulation**, that is, the modulating control of a neural signal rather than an increase in neural activity per se as "stimulation" might imply. Today, pain neuromodulation is a successful and growing field that may establish itself as a first-line treatment for chronic pain disorders. Current-generation devices use either invasive or non-invasive modulation approaches as well as either electrical or non-electrical modulation paradigms (e.g., ultrasound; see **Chapter 16**). In the next section, we further examine invasive electrical neuromodulation and outline the basic principles of operation useful for understanding the range of suitable approaches used in clinical devices today.

Basic principles of operation

As discussed in the previous section, neuropathic pain can induce hypersensitive function at all parts of the pain pathway. Dysfunction can occur at the nociceptive/somatosensory receptive terminals, the afferent nerve, pain processing at the dorsal horn, or centrally within the brain. Of these locations, implantable neuromodulation has focused on stimulation of the afferent nerve and, particularly, stimulation at the dorsal column to modulate the conduction of the pain information to the brain. While some approaches have focused on deep brain stimulation, this is less common due to the additional associated surgical difficulty. Neuromodulation of sensory endings near the skin is much easier to achieve with non-invasive approaches, making implantable devices less appealing in this context. Implantable technologies have focused on the segments of the pain pathway that are relatively straightforward to access surgically, but too deep to be easily modulated non-invasively. As discussed, most neuromodulation implants are designed to treat neuropathic pain, particularly **failed back surgery syndrome (FBSS)**, as this condition is relatively common and in many cases has few or no alternative treatment options.

Neuromodulation implants generally follow a basic design pattern that they share with other neural stimulation devices. Current FDA-approved devices[b] consist of an **implantable pulse generator (IPG)** implanted subcutaneously, a **lead wire**, and an **electrode** or **electrode array** that interfaces electrically with the target neural tissue (Fig. 14.7). Electrode arrays placed in the spinal cord typically have a flat paddle-like shape, while arrays that interface with peripheral nerves are ideally embedded in a cuff that surrounds the nerve. This is to increase surface area of the contact and minimize mechanical damage. However, both surgical positions have seen use of straight but flexible arrays similar in design to a cochlear implant. Electrode contact material is almost invariably platinum or a platinum/iridium alloy and has no notable difference from other electrode contact designs discussed in previous chapters in this book.

The majority of devices have an internal battery similar to pacemaker designs (**Chapters 2 and 13**), which is either replaceable or rechargeable, depending on power requirements. Power can also be supplied using a transcutaneous RF receiver as with a cochlear implant, although this is less common. More sophisticated devices contain

[b] Many companies produce devices that are undergoing FDA approval as neuromodulation implants. Companies with a significant market presence in this field include Medtronic and Boston Scientific.

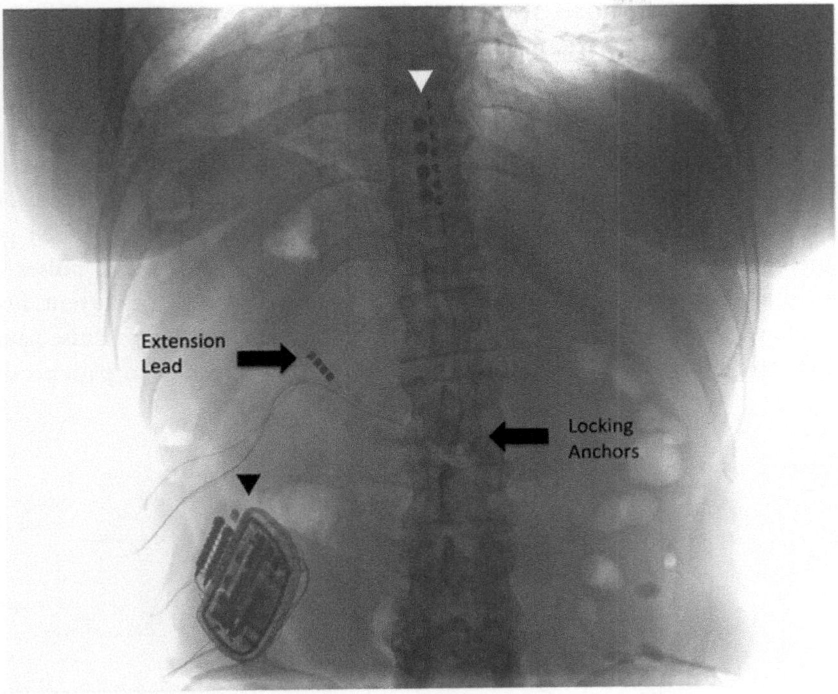

Fig. 14.7 Fluoroscopic image showing a spinal cord stimulator (SCS) with the IPG and power source *(black arrowhead)*, lead *(black arrows)*, and electrode array implanted in the spine *(white arrowhead)*. *(Figure adapted from Bunch et al. (2015).)*

recording electrodes and electronics to allow for closed-loop feedback control of the stimulation signal using compound action potential (CAP) measurements. It is also common for devices to have a wireless control system so that stimulation can be turned on/off or the intensity of the stimulation controlled directly by the patient. Patient control and closed-loop feedback systems are important because the threshold for therapeutic effect can vary over short time frames or due to physical factors such as whether a patient is upright or prone. The biggest difference compared to cochlear implants is that neuromodulation devices don't have any "capture" device: as there is no sensory information being conveyed, there is no need for an equivalent to a microphone or camera. Rather, the electrical waveforms follow set, pre-programmed patterns that are intended to inhibit or modulate pre-existing sensory processing at the target stimulation site, similar to deep brain stimulation (**Chapter 13**). There are several neuromodulation paradigms that each use a unique approach and mechanistic justification for the perceived pain relief.

Low-frequency spinal cord stimulation

Implanted at the spinal cord, the original neuromodulation devices used the basic principle of **gate theory** to explain their therapeutic effect. The proposed mechanism of operation in these devices is the indirect antidromic modulation of WDR neurons in the dorsal horn via excitation of dorsal column Aβ fibers, inhibiting co-processing of nociceptive information in the spinal cord and generating a "masking" somatosensory percept or **paresthesia** (Fig. 14.8). These **spinal cord stimulators (SCS)** generate low-frequency (~40–60 Hz) sinusoids, monophasic pulses, or biphasic pulses. Waveforms are usually generated via a current source to maintain a constant current; however, constant voltage sources have also been used, owing to their simplicity. Pulse parameters used in low-frequency spinal cord stimulators are usually matched to patients during a

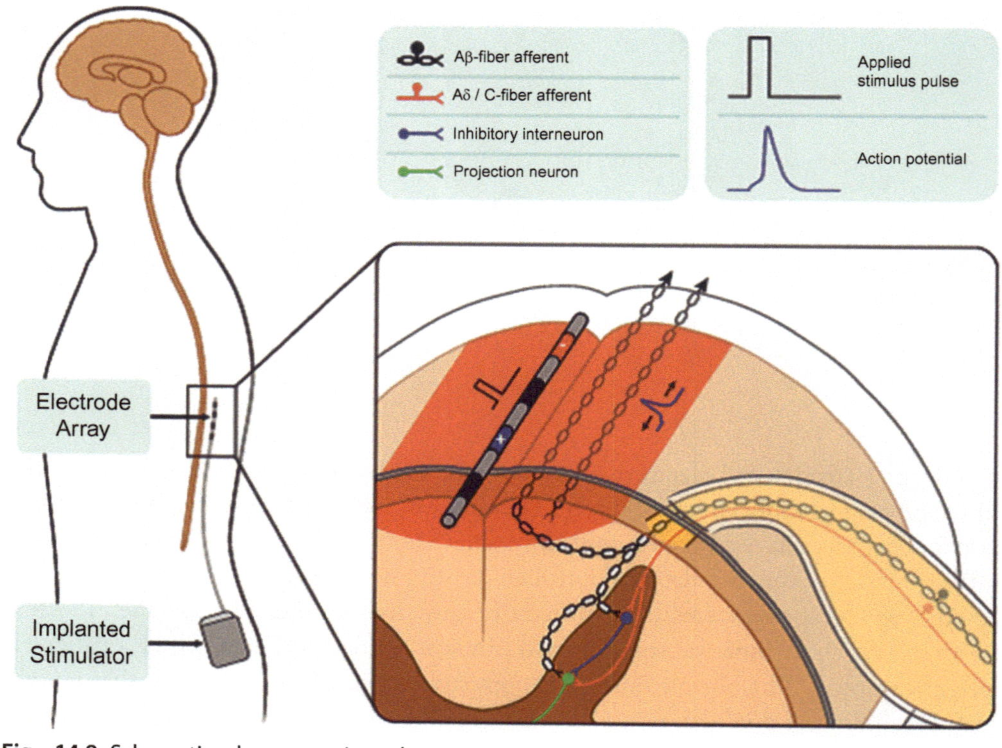

Fig. 14.8 Schematic demonstrating the most commonly accepted mechanism of action for conventional spinal cord stimulators. The electrode array in the epidural space delivers low-frequency (~40–60 Hz) pulses or sinusoids that primarily stimulate the large diameter (and so low threshold) Aβ fibers in the dorsal columns. Antidromic (back-propagating) action potentials generated by these fibers travel to the dorsal horn, where they activate inhibitory interneurons to prevent the transmission of peripheral nociceptive signals to the brain. Orthodromic action potentials travel to the brain where they generate a somatosensory percept called paresthesia. *(Figure from Lempka and Patil (2018).)*

post-implantation fitting session. Pulse durations are typically within the range of hundreds of microseconds to milliseconds. Voltages lie within the range of millivolts to volts, while current amplitudes range from microamps to milliamps.

While these basic spinal cord stimulators are still clinically implanted today, their usage has been slowly phased out in preference of more sophisticated stimulation paradigms (see Fig. 14.9). This is because low-frequency stimulation comes with significant drawbacks. Firstly, for many patients, paresthesia generation can often be inherently uncomfortable/painful on its own, which invalidates the use of these devices for those patients. This is a problem for patient selection as it is not always easy to determine which patients will respond well to paresthesia sensations. Sensory masking also interferes with the normal somatosensory function of the affected area. Over time, the masked area can drift, leading to a complete loss of therapeutic benefit if the paresthesia is no longer co-located with the pain. In many cases and especially for voltage sources, deformation of the tissue around the spine (such as when bending or lying down) can change the electrical properties of the tissue around the stimulator and interfere with the masking effect.

Burst stimulation

Novel stimulation patterns have more recently been developed to overcome the limitations associated with traditional neuromodulation waveforms discussed previously. **Burst stimulation** is a stimulation pattern that is similar to traditional SCS except that it uses repetitive pulse trains at a higher base frequency, separated by gaps in stimulation (e.g., a train of 1 ms mono- or biphasic pulses at 500 Hz, separated by a burst frequency at 40 Hz; Fig. 14.9B). This paradigm is intended to mimic neural bursting patterns that are a common information coding mechanism in the nervous system, and have been recorded in ascending pathway dorsal horn network activity. The advantage of burst pulse trains is that they appear to produce an equal or greater analgesic effect than standard SCS stimulation paradigms, with a reduction in the percept of paresthesia. Burst pattern firing is thought to modulate synaptic plasticity in the dorsal horn via activation of timing-dependent LTP mechanisms, although this has not been conclusively shown. Burst activity also appears to selectively target some neurons in the dorsal horn, such as WDR neurons, over other neurons in the dorsal column nuclei, which may explain the reduced sensation of paresthesia.

High-frequency spinal cord stimulation

Dorsal horn stimulation has also been tested using pulse train or sinusoidal stimulation at high frequencies in the 1–10 kHz range, called **high frequency stimulation (HFS**, Fig. 14.9C**)**. Due to high-frequency stimulation, only charge-balanced waveforms such as biphasic pulses or sinusoids are used to provide safe charge delivery. The resulting effect on the dorsal column is a reduction in activity, even with charge delivery well above standard SCS thresholds. This is likely because voltage-sensitive channel kinetics in

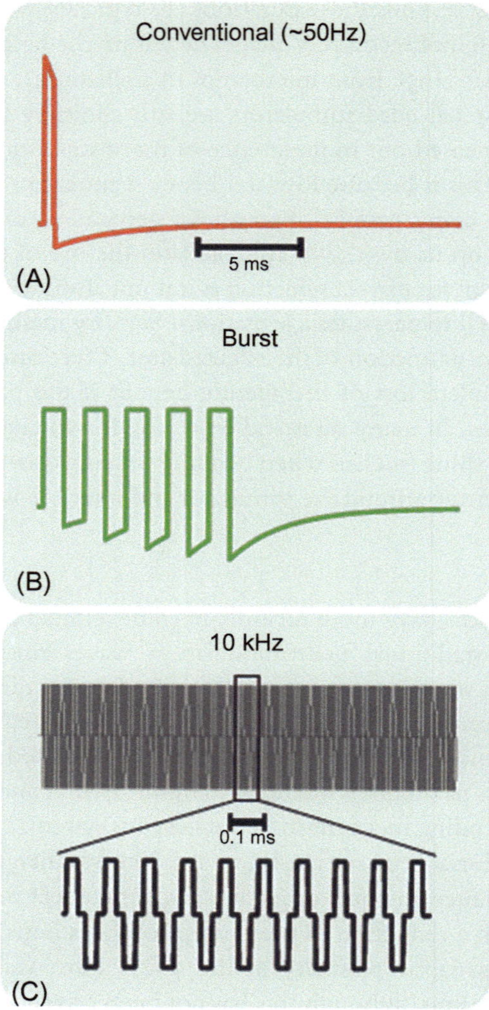

Fig. 14.9 Visual example of stimulator waveforms used in spinal cord stimulation. Conventional waveforms (A) are low (~40–60 Hz) frequency pulses (or occasionally sinusoids). Burst waveforms (B) deliver repetitive pulse trains at a higher frequency (~500 Hz), which are separated by longer burst frequencies at a similar range to conventional waveforms. High-frequency waveforms (C) deliver alternating biphasic or square wave pulses at very high frequencies, such that the interpulse gap is often shorter than the pulse itself (~1–20 KHz). The therapeutic mechanism of action is likely different for each waveform, and remains poorly understood, especially for burst and high-frequency stimulators. *(Figure from Lempka and Patil (2018).)*

the dorsal horn are not conducive to action potential initiation at such high frequencies. The mechanism for analgesia HFS is substantially different from conventional SCS. The effect is due to modulation of dorsal horn excitability, but the exact mechanism is poorly understood. HFS has distinct advantages over low-frequency pulse trains. Firstly, due to the lack of broad stimulation in the dorsal column, there is very little or no paresthesia associated with HFS at clinically effective current amplitudes. This means that a broader area can be modulated without risk of unwanted paresthesia in the normal-functioning sensory regions. As a consequence, the HFS lead can be implanted to modulate neurons over a larger spinal region, increasing the likelihood of therapeutic benefit, removing the need for intraoperative paresthesia mapping and decreasing the possibility that post-operative slip of the lead position will disrupt the analgesic effect.

Peripheral nerve block

An alternative site of neuromodulation for control of pain sensation is the peripheral afferent nerve. **Peripheral nerve block** seeks to disrupt the nociceptive stimulus before it can reach the spinal cord, providing analgesic relief. Peripheral neuromodulation is an attractive alternative to SCS because the surgical risk associated with peripheral nervous system implantation is significantly less than that of spinal cord surgery. This lowers the regulatory bar necessary to approve peripheral neuromodulation therapies, and opens up a pool of patients where spinal surgery would be considered too risky for the perceived therapeutic gain. However, peripheral nerve block and SCS are delivering different forms of therapy and thus are not directly comparable. Rather than central masking or reduction of sensitivity, peripheral implants are blocking sensory input entirely, often of the entire affected nerve. Because nociceptive Aδ and C-fibers have small axon diameters, they have greater thresholds for electrical stimulation/modulation than somatosensory and motor fibers. As such, it is currently not possible for peripheral block to target *only* nociceptive inputs; instead, they provide general sensory (and, in mixed nerves, potentially also motor) inhibition. The ideal output of a peripheral implant would block only the nociceptive fibers; so far no clinical device has achieved this goal.

Down-modulation of peripheral afferents requires an electrical waveform that can directly inhibit action potential propagation. Normally, pulses generated via an internal pulse generator (IPG) can only excite neurons and very rarely suppress them (see also **Chapters 4**, **7** and **13**; downmodulation in the spinal cord is achieved indirectly via the excitation of inhibitory interneurons, which is not possible in afferent fibers). Non-standard waveforms are thus required to achieve inhibition of the afferent nerve. The first stimulation paradigm is **charge-balanced kilohertz frequency alternating current (KHFAC)**. Superficially similar to HFS in the spinal cord, KHFAC uses a 1–100 kHz sinusoidal, square current, or voltage waveform at amplitudes on the range of 1–10 mA/2–10 V in the sciatic nerve. Amplitudes above block threshold result in a brief period of intense excitation followed by a total propagation block of the afferent nerve (i.e., APs generated in the sensory periphery can no longer be transmitted to the spinal cord). Modeling and experimental work suggests that the mechanism of block is the holding of voltage-sensitive sodium channels in a constant state of inactivation (depolarization block; see **Chapters 4 and 7**). The onset excitation is a limitation for this approach, although there have been recent strategies proposed to mitigate this effect.

The second peripheral modulation paradigm is direct current block (**DC block**). DC blocks are constant current waveforms, usually stepped or ramped and held at a static value. DC block thresholds are variable depending on the strength of the electrical contact to the nerve, but have been reported in the range of 50 μA to 1–2 mA in the sciatic nerve. DC block can be either anodic (+) or cathodic (−). Anodic block works by hyperpolarizing the tissue until APs can no longer drive enough membrane potential shift to open voltage-gated sodium channels. Cathodic block works similar to KHFAC in that it causes tonic inactivation of voltage-gated sodium channels due to highly depolarized membrane potentials, also preventing AP propagation. Cathodic block normally has a lower threshold than anodic block. A significant advantage of DC block is that sub-block amplitudes also have physiological interactions that can be exploited, such as amplitude-dependent inhibition/excitation and subthreshold spike latency/sensitivity modulation. The biggest drawback of DC waveforms is that they are difficult to "charge balance"; a true DC waveform is inherently not charge balanced and thus chronically unsafe. There are several technologies that can work around this problem. Common solutions are to design an implant so that multiple electrode contacts are "cycled" (with one electrode providing current to the nerve while others are in a recovery phase) or else to physically separate the DC electrodes using a fluidic conduit and replace them before toxic electrochemical byproducts can diffuse to the nerve. DC is also used extensively in non-invasive therapies for pain where charge balance is much less important. DC block and KHFAC can even be combined so that DC provides an initial, onset response-less inhibition that can be followed by KHFAC while the DC electrodes recover charge. This strategy potentially mitigates the primary drawback of both approaches. Both KHFAC and DC block are relatively new approaches that have shown promising preclinical and early clinical results; however, neither have yet seen full commercial translation. Their most immediate application is for post-surgical acute pain but also chronic peripheral pain in, for example, amputees.

Alternative targets for peripheral neuromodulation

While the majority of stimulation for pain neuromodulation has focused on the spinal cord and accompanying peripheral nerves, these therapies are not useful for cranial pain (most commonly, chronic headache or migraine), which does not pass through the spinal ascending pathways. **Cranial neuromodulation implants** instead focus on neuromodulation of pathways in the cranial nociceptive system: the *sphenopalatine ganglion*, the *trigeminal nucleus caudalis*, and the *occipital nerve*. These approaches are relatively new and so far have only been tested with simple SCS-like pulse train waveforms. Clinical devices that modulate these targets have shown varied but generally positive patient outcomes. However, there is a limited understanding of the mechanisms of action for this approach and active research is needed to properly understand the physiology behind the published results.

Another rapidly growing area of research is **vagal nerve neuromodulation**. The vagus nerve contains fibers that provide parasympathetic control of the heart, lungs, and digestive tract, as well as contributes to immune system response via an inflammatory reflex. Stimulation of the vagus nerve could potentially lower inflammatory responses that play a role in the onset and maintenance of not only neuropathic pain but also auto-inflammatory diseases such as inflammatory bowel disease and arthritis. Vagus nerve stimulation is also a target for headaches/migraines due to a secondary interruption of the spinal trigeminal nucleus. Beyond the scope of chronic pain, the vagus nerve also holds potential for the modulation of autonomic functions (e.g., for the treatment of lung and heart conditions). These applications are complicated by the multiple conflicting functions of the vagus and the possibility of inappropriate stimulation/inhibition of vital parasympathetic functions. Finally, very recent approaches used spinal stimulation as a method for alleviating motor consequences of spinal cord injury on stand and walking. This new experimental approach bears promise for future new therapies of paraplegia.

Measuring clinical outcomes

The sensation of chronic pain is fundamentally and physiologically intertwined with subjective conscious perception. Patients can report very different magnitudes of pain for the same magnitude of nociceptive input, and this reflects a real and physiologically grounded subjective difference in the *percept* or *experience* of that pain. This is a fundamental property of pain perception that cannot be "filtered" out as noise or otherwise ignored when pain management outcomes are considered. After all, central in many forms of chronic pain is the presence of pain percepts that are inappropriate to the magnitude of the nociceptive stimulus.

The subjective nature of pain perception makes measurement of patient outcomes in chronic pain management difficult to achieve. Currently, there is no quantifiable physiological measure of an individual's pain percept. Instead, clinicians primarily rely on **self-reporting** to determine clinical outcomes in pain therapies. Self-reporting does not mean unquantifiable. A number of scientific tools and approaches can be used to better standardize self-reporting assessments between studies to allow for useful comparisons of efficacy. These tools allow for a final pain-reduction quantification, which can then be used with a cutoff value to assess efficacy. The most commonly accepted cutoff threshold for clinical significance is a 30% reduction in self-reported pain.

The most common form of pain measure is via **questionnaires**. These are standardized forms that allow a patient to self-report in a way that can more easily be compared between patients. Pain questionnaires come in two main forms: **unidimensional scale** questionnaires and **multidimensional scale** questionnaires. Unidimensional questionnaires are very simple and straightforward measures that rank outcomes on a single discreet scale, such as "0–10" or "very much improved" to "very much worse." They typically involve only one or few items (questions). Unidimensional self-reporting scales are fast and, due to their ubiquity in modern life beyond the medical context, easily understood by patients. Due to their simplicity, many unidimensional questionnaires can be administered to patients verbally (i.e., the doctor asks the questions rather than the patient marking their responses on a sheet), which is important when patients have low or no mobility (common for severe chronic pain). The primary limitation of unidimensional scales is that they provide only coarse data that has low statistical power and must be carefully controlled for bias. For example, different cultures can have systematic differences in how they respond to questions about pain. Some examples of unidimensional scale questionnaires used in pain management include the numerical rating score (NRS), the visual analogue scale (VAS), verbal rating scale (VRS), and patient global impression of change (PGIC).

Given the complexity of the pain percept, more sophisticated self-report measurements are often required alongside the simple unidimensional scales. When many different dimensions of subjective experience are reported (such as pain intensity, frequency, functional impairment, general quality of life, etc.) a questionnaire becomes a **multidimensional scale** questionnaire. By increasing the complexity of the self-reported assessment, multidimensional scales have greater statistical power, can better control for patient bias, and allow for a comparison between reported pain intensity and reported functional disability. However, they are often lengthy and difficult to conduct verbally, which is a consideration for patients with a high degree of functional disability. Moreover, quantitative comparisons between different multidimensional questionnaires can be difficult. Common multidimensional questionnaires include the short-form McGill pain questionnaire (SF-MPQ), the brief pain inventory short form (BPI-SF), the West Haven-Yale multidimensional pain inventory (WHYMPI), and the treatment outcomes of pain survey (TOPS).

Finally, when patients are incapable of reliable self-reporting (such as infants), or when used in conjunction with questionnaires, qualitative measurements can be taken by assessing behavioral responses of individuals, such as posture, gait, and object manipulation. Behavioral responses are qualitative and can be unreliable. They are only used to support quantitative measures unless other assessments are impossible to administer in specific cases.

No currently available neuromodulation implant has shown consistently high (>70%) reductions in measures of chronic pain. More typically, pain reduction measures in clinical trials have hovered around the cutoff for clinical significance (>30%). SCS trials commonly report a loss of therapeutic effect over time, either due to habituation to the electrical stimulation or a progression of the underlying disease state. However, given the dearth of available therapies for chronic neuropathic pain and the dramatic impact it has on quality of life, even marginal clinical significance is considered ethically justifiable (and economically viable) for the commercial translation of neuromodulation devices. The desire for better patient outcomes and a more consistently reliable intervention continues to actively drive scientific, technological, and commercial innovation in this field.

Brief summary

- Pain is distinct from nociception. Nociception is the physical detection of potentially injurious forces by the peripheral nervous system. Pain is the interpretation of those signals by the central nervous system.
- Somatosensory (touch) and nociceptive (pain) systems have overlap in function, with some receptors encoding both injurious and non-injurious forces.
- The spinal cord is where most nociceptive and somatosensory information is first centrally processed. Synaptic inputs between first- and second-order neurons are located with a laminar structure called the dorsal horn.
- There are feedback and feed-forward projections from the spine to the brain, which modulate the function of spinal processing and peripheral sensitivity.
- Neuropathic pain is the chronic malfunction of the processing or perception of pain even when there is no underlying tissue damage.
- Electrical neuromodulation attempts to block pain signals or else reduce their intensity using electrical currents delivered externally or with an implant.
- The most common implants are spinal cord stimulators (SCS), which use pulsed current or voltage waveforms to generate somatosensory sensations (paresthesia) that "mask" the painful stimuli.
- More recent implants have delivered pulses in a burst pattern or at very high frequencies. It is also possible to deliver DC waveforms rather than pulses.
- Neuromodulation has demonstrated clinical efficacy, but the magnitude of the therapeutic benefit remains mild. Continued research aims to improve these outcomes.

Key literature and further reading

Alles, S.R.A., Smith, P.A., 2018. Etiology and pharmacology of neuropathic pain. Pharmacol. Rev. 70, 316–347.

Basbaum, A.I., et al., 2010. Cellular and molecular mechanisms of pain. Cell 139 (2), 267–284.

Bunch, J.R., Goldstein, H.V., Hurley, R.W., 2015. Complete coverage of phantom limb and stump pain with constant current SCS system: a case report and review of the literature. Pain Pract. 15 (1), 20–26. https://doi.org/10.1111/papr.12226.
Campbell, J.N., Meyer, R.A., 2006. Mechanisms of neuropathic pain. Neuron 52 (1), 77–92. https://doi.org/10.1016/j.neuron.2006.09.021.
Delmas, P., Hao, J., Rodat-Despoix, L., 2011. Molecular mechanisms of mechanotransduction in mammalian sensory neurons. Nat. Rev. Neurosci. 12, 139–153.
Fishman, M.A., et al., 2019. The evolution of neuromodulation in the treatment of chronic pain: forward-looking perspectives. Pain Med. 20, S58–S68.
Hofmeister, M., et al., 2020. Effectiveness of neurostimulation technologies for the management of chronic pain: a systematic review. Neuromodulation 23 (2), 150–157.
Koch, S.C., Acton, D., Goulding, M., 2018. Spinal circuits for touch, pain, and itch. Annu. Rev. Physiol. 80, 189–217.
Lempka, S.F., Patil, P.G., 2018. Innovations in spinal cord stimulation for pain. Curr. Opin. Biomed. Eng. 8, 51–60. https://doi.org/10.1016/j.cobme.2018.10.005.
Lind, et al., 2016. Spinal cord stimulation alters protein levels in the cerebrospinal fluid of neuropathic pain patients: a proteomic mass spectrometric analysis. Neuromodulation 19 (6), 549–562.
Montomery, K.L., et al., 2016. Wirelessly powered, fully internal optogenetics for brain, spinal and peripheral circuits in mice. Nat. Methods 12 (10), 969–974.
Neligan, P.C., Chang, J., 2013. Plastic Surgery. Third ed. Vol. 6. Elsevier, pp. 694–718.
Sneddon, L.U., 2018. Comparative physiology of nociception and pain. Physiology 33, 63–73.
Smith, E.S.J., 2018. Advances in understanding nociception and neuropathic pain. J. Neurol. 265, 231–238.
Todd, A.J., 2010. Neuronal circuitry for pain processing in the dorsal horn. Nat. Rev. Neurosci. 11 (12), 823–836. https://doi.org/10.1038/nrn2947.
Turk, D.C., Melzack, R., 2001. Handbook of Pain Assessment. Guildford Press, New York.
Wagner, F.B., et al., 2018. Targeted neurotechnology restores walking in humans with spinal cord injury. Nature 563, 65–71.
Yu, K., Niu, X., He, B., 2020. Neuromodulation management of chronic neuropathic pain in the central nervous system. Adv. Funct. Mater. 1908999.

CHAPTER 15

Sensing implants

While sensing the environment through the sensory systems (e.g., sight, hearing, and touch), we can actively modify our environment using the motor system. Such active interaction not only allows us to live in the environment but also helps to verify the internal model of the world we construct based on sensory input. Furthermore, the motor system allows us to speak and breathe. Therefore, functionality of the motor system is essential for life. For the motor system to be effective, it requires information on the position of the parts of our body and the body's relation to space and objects. For the former, proprioception (i.e., information on the state of the muscles and joints) is key. A large number of proprioceptors in our body are dedicated to this function. For registering the position of the body in space, the vestibular system, as discussed in **Chapter 16**, is vital. All these systems provide input to the motor system.

Injuries (e.g., spinal cord injury, SCI), strokes, and central nervous diseases (degenerative diseases including, for example, amyotrophic lateral sclerosis (ALS)) can impair the motor system. This leads to partial or complete inability of active interaction with the environment. Hence, restoration of the ability to carry out movements is an urgent need if the brain is disconnected from the muscles. Similar, this holds true for conditions where the effector is damaged, as is the case in amputations.

To drive muscles artificially if body parts are disconnected from the central motor system, the control signal first has to be extracted from the motor system. This requires a detailed knowledge of the codes used in the motor system. In general, two possibilities for such registration of motor commands can be used:

1. Signals generated from the spared muscles. For example, in hand amputations where the final effector (the fingers) is not preserved, the forearm (containing the muscles for moving the fingers using long tendons) is still functional. In such a case, the electrical signals of the muscles can be registered from the skin surface. With an array of skin sensors an artificial neuronal network can be trained to disentangle the individual movement of the amputated organ. To train the network the subject is asked to imagine movements of the amputated hand in a certain direction. This activates the muscles in a defined spatio-temporal sequence corresponding to the intended movement. A computer can be trained to discriminate between intended movements using the sensor signals and an artificial neuronal network. Such devices are already available on the market. They do not require implants and thus will not be considered in detail here.

Prostheses for the Brain
https://doi.org/10.1016/B978-0-12-818892-7.00015-8

2. Signals from the nervous system. They can be recorded directly at several locations: in peripheral nerves but also more centrally, best accessible in the motor cortex. The motor cortex provides a large volume of neural tissue. Since movements, as will be shown later, are coded by position of the active neurons there, and this is topologically coded (in line with the sensory systems; see **Chapter 9**), the motor cortex is well suited to provide signals to decipher intended movement from neuronal activity. Using these signals a device can drive paralyzed muscles by electric stimulation, robotic prostheses that replace limbs can be controlled, or robots can be commanded to perform the necessary tasks. However, motion is a complex process requiring accurate control of position in space, timing, velocity, and acceleration.

Movements of the body and limbs have many degrees of freedom. In contrast to an octopus, the skeleton of mammals contains a set of rigid elements (bones) connected by joints. Each of the joints provides specific degrees of freedom for angular and rotational movements within a limited range. For example, the knee and elbow joint permit no rotational movements but can be flexed in one dimension. In contrast, the shoulder joint is able to move in two angles and can be rotated in a certain range. Robots can be designed with more elements and movement ranges that can easily exceed the possibilities of joints. However, they have their own limitations. For example, it is difficult to design a mechanical joint that permits rotations and angulations around the same point. Hence, even anthropomorphic prostheses and externally worn robotic exoskeletons cannot support and copy the movement of human joints one to one.

For each movement, there is a group of muscles facilitating it (agonists) and a group of muscles opposing it (antagonists). The movement of a body part therefore requires the activation of agonists and the relaxation of antagonists. Synchronized contraction of agonists and antagonists causes stiffening of the joint. Physiologically, the coordinated action of agonists and antagonists, and the integration of proprioceptive signals from the muscles, is provided by circuits in the spinal cord (**Chapter 13**). If these circuits are bypassed, the procedure of stimulation needs to consider such relations, too.

Any movement requires the planning and calculation of the position, direction, velocity, and acceleration of an intended move. For example, the acceleration and deceleration of a limb requires the proper timing of opposite forces and the knowledge of the finite counterweight and position of the body and limbs. As described in **Chapter 13**, this involves innate reflexes of the spinal cord as well as flexible adaptation of the implicit (motor) memory. This implicit memory without conscious awareness adapts the movement to previous experiences and improves the performance of motor tasks. Unknown movement sequences are acquired slowly, but continuously speed up during training. The cerebellum plays a key role for the training of motion sequences that can be recalled later automatically, particularly for temporal coordination and fine motor acts. Although comprising only 10% of the weight of the human brain, the cerebellum contains 70% of all neurons. One part of the cerebellum (vestibulocerebellum) receives input from the

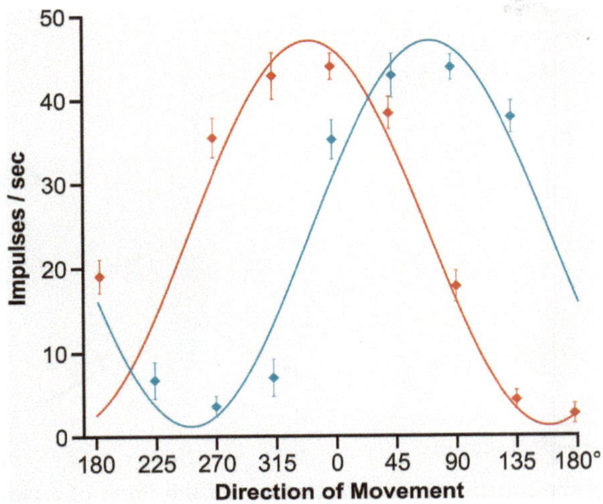

Fig. 15.1 Tuning of a neuron in M1 to movement direction. The activity of the recorded cell (red) is approximated by the function in Eq. (15.1) resulting in broadly tuned directionality. Adding another unit (blue) with different preferred direction leads to a better resolution and disambiguates the discharge rates as a code of movement direction. *(Adapted from Georgopoulos et al. (1982).)*

vestibular organ and uses it for body balance and fine-tuning of eye movements. Another part receives proprioceptive input from the spinal cord about the position of the body and limbs and regulates afferent and efferent input in a servo loop (spinocerebellum). The pontocerebellum is involved in planning movement. It receives input from motor areas of the premotor cortex and supplementary motor area (SMA; Fig. 13.1). Here coarse spatio-temporal plans of movements are fine-tuned and matched to previous experiences and are finally sent via the thalamus to the motor cortex.

In essence, this distributed network is a highly advanced real-time computer with the aim to plan and coordinate spatiotemporal motion patterns. But how can such a motion-computer be recorded to control a robotic prosthesis even in the absence of proprioceptive input?

A key factor to establish a brain-machine interface (BMI)[1] to connect the brain to an artificial external actuator is the findings in primates that neurons in the primary motor cortex M1 are sensitive to the direction of arm movement (Fig. 15.1). In contrast to passive movements, for volitional movements in two and three dimensions, the M1 cell firing rates are tuned to movement in one specific direction. As can be seen in Fig. 15.2, individual cells are broadly tuned to one "preferred" movement direction following a function in Eq. (15.1).

[1] Also known as Brain Computer Interface (BCI), see, e.g., Birbaumer, N., Ghanayim, N., Hinterberger, T., Iversen, I., Kotchoubey, B., Kubler, A., Perelmouter, J., Taub, E., Flor, H., 1999. A spelling device for the paralyzed. Nature 398, 297–298.

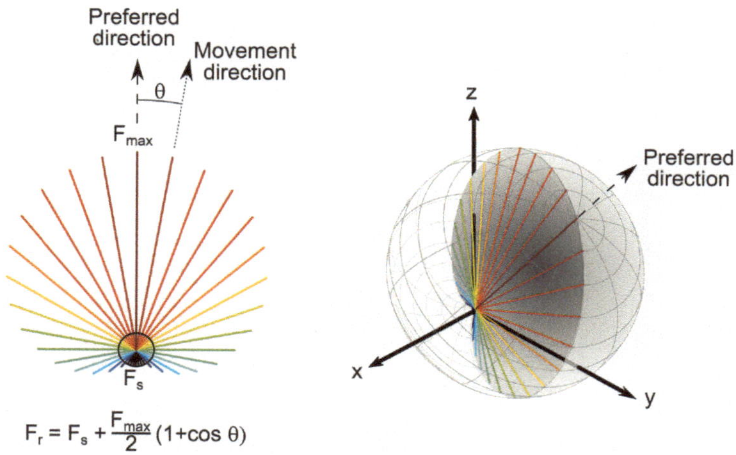

Fig. 15.2 Schematic of the broadly tuned directionality of the firing of a neuron. Cross-section of tuning in the preferred direction is shown on the left side. The length of a line indicates the normalized discharge rate of the neuron for multiple directions. A single tuning function to movements has an ambiguity at mid-level discharge rate that may decode for any direction with the same angle between the preferred direction and the motion. This can be addressed by adding more units with different preferred directions.

$$F_r = F_s + \frac{F_{\max}}{2}(1 + \cos\Theta) \tag{15.1}$$

Here the firing rate is F_r, the spontaneous rate is F_s, maximum increase of the rate is $F_{\max}$, and Θ is the angle between the preferred and the direction of the movement. Although the cosine function is only broadly tuned, neuron populations from M1 can be pooled to calculate the direction of a movement with much greater accuracy (Fig. 15.2). It thus requires several cortical neurons to code a given movement. In other words, there is a population code in the cortical area M1.

Subsequently these observations on motor coding in M1 have been extended to continuous movements in three-dimensional space encompassing action across multiple joints. It has been demonstrated that not only is direction encoded by one neuron but velocity and inertia are encoded in M1 as well. Robust extraction algorithms of information from distributed neuronal populations can be used to decode movement intent. The ability to decode intended movement (as opposed to an actual activation pattern of the muscles) reduces the complexity of the mechanical task with a multitude of degrees of freedom of joints and separate muscles substantially. Thus this coding in the M1 field simplifies the computational demands required for prostheses. Encoding of the dynamic movement parameters (and not the action of a multitude of separate muscles) therefore provides the optimal basis for neural prosthetic devices. For example, the movement of an arm from a starting point to a target in a reach-and-grasp experiment is simplified from a complex pattern of individual muscle movements specific to the limb to a simple direction and trajectory intention. Such experimental data were obtained by matching cortical activity recorded during animal experiments to actual movements performed by the limb. The discharge rates can be correlated with observable movements and a decoder can be trained to determine the intended movement from the recorded brain activity. This process, called "decoder training," is required to adapt a computer algorithm for an individual patient to interpret what motion is encoded by the neurons of the brain that are recorded. However, in paralyzed patients who are unable to move or in those with missing limbs that have to be substituted, the observation of the movement is not possible. In those subjects, it is only possible to use the recording of neuronal activity during imaginary movements for decoder training. Brain activity recordings during video presentation of a motion, when the patient was asked to imagine performing the motion, were successfully used to train decoders. In the following operational phase these patients were able to control an actuator or artificial limb with the so-trained decoder. This demonstrates that the actual movement is not encoded on the cortical level, but rather the intent for a movement is encoded, making decoder training feasible even in paralyzed subjects (Fig. 15.3).

In summary, the prerequisites for successful design of brain-controlled motorized prostheses for paralyzed human subjects are:

1. Movements are encoded in widely distributed neuronal populations of cells broadly tuned to a preferred direction. Rather than neurons exclusively specialized for a single function, each neuron is involved in multiple functions in form of a population code, and optimal decoding requires the readout of large neuron populations simultaneously. Hence, sensors to record large-scale brain activity with sufficient time resolution and real-time decoding algorithms are required.
2. The complexity of multiple muscle actions for a movement is implemented on subcortical levels. The cortex codes the intended movement, and since motorized prostheses have a slightly different arrangement of movable parts, it is a simpler task to implement the intentional cortical signals than detailed dynamic muscle patterns represented at lower levels of the motor system.
3. The interpretation of cortically recorded cell signals can be accomplished by matching the volitional movement to the discharge rates within a large ensemble. For this purpose, a calibration procedure is required to interpret the cortical signal and to determine, for example, the preferred directions of neurons in an ensemble.
4. Normal physiological processing and generation of intention of motion are based on proprioceptive and vestibular input that is not present in this code and requires further adaptations.

But how many neurons have to be recorded to supply sufficient information for accurate motion control? Single neuron recordings are not sufficient to predict movements

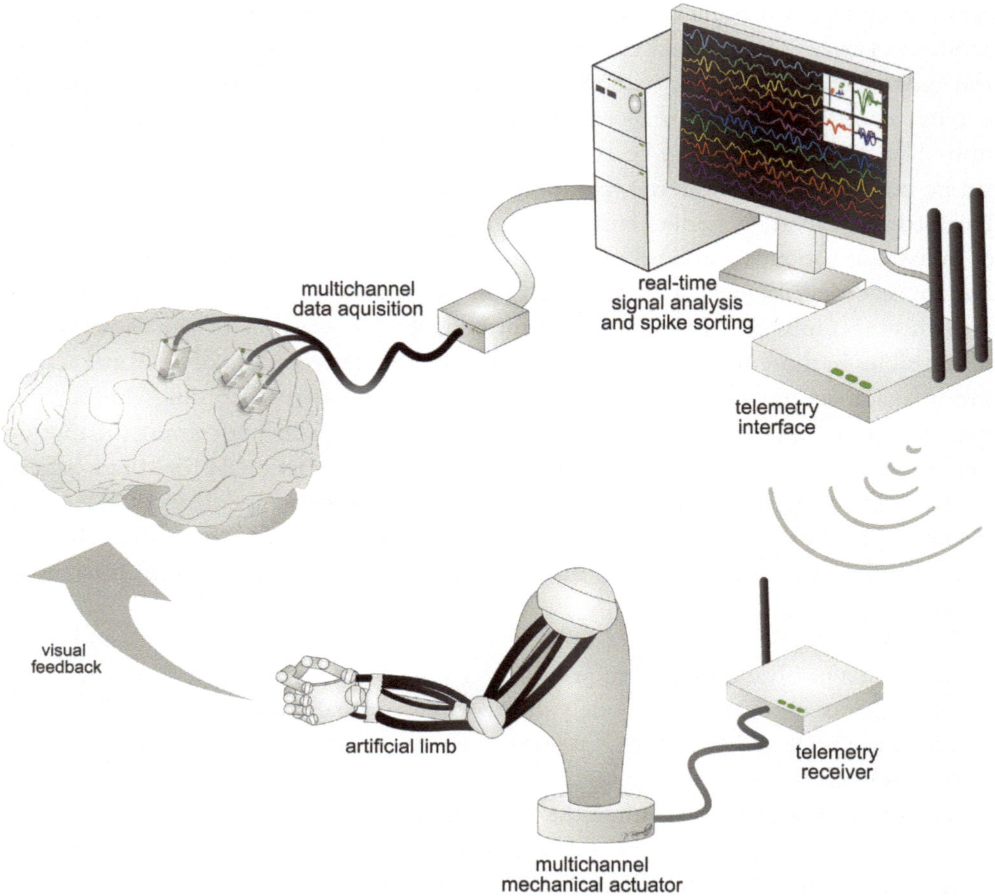

Fig. 15.3 Schematic of the principal components of a BMI controlling an artificial arm. A large population of neurons in one or more relevant areas (e.g., M1) is recorded with a large number of electrodes and single unit spike activity is extracted real time. A trained decoder extracts the motion intent in terms of position, velocity, and gripping force, and the result is transmitted to an effector. The artificial limb is controlled by the motion intent and carries out the intent providing visual feedback. Additional "tactile" and "proprioceptive" feedback from within the prosthetic limb can be added.

accurately. The trial-to-trial variability of their firing rates, the neuronal noise, can be significantly reduced by recording simultaneously from ensembles of neurons. This allows more reliable single-trial predictions of intentions for actual movements. Owl monkeys implanted with microwire arrays in several cortical areas were simultaneously recorded while the monkeys performed one- and three-dimensional movements (lever left/right and reach-and-grasp experiments). The data obtained were decoded using a linear prediction algorithm and an artificial neural network to derive predictions of the motion that were used to real-time control a robotic device (locally and remotely transmitted through the Internet). The initial training phase was terminated when the correlation coefficient R^2 between the prediction and the actual movement reached a plateau. The correlation of the prediction was optimal when the maximal number of recorded neurons was used, and it decreased when fewer recordings for the prediction were used. By reducing the number of neurons for the linear prediction artificially, a **neuron dropping curve** (NDC) (Fig. 15.4) was plotted and can be fitted by a hyperbolic function

$$R^2 = \frac{Nc}{1 + Nc} \tag{15.2}$$

where N is the number of used neurons and c is a constant determined from the fitted data. From this approximation in Eq. (15.2) it follows that reducing the number of recorded neurons results in a lower correlation between the prediction and the actual movement. Alternatively, increasing the recorded neuron population number leads to an increase in accuracy, but to a lesser extent.

Although the number of recorded neurons in the original experiment was relatively small, the good approximation by the hyperbolic function permits the extrapolation and estimation of the number of neurons needed to obtain predefined accuracy. Movement prediction is possible with 30 to 40 neurons, but more than 100 neurons are required for an acceptable accuracy. Similar counts are required for prosthetic limb controls. Equally important, the extrapolations of the hyperbolic curves revealed that beside recordings from the primary motor cortex (M1) recordings from the posterior parietal cortex (PP) and dorsal premotor cortex (PMd) yield equally good or better predictions. Using NDC analysis, the relative importance of cortical areas for a specific action can be quantified. Moreover, sensitivities to features additional to movement direction, such as velocity, position, and gripping force, can be identified in the neuronal activity.

Multiple BMIs have been developed and used to control a large variety of computer cursors, actuators, robotic limbs and exoskeletons, avatar bodies, and wheelchairs. Additionally, BMIs were used for functional electrical stimulation (FES) of muscles allowing paralyzed patients to control their bodies. Recordings of brain activity can be performed either non-invasively (from the skin surface using large-scale electroencephalographic electrodes) or invasively (either from the surface of the cortex or with penetrating electrodes from the neuronal tissue). Each of these approaches has its advantages and disadvantages in terms of the associated risk, time resolution, and spatial resolution (Fig. 15.5).

Non-invasive BCI

Non-invasive brain-computer interfaces (BCIs) are currently the method of choice in clinical applications as they employ extracorporeal electrodes for recording. However,

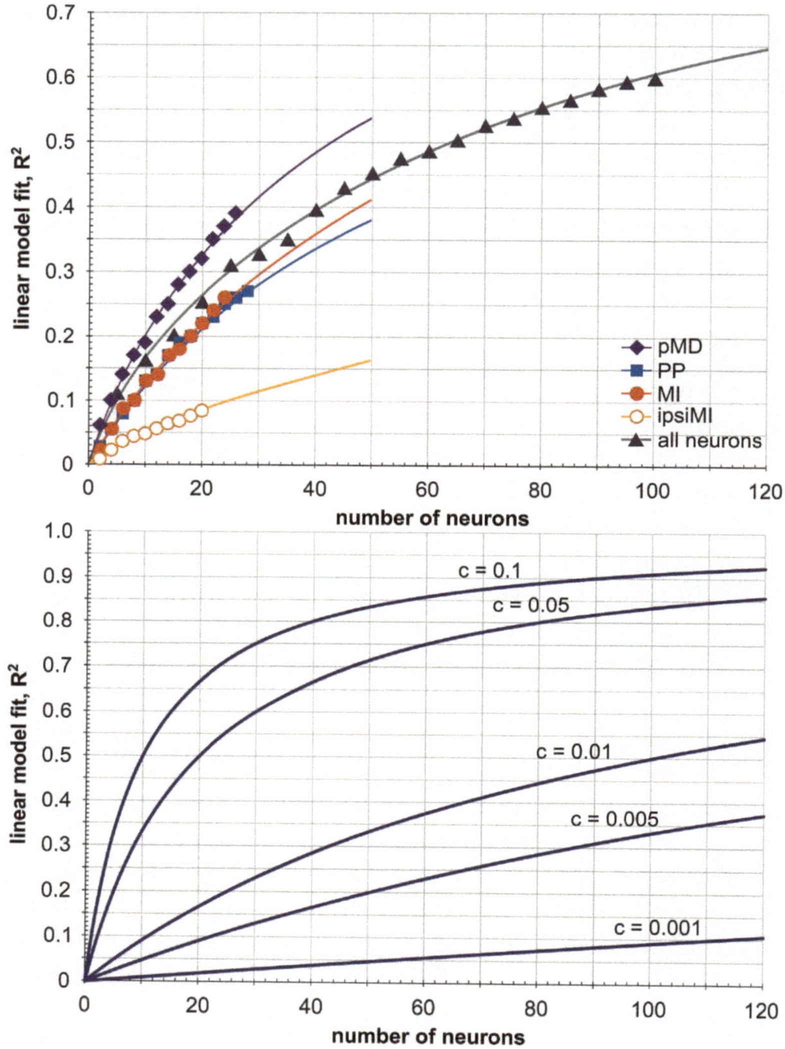

Fig. 15.4 Neuron-dropping curves (NDCs). *Upper panel*: Experimental data from a single recording session in a monkey: recordings from primary motor cortex (MI), posterior parietal cortex (PP), and dorsal premotor cortex (PMd) The correlation coefficient R^2 of actual movement with the linear prediction model for decreasing numbers of neurons was calculated, demonstrating that R^2 can be approximated with a hyperbolic function. For better visibility only every fifth data point is shown. *Lower panel*: The hyperbolic function (15.2) for different constants *c*. *(Adapted from Wessberg et al. (2000).)*

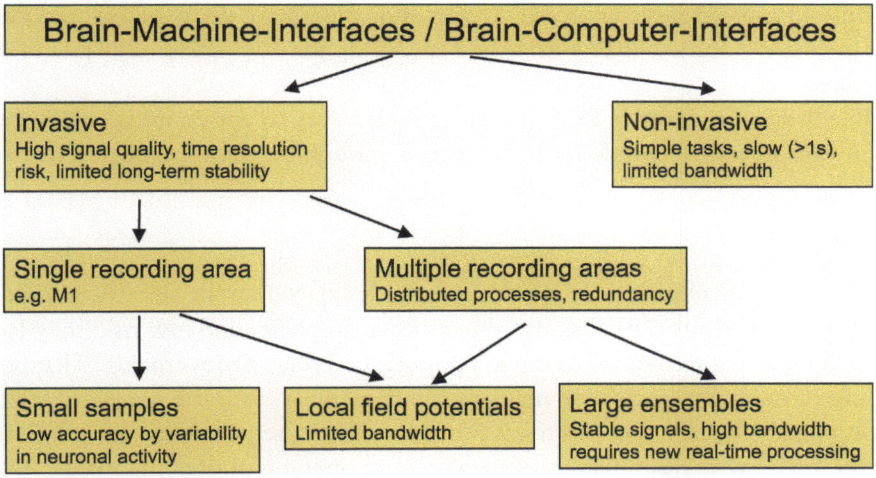

Fig. 15.5 Overview of non-invasive (skin surface) and invasive (from neuronal tissue with surface recording electrodes or penetrating electrodes for recordings from individual neurons) BMIs.

electroencephalography (EEG) provides only low spatial resolution and due to low-pass-filtered signals, lower temporal resolution compared to invasive recordings as well.

Complete paralysis with intact sensory and cognitive functions is a condition that may occur in patients after a stroke or a later stage of progressive degenerative neurological diseases. Some of them ultimately become "locked-in" patients unable to control the majority of their muscles and thus may be unable to communicate. In the 1990s BCIs on the basis of noninvasively recorded cortical potentials were developed, allowing locked-in patients to write messages on a computer screen. More importantly, this work demonstrated that patients are able to acquire the skill to voluntarily control their EEG signals during a training phase to finally use it for yes/no decisions. To increase response performance in paralyzed or locked-in patients that cannot communicate, "dependent" BCIs are used. Following training the subject can use their EEG signals to intentionally position the cursor left or right, providing yes/no responses. The software that reads out the EEG signal can in this paradigm be triggered to the time window after stimulus presentation, making the neuronal read-out more reliable.

A similar system can be used in patients within a partial locked-in state where voluntary eye movements and blinks are still possible. For these subjects a message system based on the electrical signals of the eye muscles recorded from the skin surface near the eyes (an electrooculogram; EOG) can be used. While the EOG responses were smaller than in normal subjects, most could select letters from an auditory speller system in a 5-s recording window. However, how long such a system can provide a means of communication in patients with progressive neuronal diseases and consequent decay of the amplitudes of the electrooculographic signals with time depends on the etiology and the rate of disease progression.

While these non-invasive BCI systems provide a way to communicate with the subject, they are not yet technologically advanced enough to control a prosthetic limb.

Invasive BCI

Non-invasive BCIs require only external electrodes placed on the skin. Although this is the first choice in clinical applications due to their simplicity and low risk, they lack the spatial and temporal resolution to tap the population code of movements. That requires recording of many isolated single neurons simultaneously with the necessary selectivity and minimized crosstalk. The alternative, invasive BMIs, require a surgical procedure to access the brain, with trephination of the skull and opening of the dura mater. Potential complications include infections, leakage of cerebrospinal fluid and bleeding. Penetrating electrodes or electrode arrays (i.e., electrodes that enter the neuronal tissue) additionally carry the risk of tissue damage and induction of fibrotic tissue growth that decreases the number of recordable neurons over time. Removal or re-implantation of penetrating electrodes brings further risk of damage. Electrocorticography (ECoG) with pliable electrode grids placed on the cortex surface is a less invasive solution since it does not penetrate into the tissue. Recording extracellular potentials from the surface of the brain is not as invasive as penetrating electrodes, provides better spatial and temporal resolution and signal-to-noise ratio than non-invasive recordings, and is often stable over years in animals and humans. Thus it is used as a less invasive alternative to penetrating electrodes.

Electrocorticographic and endovascular recording

Due to the electrode placement on the surface of the brain, ECoG lessens the risks of medical complications compared to other invasive methods. In clinical practice, a standard application is the preoperative cortical mapping in epileptic patients to identify affected cortical areas. Electrode grids can be placed either on the dura mater, which is the safer option, or underneath the dura directly on the surface of the brain (subdurally) on top of the pia mater. As percutaneous cable connections are associated with an infection risk, wireless fully implantable recording devices with data transmission have been developed, reducing the risk of infection in chronic monitoring of epilepsy patients or BMI applications. The mechanical mismatch between soft neural tissues and stiff neural implants decreases long-term stability and performance. This issue can be experimentally addressed by a soft neural implant with the shape and mechanical properties of dura mater called e-dura. This electronic dura mater contains electrodes, interconnects, chemical sensors, and chemical injectors to deliver combined electrochemical neuromodulation. The e-dura is made of a silicone substrate with stretchable gold interconnects and platinum contacts with a diameter of 0.3 mm.

Typical ECoG electrode arrays in clinical practice are usually small rectangular grids of 10 to 100 Pt or PtIr electrodes. Common spacing is from 10 mm to a few millimeters, as the physical limit for resolution is approximately 1.5 mm (this compares in extent to approximately five cortical columns). The task with these recorded signals is to decode the intention of the subject; therefore the computer software focused on this task is called a **decoder**. Using high-resolution ECoG grids and dedicated decoder software, an appropriate classification of finger movements and hand gestures has been achieved that could be used to control an artificial hand. First, during an "**observational phase**," the most prominent features of the recorded signal are identified and their discriminative power between the intended movements is defined. This information is subsequently used for BMI control of actuators during the "**operational phase**" (i.e., during the use of the prosthetic device). Errors in the operational phase can be fed back to the decoder to further improve precision.

In locked-in patients, selected ECoG components were used to steer the cursor in a two-dimensional computer cursor movement task. After a training period of 12–26 min, five subjects were able to achieve up to 70% accuracy in a four-target task. Other experiments have demonstrated that classification can be performed with high accuracy based on ECoG recordings from the hemisphere contralateral to the working hand. Decoding of continuous movements is also possible, such as producing hand gestures ("scissor," "rock," and "paper") with an online-controlled hand prosthesis achieving approximately 80% accuracy. Recently a practical, fully implantable ECoG BMI was introduced that enabled an amyotrophic lateral sclerosis (ALS) patient to control a typing program by imagining voluntary hand movements at a rate of two letters per minute. While slow, this device offers a practical solution for severely impaired patients to restore communication.

In conclusion, ECoG is suitable for BMI applications where the classification and reproduction of a limited set of motor outputs is sufficient. Many of the ECoG systems (e.g., for identification of epileptic loci) are in clinical use.

Common ECoG grids require the surgical opening of the skull and implantation into the cranial cavity bearing the risk of inflammations, brain trauma, and other severe complications. One experimental way to simplify the positioning of electrode arrays is a minimally invasive approach by placing a passive stent-type of an electrode array (*stentrode*) within a *vein*. Stents are being used in cardiovascular medicine to extend a narrowed portion of a vein by a mechanical frame that keeps it in desired shape. In neuroprosthetic application, this is performed by implantation of a similar device, but this time equipped with recording electrodes. The stentrode is placed into a superficial cortical vein over the motor cortex via catheter angiography. ECoG recordings were shown to be comparable to epidural surface grids without blood flow impairment. Successful recording was possible over a half-year in an animal experiment. So far, there has been no clinical translation of this technique.

Single-unit recording arrays

For the extraction of accurate information on intended movement, the simultaneous registration of the activity of large distributed neuronal populations relevant for a specific task has to be performed in real time or close to real time. For this purpose, usually several hundred or thousands of neurons in a single area or multiple areas have to be recorded reliably, stable over years. Placing the electrodes into cortical or subcortical structures has to be as atraumatic as possible and should preserve the neural tissue and its axonal connections maximally. Longevity of the electrode-tissue complex and its electrical connection is essential as re-implantations constitute additional risks and may not be possible. Although re-implantations of other implants, such as cochlear implants, is possible, this may not apply to brain tissue electrodes where extraction of the electrode, particularly for electrode arrays, is highly problematic. Usually, the neuronal tissue generates a foreign body reaction (**Chapter 8**) and adheres to the electrodes. Therefore their removal is associated with significant tissue damage. Bleedings are common when removing such electrodes, leading to further damage. Re-implantation at the same place may thus find damaged tissue with poor signal quality.

Silicon microarrays

The **Utah array** (Fig. 15.6) developed at the University of Utah (USA), is the only micro-electrode array that is approved for use in humans by the Food and Drug

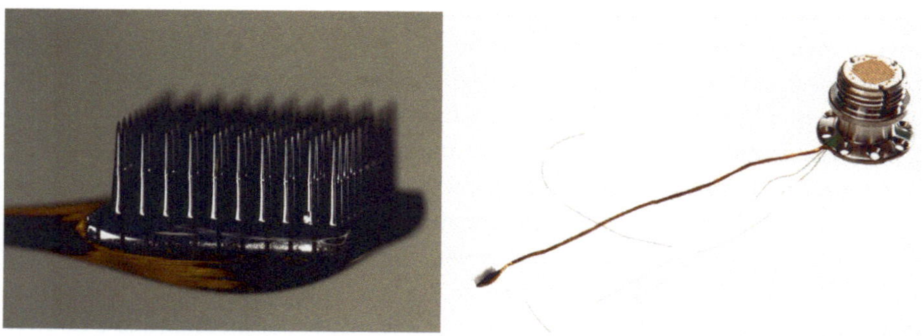

Fig. 15.6 The planar 10×10 electrode array for neural recording (Utah Array™—© 2020 Blackrock Microsystems, LLC, *left side*). In the NeuroPort Array™—© 2020 Blackrock Microsystems, LLC for human use, the 4×4 mm array is connected by a 13 cm ribbon cable to the percutaneous titanium pedestal *(right side)* containing the percutaneous connector, which can be mounted to the skull bone penetrating the skin.

Administration (FDA). The recording array consists of a 10×10 microneedle array with a spacing of 0.4 mm and a depth of 1.5 mm. The three-dimensional microstructure is made from silicon by sawing trenches and rounding and sharpening the needles by etching, forming conical microneedles. The rigid needle shafts are polyimide coated for isolation, having platinum-coated tips for recording/stimulation. Ninety-six electrodes of the array are available for recording. They are electrically connected to gold microwires at the rear-side of the planar carrier. The microwire bundle is several centimeters long and can be contacted by a percutaneous titanium multi-contact connector mounted to the skull bone. More recent developments allow multiple contacts at the tip and along the sides of each needle to increase the number of contacts.

As the rigid array has a relatively homogeneous distribution of needles/electrodes over an area of 4×4 mm, slow insertion of the array leads to a **bed-of-nails effect**, indenting the cortex surface without penetration. To avoid such *dimpling* of the soft brain tissue the array has to be inserted into the cortex ballistically using a pneumatic device, exploiting fast velocity to insert the electrode into the brain. Although the insertion causes trauma (it is difficult to impossible to avoid vessels due to the size of the device and the rigid spacing of the electrodes; vascular damage and bleedings are a regular consequence) and fibrous encapsulation has been reported in cats, enough active recordable neurons were available 5 years after implantation in a tetraplegic human subject to control a robotic arm in a reach-and-grasp experiment.

In contrast to microhemorrhages that are probably limited to a short time after insertion, chronic inflammatory reactions can negatively impact neurons and microelectrodes by activation and migration of microglial cells towards the microelectrodes (**Chapter 8**). Micro motions of the array relative to the surrounding neurons can also produce (sometimes reversible) changes in properties of the recorded signals as well as provide irritation and further foreign body reaction. Both effects result in variability and long-term reduction of viable neuron channels making adaptive spike identification and continuous recalibration necessary. Another limitation arises from the insertion technique and the planar form of the array as they limit the insertion into curved surfaces and sulci. Finally, the brain is in constant movement even at rest due to heartbeat and respiration; thus rigid arrays with rigid wire leads may cause constant irritation and facilitate further inflammatory reactions. Even silicone is more rigid than the brain tissue, and therefore new conductive and insulating materials are under investigation.

Even with these restrictions, the Utah array has been successfully used in humans, initially enabling a paralyzed patient to neuronally track a fast-moving cursor of changing directions that was steered by a technician. Later, using recordings from a small population of neurons in the motor cortex (M1) arm area, drinking coffee from a bottle was possible with a DLR Light-Weight Robot III. For the decoder training (observational phase) neuronal recordings during intended hand states were used. The subject imagined movements and squeezing of her hand during the training phase of a linear decoder to generate hand-state and velocity commands for the operational phase.

In another experiment the control of more complex movements of an anthropomorphic arm, a prosthesis with seven degrees of freedom (three-dimensional translation, three-dimensional orientation, one-dimensional grasping) allowed a tetraplegic patient to perform coordinated reach-and-grasp movements with the artificial arm. The experimental application in completely paralyzed human subjects enables new insights into mechanisms and usability of other cortical areas. Here again, recording neural population activity during imaginary motion can be successfully used to train decoders in an observational phase. Other than the primary motor cortex, areas such as the posterior parietal cortex (PPC) that process high-level, cognitive aspects of action planning can be efficiently used for "thought-reading" intentions and to control devices.

To control artificial limbs, the brain-derived decoded information of intended or imagined motion can be used to re-activate the paralyzed limbs by functional electrostimulation (FES). In a 24-year-old patient with tetraplegia from a spinal cord injury, signals derived from the primary motor cortex microelectrode array could be used to control a custom-built electric stimulation system. After identification of primary motor cortex areas for hand movements by fMRI imaging preoperatively, mirroring videos of hand movements, and implantation of the recording array, the patient was able to perform different wrist and hand movements using the stimulation system, even for functional tasks in daily life. Also this technology provides promise for future clinical tranlsation.

The University of Michigan developed an alternative product for experimental use: the "Michigan probe" (recently also called the **NeuroNexus probe**, named after the spin-off of this development, the NeuroNexus company) based on silicon technology used in microchip design, with microelectrode contacts made of iridium and placed on a carrier in a customized way. The electrodes are placed on one or several shanks of a comb-like structure that can record from all layers in the cortex using one such electrode. The fabrication technology provides a large flexibility in design at reasonable costs. This alternative product has become the most popular in research, but has not yet found a clinical application.

Both, the NeuroNexus probe and the Utah array approach are combined in a concept for a silicon-based planar electrode array with multiple recording contacts per shank. In the future this can potentially be used for recordings from different cortical layers simultaneously.

Microwire recordings

Microwire penetrating electrodes were a standard technique for recording brain activity in animals before being largely replaced by the Utah and NeuroNexus multielectrode

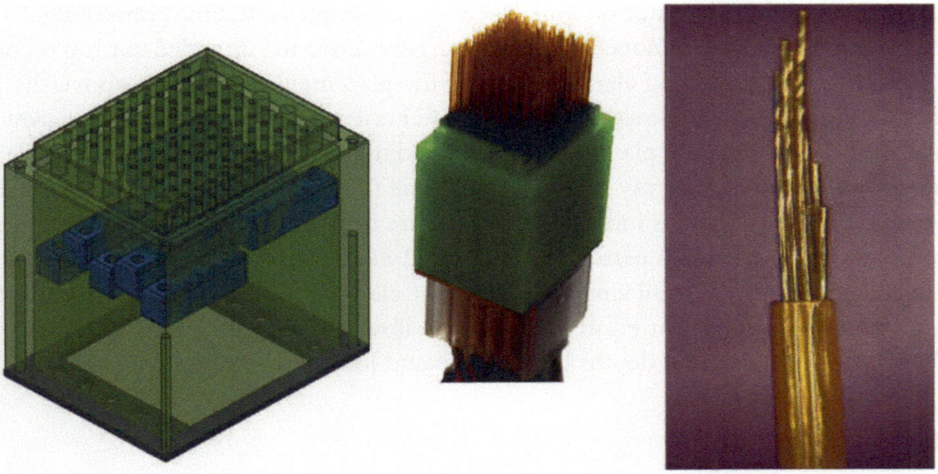

Fig. 15.7 *Left*: Micro-wire array (cube) with 10 × 10 guiding tubes and individually adjustable wire holders. The array covers an area of 10 × 10 mm. Center: Assembled micro-wire array. *Right*: Bundle of staggered micro-wires in a guiding tube. Wires usually have a diameter of 12–50 μm. *(Figures from Schwarz et al. (2014).)*

arrays. Microwire electrodes consist of microwire bundles of usually up to 10 isolated wires staggered appropriately to the depths required. They are usually made from tungsten or stainless steel and tips that can be gold plated for better biocompatibility. Carbon nanotubes can also be used to decrease impedance and to improve signal-to-noise ratios. The common wire diameters are 10–50 μm and each bundle is guided by a polymer tube (Fig. 15.7). Guiding tubes containing the bundles are arranged in either one-dimensional ("*combs*") or two-dimensional ("*cubes*") arrays, typically with 1 mm spacing to avoid brain surface dimpling and tissue damage. As each contact commonly records one to two neurons per contact, an array with 10 × 10 guiding tubes is able to record from one to 2000 neurons, covering an area of approximately 1 cm^2. Depending on the brain size, multiple cubes can be combined to tap multiple areas of interest.

Although built from standard elements, the concept of microwire arrays has many advantages, is versatile, and can be used in different applications. Subsets of the array can be adjusted to different depths and the maximal length of the wire bundles can be up to 5–15 mm. Hence, both cortical and subcortical structures in an extended depth range can be accessed too. As individual wires are directly connected, each wire can be used for either recording or stimulation. Most importantly, these implants provide longevity with reliable recordings over 4–5 years in free-moving monkeys with little loss of active neurons over time. This is likely given by the fact that the thin wires do not provide much mechanical resistance against the brain tissue, minimizing relative movements.

On the downside, the implantation procedure is complex and time consuming. Skull bone and dura mater are removed in a sterile surgery above the intended cortical recording area, as in all penetrating electrodes. After the placement of the array above the pia mater, the surgical area is allowed to recover. After one week of recovery, the microwire arrays are inserted into the pia mater with fine adjustments. To avoid the bed-of-nails effect only a subset of the array is inserted at a time (Fig. 15.7 left) that can be manually lowered while the activity is monitored. The entire insertion of all bundles to their final position in the brain tissue is performed over a 1–2 week period. Following surgery, dura mater and bone regrow, stabilizing and sealing the electrodes. Although this procedure is complex and requires major effort and time, it allows for the controlled insertion into different target regions and depths being stable and long-term viable for recording.

Future concepts

One advantage of microwire arrays is the compliance of the fiber bundles that compensates for micromovements and thus possibly contributes to the longevity of the recording array. To decrease the relative shear motion between cortex tissue and the microelectrodes, **polymer microelectrodes** have been developed (Fig. 15.8). They are more compliant than wires and exert less strain on the nervous tissue during micromovements. By hooking flexible carriers with multiple electrode contacts and a loop at their tip to a guidance needle, they are pulled into the tissue. An alternative way to insert a soft electrode into the tissue is to increase its stiffness temporarily. For example, this can be obtained by temporarily attaching the soft array to a stiffener with dissolvable glue (e.g., poly-ethylene-glycol (PEG)) that detaches from the polymer electrode after insertion and can be retracted afterwards. A historic approach used a hard coating by sugar

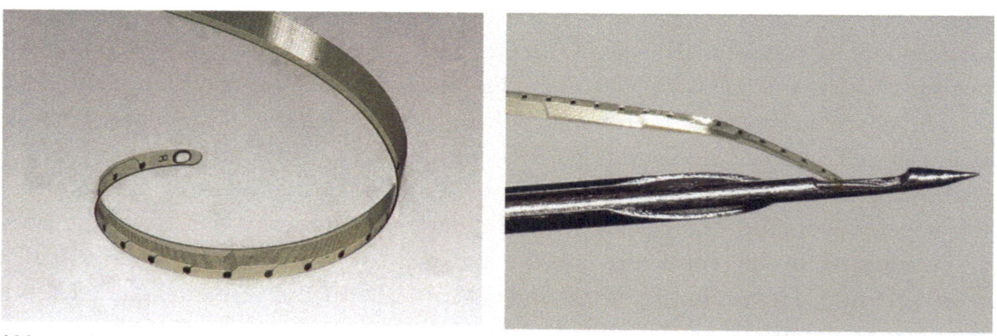

(A) (B)

Fig. 15.8 (A) MicroFlex Array™—© 2020 Blackrock Microsystems, LLC microelectrode array on a polymer flexible carrier with the loop for tissue insertion at the tip. Depending on the application, arrays may have 12–24 electrodes with diameter of 15–100 μm and spacing of 10–500 μm on a 10 μm carrier. The electrode array can be up to 67 mm long with a width of 200 μm, tappering down to 100 μm at the tip. (B) Electrode array hooked to the insertion needle.

(e.g., dextrose) that is spontaneously dissolved after insertion into the brain (and is, of course, biodegradable).

In contrast to predefined silicon or wire bundle arrays, single electrodes have the advantage that predefined sites can be precisely accessed even on curved surfaces or in sulci, and overlying vessels can be avoided. Nevertheless, precise placement of multiple probes would be too time-consuming. One possibility to combine large numbers of recording sites with enabling micro-movements is the **robotic placement** of large numbers of fine and flexible polymer probes. By hooking flexible polyimide carriers with up to 96 PEDOT (Chapter 6) electrode contacts with a loop at their tip to a tungsten needle, they can be pulled into the tissue similar to a sewing machine. Whereas the insertion speed is variable, the needle can be retracted with a high speed, disconnecting the tungsten needle from the tip leaving the soft electrode array (thread) in the tissue. With a neurosurgical robot it is possible to position precisely up to six threads per minute into preplanned cortical tissue locations across multiple brain regions, avoiding vessels.

An entirely different experimental concept is followed in **neural dust electrodes**. Here the wire-bound access to the recording electrodes is entirely eliminated by using ultra-sound powered, free-floating, independent 10–100 μm sensor elements. The low-power electronic sensors are coupled by ultrasonic power delivery and backscatter communication to a sub cranial receiver/transmitter outside the brain. In contrast to radiofrequency transmission that suffers from high inefficiency, ultrasound has a greater penetration depth in tissue. To increase energy efficiency in both technologies, beam steering can be used to locally increase the energy supply to the elements. Although neural dust electrodes have been successfully used to record high fidelity electromyogram (EMG) and electroneurogram (ENG) signals from anesthetized rats, the targeted placing, localizing, and tracking over time of a sufficient number of sensor elements still needs to be developed. Additionally, for electrical stimulation more energy than is currently available for the sensor elements may be required.

Instead of placing the recording electrode accurately into a target structure, which is sometimes a difficult problem, this issue can also be solved by attracting the fibers of interest to the electrode using **neurotrophic factors**. In an early attempt, a piece of the sciatic nerve was placed into a hollow glass cone containing four gold wires for recording. After implantation into the cortex single- and multi-unit activity could be recorded for several months and newly ingrown neurites were confirmed later with histology. In a paralyzed human this type of electrode was later used for a BMI to spell letters on a computer screen with up to three letters/minute. A two-channel neurotrophic electrode implanted in a speech related region of the precentral cortex was used later in a real-time vowel production task in another locked-in subject. Here recording of 56 distinguishable units were decoded by a decoder (Kalman filter-based) translating the neural signals into continuous parameters for controlling a synthesizer. The speech synthesizer provided within 50 ms acoustic feedback of the formants F1 and F2. After a neurite growth period of 3–4 months facilitated by neurotrophic factors released from the glass cone, a limited set of vowels (A, OO, IY, UH) could be produced by a speech synthesizer with a hit rate of 70%. A maintained signaling pattern over 4 years demonstrates the longevity and viability as chronic BCI of this neurotrophic factor concept.

However, extracting neuronal activity from the brain of a large population of neurons across multiple areas is only one aspect of controlling speech synthesis or the movement of artificial limbs. Equally important is the interpretation of the brain-derived multi-unit activity with robust and fast extraction algorithms that are able to translate the movement intent into an execution. Matching cortical activity to actual movements is a non-trivial task that requires algorithms that can be carried out in real time and that can be trained to interpret the available activity of an individual with sufficient speed and acuity. These algorithms are called "decoders" and will be introduced in the following.

Decoders

Movements are encoded by large distributed neuronal population of cells that are broadly tuned to specific independent qualities such as movement direction, force, or acceleration. Using arrays of electrodes, large subpopulations of neurons in one or more relevant areas can be accessed and single-unit spike activity from them can be recorded. However, the main task remains the interpretation and translation of the activity of the recorded cells to extract the intended movement. This is the most crucial step for all neural prosthetic devices with BCIs: the conversion of the measurable information from the brain to meaningful intended real-world action. Real-time decoders (i.e., fast and reliable computational algorithms) are required to interpret a subject's brain activity and to convert it into commands suitable for artificial actuators. Multitudes of mathematical and computational approaches have been proposed as decoders of motor activity generated by the brain. All decoders derive from a set of brain recorded input channels another set of output variables that correspond to the motion variables of the actuators in the real world. These multiple-input multiple-output (MIMO) models are described as a vector (set) of inputs of size N and a vector (set) of outputs of size M. Usually the size of recorded neurons is bigger than the number of outputs ($N > M$), and BMIs require the near-real-time interpretation of multiple noisy neuronal inputs and extraction of a few condensed output parameters to control the actuators.

Initially such algorithms were developed to match offline experimentally recorded multiple-input information from the brain to an output that was observable, such as a movement. Discharge rates were correlated with observable movements offline and an algorithm (decoder) was trained to determine the intended movement from the recorded brain activity. This "decoder training" is also required in BMIs to adapt a computer algorithm to the individually recorded brain activity of a patient and is a necessary step in the interpretation of the brain-encoded motion. Such a calibration procedure is required in all BMIs to control an actuator. However, the input-output relationship is not stable over time, and the decoder has to be recalibrated periodically or continuously while working. The reasons are manifold: recorded neurons get lost, physiological changes such as scar tissue growth may occur and can affect the recorded signals, and so on. Moreover, brain plasticity and adaptation (**Chapter 9**) can change the cortical signal. In current devices visual feedback of the movement actually carried out provides the strongest backward input to the brain, but tactile and proprioceptive feedback is also feasible and may add independent feedback pathways in future applications.

Since the 1970s, many decoding algorithms have been developed and tested in a multitude of applications. The development of efficient and fast computer algorithms has become its own extended field. Here we introduce a few analytical concepts that are used today: **population vector**, linear **Wiener filters**, and **Kalman filters**. **Artificial neural networks** are also successfully applied in real-time interpretation of brain-derived movement control, but the concepts in such networks differ in too many aspects to be discussed in detail here. Each of these approaches has advantages and more concepts will appear in the future that will have to be investigated. In the following section we describe only the principal concepts.

Population vector

As already mentioned (see Figs. 15.1 and 15.2) the discharge rate of broadly tuned neurons was found sensitive to the direction of movement. To reconstruct movement parameters the spikes counted in a time window are used to generate an input vector of size N with continuous firing rates $\vec{x}(t)$ of each neuron. In the population vector model an output vector $\vec{y}(t)$ of size M is generated representing the output components. In the population vector model a linear dependence is assumed and the components $y_i(t)$ of the output vector can be written as:

$$y_i(t) = b_i + \sum_{j=1}^{N} a_{i,j} x_j(t) \quad i = 1 \ldots M \tag{15.3}$$

where the constants b_i correspond to the weighted spontaneous rates and outputs at time t can be calculated from inputs $\vec{x}(t)$ at the same time. In the original population vector model that decodes output variables from a set of input variables, the factors $a_{i,j}$ would correspond to the cosine between the "preferred direction" of neuron j and the movement direction of the actuator Eq. (15.3) can be rewritten in a matrix form as

$$\vec{y}(t) = \vec{b} + \vec{x}(t)A \tag{15.4}$$

For example, in the simple case of the preferred direction model, the matrix A would have N rows for the number of recorded neurons and M columns coding for the movement directions (e.g., Cartesian coordinates x, y, z in three dimensions). This approach is not restricted to "preferred directions" and can be extended to other independent output dimensions, such as velocity, gripping force, or rotation. In this case the elements of the matrix are not as intuitive as in the population vector model. Only for motion directions can the determination of matrix elements be easily calculated, and in a generalized form a systematic method to determine the matrix factors $a_{i,\,j}$ is not straightforward. Moreover, the application in BMI of simply relating inputs at an instant linear to outputs is limited.

Wiener filter

Another linear decoding algorithm, the discrete Wiener filter, is a more general approach than the simple population vector model described before. It has been successfully employed in many BMI applications and uses not only the input information at the same instant but also the precedent neuronal activity. Additionally, it includes an optimization procedure to minimize mean square errors. The output vector $\vec{y}\,(t)$ can contain many independent static and dynamic modalities, for example position, velocity, acceleration, rotation, and gripping force, and is modeled as a weighted linear combination of the neuronal activity in the preceding time. For this purpose, the time of the recording is divided into discrete windows preceding t, called "taps," and the neuronal average discharge rate within each of the windows for each neuron is calculated. A typical choice is to use 10 windows of 100 ms length. The basic form of a Wiener filter for causal processes (only states in the past can have an effect on the present state) can be written for T discrete time lags as:

$$\vec{y}\,(t) = \vec{b} + \sum_{u=0}^{T} \vec{x}\,(t-u)A(u) \tag{15.5}$$

In Eq. (15.5) $\vec{x}\,(t,\,u)$ are the discharge rates at a time $t-u$, $A(u)$ is the matrix of weights, $\vec{b}$ is a constant vector, and $\vec{y}\,(t)$ is the state vector at time t. Using an input matrix X that contains in its columns the discharge rates of the N neurons for each of the T taps and an additional prepending column of ones for the y-intercepts $\vec{b}$ ($NT+1$ columns), Eq. (15.5) can be reformulated as

$$Y = XA \tag{15.6}$$

In this form the matrix A can be determined using the pseudo-inverse matrix $inv(X^T X)$ that additionally solves the optimization problem and minimizes the mean square error.

$$A = inv\left(X^T X\right) X^T Y \tag{15.7}$$

In the easiest case the parameters in matrix A are calculated from the neuronal inputs and the observed behavioral parameters Y in a training phase of the decoder. Subsequently when the decoder has achieved a sufficient accuracy in performance, this parameter set is used in an operational mode to control the BMI.

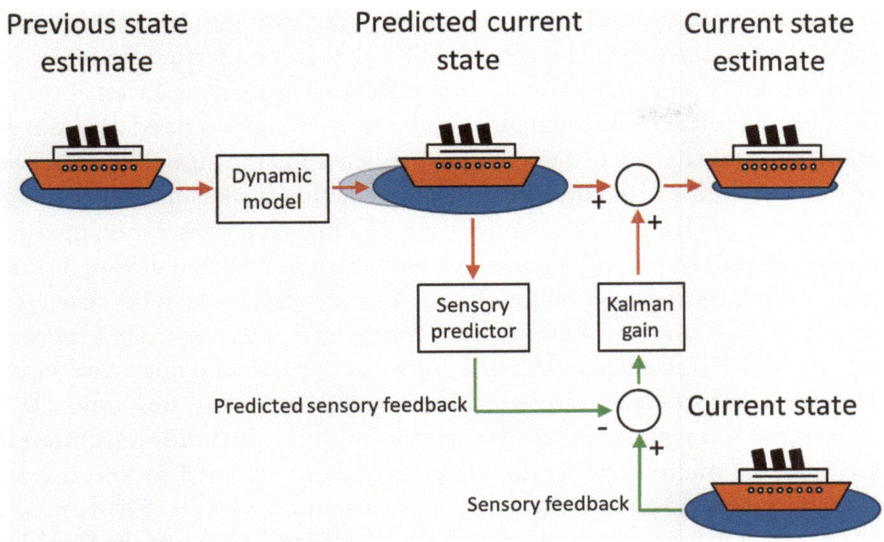

Fig. 15.9 Schematic of one recursive Kalman filter step to obtain the new state estimate. Possible position (state) and uncertainties are indicated by the size of the blue circles. When the predicted new state is calculated from the previous state the uncertainty is increased (predicted current state). A possible sensory input is calculated from the predicted state and the difference to the actual sensory input (that also has an uncertainty) is used to refine the current state estimate. The Kalman gain converts the sensory difference into state errors by weighting the inputs by their respective uncertainties. Sensory and state signals are shown as *green* and *red arrows*, respectively.

Kalman filter

Like the Wiener filter the Kalman filter (KF) is a MIMO model that estimates the state of a linear dynamic system from multiple measured inputs. It produces an estimate of state as the weighted average of the predicted state, from a dynamic model of the previous state and the measurement of the current state (Fig. 15.9). KFs are an important element of control theory. As an easy example we consider a ship or airplane with constant velocity. Knowing the previous position with a certain precision we can estimate the current position by adding the covered distance (physical model). This corresponds to the "prediction phase" in the recursive update of the KF. However, over time inaccuracies will sum up and external disturbances such as drift will decrease the exactness of our new position. In the "update phase" of the KF the new position is determined again with some uncertainty and the inaccurate (noisy) predicted position is compared with the inaccurately (noisy) determined new position to improve the prediction.

The KF is an efficient recursive filter that estimates the state of a linear dynamic system from a series of noisy measurements and inaccurate predictions. It calculates in discrete time steps a prediction of the current state from a previous state based on a dynamic model. Together with the conversion of this predicted state into its sensory equivalent this is called the "update step." The strength of KFs is that the uncertainties of the sensory input and the prediction are taken into account. Depending on their uncertainty in terms of covariance, the relative sensory inputs and predictions are weighted accordingly and the current state estimate will be between the predicted and the measured state. The certainty of the measurement and the current state prediction is taken into account by their relative weight in the KF gain. By choosing a high filter gain, the sensory input is more closely followed and sensory input noise will result in a noisy state prediction. In contrast, a low gain will put more accent on the prediction and will smoothen the state response. By tuning the "gain," the KF can be adjusted for optimal performance in a specific task.

Although the KF is an efficient recursive filter that can deal with noisy data, inaccurate measurements, and to a certain degree with external disturbances, it is limited to linear dynamic systems. As many biological systems are non-linear, **extended Kalman filters** (EKFs) employing multivariate Taylor series expansions are used to linearize models locally around a working point to treat non-linear systems. However, EKFs can be computationally cost-intensive and may suffer from instabilities. One non-linear KF that is promising for BMI applications is the **unscented Kalman Filter** (UKF). Non-linear neuronal tuning behavior and more than one recent state have been implemented in BMI decoders using the UKF.

Artificial neural networks are also successfully used for decoding of cortical activity during observed or imagined movements in a training phase, as an alternative to the analytic modeling analyses just discussed. A broad range of network designs, for example, (multilayer) perceptrons, were successfully applied in real-time interpretation of brain-derived movement decoding and can outperform other strategies. Moreover, neural networks inherently have the potential to model non-linear behavior. Specifically, recurrent neural networks (RNNs) can learn nonlinear relations in time series with memory effects (i.e., dependencies on previous states) and provide faster learning and better performance in some tasks than other current state-of-the-art methods like UKFs. Learning speed is important because interpretation of brain activity frozen after decoder training loses relevance over time. The recording electrode position may shift, the number of active electrodes may decrease over time, and/or the brain can undergo plastic adaptation. To compensate for this, adaptive decoders are being developed that update the algorithm setting continuously. For example, in reinforcement learning, parameter sets that lead to a successful result in a task are strengthened through a scalar feedback signal. Some of these adaptive algorithms are able to improve the decoder performance starting from an initial arbitrary parameter setting.

Chronic long-term recording of large populations of neurons, the identification of the optimal cortical structures, and the improvement of decoding algorithms are crucial for the success and implementation of everyday prosthetic devices and thus they are the subject of intensive ongoing research.

Brief summary

- Sensing implants detect and decode neural information to enable movement via an artificial output (such as control of an artificial limb or computer cursor).
- Movement intentions are encoded by large distributed neuronal populations of broadly tuned neurons distributed over several cortical areas.
- To determine how many neurons have to be recorded to obtain a certain accuracy of the prediction, the NDC can be employed.
- Both non-invasive and invasive (requiring surgery) techniques are used to obtain neural recordings.
- ECoG is well established in clinical practice and can be used for classifiers and reproduction of limited sets of motor outputs.
- Penetrating electrodes such as the Utah array provide better recording fidelity, but suffer from safety and long-term stability issues.
- Micro-wire arrays and soft polymer electrodes are upcoming technologies that better match the mechanical environment of the brain.
- All BMIs rely on decoding algorithms to accurately convert neural signals into motor intentions.
- The most common decoding algorithms are population vector decoders, Wiener filters, and Kalman filters. Each has advantages and disadvantages.
- Neural networks and other artificial learning algorithms provide an additional possibility for new decoding strategies.

Key literature and further reading

Aflalo, T., Kellis, S., Klaes, C., Lee, B., Shi, Y., Pejsa, K., Shanfield, K., Hayes-Jackson, S., Aisen, M., Heck, C., Liu, C., Andersen, R.A., 2015. Neurophysiology. Decoding motor imagery from the posterior parietal cortex of a tetraplegic human. Science 348, 906–910.

Birbaumer, N., Ghanayim, N., Hinterberger, T., Iversen, I., Kotchoubey, B., Kubler, A., Perelmouter, J., Taub, E., Flor, H., 1999. A spelling device for the paralysed. Nature 398, 297–298.

Bouton, C.E., Shaikhouni, A., Annetta, N.V., Bockbrader, M.A., Friedenberg, D.A., Nielson, D.M., Sharma, G., Sederberg, P.B., Glenn, B.C., Mysiw, W.J., Morgan, A.G., Deogaonkar, M., Rezai, A.R., 2016. Restoring cortical control of functional movement in a human with quadriplegia. Nature 533, 247–250.

Donoghue, J.P., 2008. Bridging the brain to the world: a perspective on neural interface systems. Neuron 60, 511–521.

Georgopoulos, A.P., Kalaska, J.F., Caminiti, R., Massey, J.T., 1982. On the relations between the direction of two-dimensional arm movements and cell discharge in primate motor cortex. J. Neurosci. 2, 1527–1537.

Hochberg, L.R., Bacher, D., Jarosiewicz, B., Masse, N.Y., Simeral, J.D., Vogel, J., Haddadin, S., Liu, J., Cash, S.S., van der, S.P., Donoghue, J.P., 2012. Reach and grasp by people with tetraplegia using a neurally controlled robotic arm. Nature 485, 372–375.

Lebedev, M.A., Nicolelis, M.A., 2017. Brain-machine interfaces: from basic science to neuroprostheses and neurorehabilitation. Physiol. Rev. 97, 767–837.

Musk, E., Neuralink, 2019. An integrated brain-machine interface platform with thousands of channels. BioRxiv. https://doi.org/10.1101/703801.

Schwarz, D.A., Lebedev, M.A., Hanson, T.L., Dimitrov, D.F., Lehew, G., Meloy, J., Rajangam, S., Subramanian, V., Ifft, P.J., Li, Z., Ramakrishnan, A., Tate, A., Zhuang, K.Z., Nicolelis, M.A., 2014. Chronic, wireless recordings of large-scale brain activity in freely moving rhesus monkeys. Nat. Methods 11, 670–676.

Volkova, K., Lebedev, M.A., Kaplan, A., Ossadtchi, A., 2019. Decoding movement from electrocorticographic activity: a review. Front. Neuroinform. 13, 74.

Wessberg, J., Stambaugh, C.R., Kralik, J.D., Beck, P.D., Laubach, M., Chapin, J.K., Kim, J., Biggs, S.J., Srinivasan, M.A., Nicolelis, M.A., 2000. Real-time prediction of hand trajectory by ensembles of cortical neurons in primates. Nature 408, 361–365.

Wolpert, D.M., Ghahramani, Z., 2000. Computational principles of movement neuroscience. Nat. Neurosci. 3 (Suppl), 1212–1217.

CHAPTER 16

Future directions

Emerging neural interface therapies

There has been a rapid pace of innovation, translation, and commercialization of neural prostheses in recent years. An ever-increasing understanding of the nervous system in health and disease, coupled with advances in materials science, have resulted in a proliferation of neural interface designs and technologies. Although clinical translation in this field is, by necessity, a slow process (see **Chapter 3**), many of these emerging technologies are now close to commercialization. Furthermore, many novel technologies are undergoing preclinical development with the aim to overcome the technical constraints of the field imposed by current limitations in the materials, safe electrical waveforms, and surgical approaches. This chapter gives an overview of a subset of these emerging therapies and blue-sky innovations, with the intent of outlining for the reader the potential directions of neural prosthesis research and therapy in the coming decades.

Vestibular protheses

Vestibular system physiology

The vestibular sensory system detects the translation and rotation of the head in space and its orientation relative to gravity. Alongside the visual, proprioceptive, and somatosensory systems, it is a vital component of our sense of balance. Our sense of balance helps us maintain posture, move through space, adjust to sudden changes in position, and retain stable gaze fixation during head movements.

In humans and other mammals, the peripheral component of the vestibular system is contained within the inner ear. Each side of the vestibular sensory periphery contains a set of three structures called the **semicircular canals** that begin and terminate in a larger chamber called the **vestibule** (Fig. 16.1). These canals are called the **horizontal canal**, the **posterior canal**, and the **superior/anterior canal**. The bony canals and vestibule are filled with a fluid similar to cerebrospinal fluid (CSF) called perilymph. Suspended in the canals is a further division called the **membranous labyrinth**, which contains endolymph of similar composition to the cochlea. The three semicircular canals are orientated relative to the head such that any rotation of the head in three-dimensional space causes the inertial rotation of fluid within one or more canals. The membranous labyrinth in each semicircular canal terminates in an **ampulla**, where a bed of vestibular sensory cells called **hair cells** are contained within the crista ampullaris.

Prostheses for the Brain
https://doi.org/10.1016/B978-0-12-818892-7.00017-1

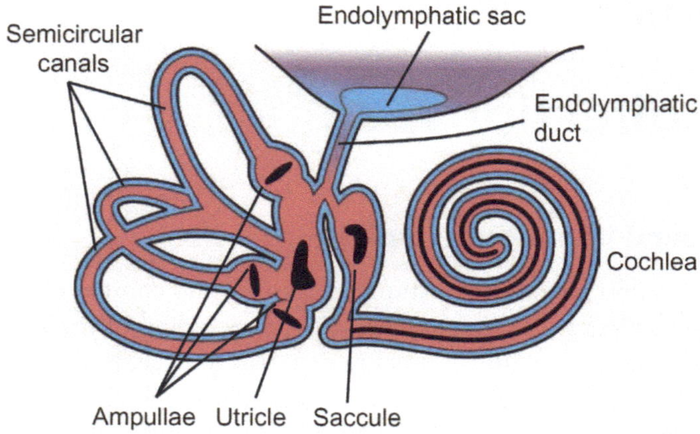

Fig. 16.1 Anatomic diagram of the inner ear, including the vestibular labyrinth and the cochlea. Within the vestibular labyrinth are three semicircular canals (Superior, Posterior, and Horizontal), which contain a sensory epithelium at the ampulla for the detection of head rotation. The canals all terminate in the vestibule. The vestibule is an open chamber that also contains the otolith organs (the utricle and saccule), which are sensory epithelia specialized for the detection of head translation and static tilt relative to gravity. *(Figure from Marcus and Wangemann (2009).)*

The hair cells of the vestibular system are mechanoreceptors that detect the deflection of the cupula, a gelatinous mass within the ampulla, in response to the motion of fluid within the membranous labyrinth (Fig. 16.2). A set of stereociliary bundles sprout from the apex of each hair cell, consisting of a kinocilium and rows of stereocilia. At the base of these bundles are mechanoreceptive ion channels that open and close in response to the deflection of the bundle. At rest (no deflection), there is high spontaneous "resting" activity at the hair cell/afferent synapse. If the bundle is deflected towards the kinocilium, this depolarizes the hair cell, leading to further neurotransmitter release and increased activation of the post-synaptic vestibular afferent. Deflection away from the kinocilium hyperpolarizes the hair cell, reducing neurotransmitter release and decreasing activation of the afferent. In this manner, rotation in either direction can be encoded by the vestibular system as an increase or decrease from a "baseline rate" of activation. Two main types of hair cells exist (Type I and Type II) that differ in their types of synaptic connections and variability in resting discharge rates. The hair cells of the semicircular canals detect **angular acceleration**, not velocity or position; over time during a constant rotational velocity, friction will eventually cause the fluid rotation to match the body rotation and the cupula will no longer be deflected.

Two additional sets of vestibular sensory organs, called the **otolith organs**, exist in the chamber of the vestibule. These two organs, called the **utricle** and **saccule**, are located within their respective vestibular maculae and their hair cells are embedded in a gel-like structure called the otolithic membrane. The otolithic membrane is seeded with calcium carbonate particles called otoconia that have a greater density than the

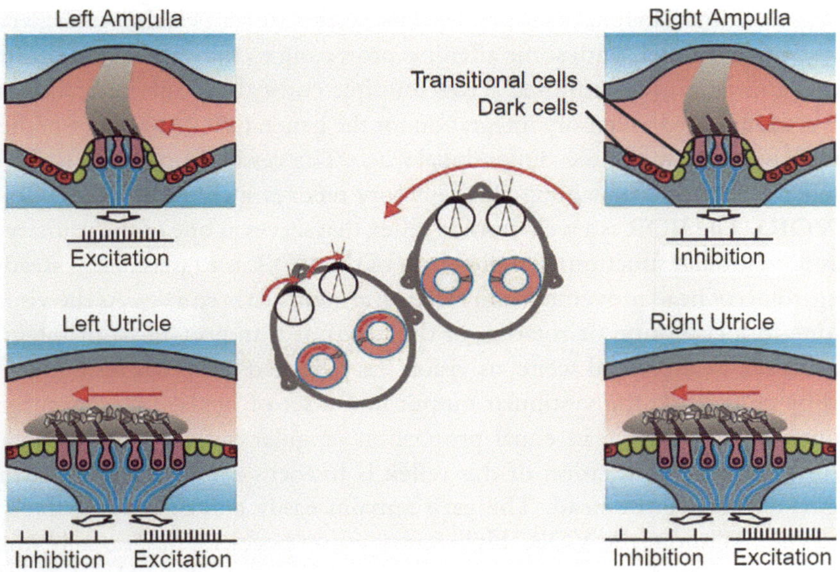

Fig. 16.2 Diagram showing the sensory mechanism of the ampulla in the semicircular canals. As the head rotates, there is counter-rotation of the fluid (relative to the head as the frame of reference) within the canals as a consequence of inertia. This imparts kinetic force on the gelatinous cupula that surrounds the hair cells in the ampulla, displacing it and subsequently bending the embedded hair cells. In the utricle the gelatinous embedding of the stereocilia contain the otoconia with a higher density than the fluid, making them susceptible to translational acceleration and gravity. The hair cells are mechanoreceptors that respond to this deflection by depolarizing or hyperpolarizing, depending on the direction of deflection. *(Figure from Marcus and Wangemann (2009).)*

surrounding fluid and provide weight to the otolithic membrane. As the head is translated or rotated relative to gravity, the otoconia have inertial drag that shifts the membrane relative to the hair cells in a similar fashion to the ampullae of the semicircular canals. The utricle is positioned so that it can more effectively detect movement in the horizontal plane, while the saccule more effectively detects movement in the vertical plane. In contrast to the semicircular canals, which primarily detect rotational acceleration, the utricle and saccule are primarily responsible for the detection of linear acceleration (i.e., translation) and the tilt of the head relative to gravity. The orientation of each end organ means that between them, the position, translation, and rotation of the head in three-dimensional space and in relation to gravity can be encoded. Each set of vestibular organs works in concert with a paired contralateral counterpart to produce a "**push-pull**" system of head rotation detection. For example, when the head is rotated so that the left anterior canal is stimulated, the same motion will inhibit the right posterior canal. This improves the signal quality via redundancy and coupled feedback. The canal pairings are referred to as RALP (right anterior/left posterior), LARP (left anterior/right posterior), and LHRH or Z (left/right horizontal).

The signals from individual canals and otolith organs are sent via the vestibular afferent to the **vestibular nuclei**, with some afferents projecting to the cerebellum. From there, vestibular information is transmitted across multiple cortical and subcortical areas, many of which are implicated in sensory integration for the generation of a percept of the body's position and movement in three-dimensional space. The vestibular pathway is also directly responsible for balance-maintaining compensatory reflexes such as the **vestibulo-ocular reflex (VOR)**. The VOR is a well-studied reflex that serves as one of the primary clinical measures of vestibular function. The function of the VOR is to maintain a steady visual image regardless of head movement and rotation around all three axes. As the visual scene moves (due to locomotion or rotation of the head), it is important to maintain an eye position relative to the visual scene, as vision has a limited temporal resolution. This is achieved by converting the vestibular output into a set of ocular muscle motor inputs that counter-rotate the eye in equal proportion (angular velocity) to the rotation of the head. A basic demonstration of this reflex is to focus on a static object (this page or a finger) and move the head. The gaze remains easily and reflexively fixed on the tracked object. Without the VOR, high-acuity vision becomes functionally impossible in many everyday situations as the visual scene is continuously shifted by the movement of the head (like when recording with a camera in absence of visual scene stabilization). Additionally, the vestibular system also exerts a constant ("tonic") drive to the muscles of the trunk (axial muscles) that stabilize the body in the upright position (the vestibule-spinal reflex). This guarantees stable standing posture that can adapt to movements sensed by the vestibular system. In absence of this reflex, standing stability is reduced and the probability of falls is increased.

Vestibular implants

Patients with bilateral loss of vestibular function suffer from crippling disabilities involving stable retinal image, balance, and locomotion. This balance deficit is particularly pronounced in absence of vision (e.g., in the dark), since the visual system can compensate the loss of vestibular function to an extent, although the control loop from the visual system is much slower. Furthermore, in some conditions loss of vestibular functions is associated with a feeling of weightlessness, spinning, or rotation, with corresponding nausea. The symptoms of an acute loss of vestibular function may reduce over time as visual adaptation occurs, but the compensation is far from complete and often symptoms persist.

This all results in a reduction in independence and quality of life, with an economic burden comparable to bilateral hearing loss. As individuals age, loss of vestibular function greatly increases the chance of falls, which are a primary contributor to morbidity in the elderly. Vestibular dysfunction can be partly compensated for with the help of rehabilitation therapy, particularly in children, but severe bilateral vestibular loss remains a permanent and untreatable condition. Vestibular implants are one solution to this problem

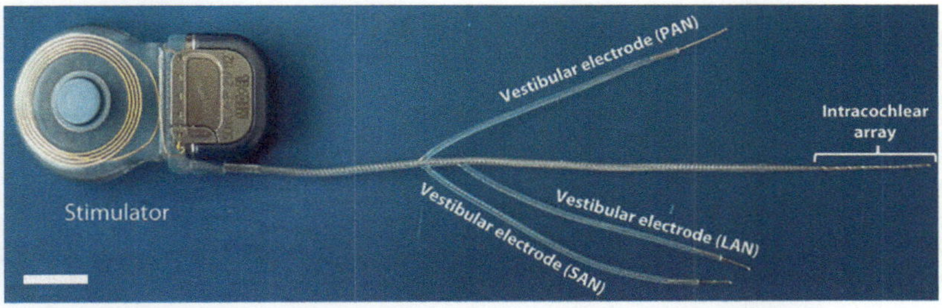

Fig. 16.3 Example of a vestibular prosthesis design for human implantation. This design integrates a cochlear implant and three vestibular electrodes for patients with combined hearing/vestibular loss. All vestibular implant designs have similarities such as a flexible, bifurcated approach and the adaptation of preexisting cochlear implant electronics. Scale bar is 1 cm. *(Image from Perez Fornos et al. (2014).)*

and there has been a concerted effort to develop vestibular prostheses that can artificially restore function in this population of patients.

Due to the physiological similarities between the two sensory systems, vestibular prostheses are similar to and originally modified from cochlear implant designs. They consist of a trifurcated platinum or platinum-iridium electrode array positioned on flexible wires that can be inserted into each of the three semicircular canals (Fig. 16.3). The encapsulated electronics and inductive power/control transmission from external components are all similar to cochlear implant technologies discussed previously in **Chapter 11**, except that the input is rotational/translational information captured with motion sensors rather than auditory information captured with microphones. The components and requirements are similar enough that it is possible to modify a cochlear implant to provide both cochlear stimulation *and* vestibular stimulation on different electrodes.

Vestibular physiology has a resting **spontaneous baseline** of activity required for the aforementioned vestibulospinal reflex. It further encodes the direction of head rotation as changes both above and below this baseline. To maintain strict safety criteria, vestibular implants must deliver charge-balanced, biphasic pulses (similar to cochlear implants), which can excite neurons but cannot easily inhibit them (see **Chapter 6**). To compensate for this, pulses are delivered constantly at rest (0 degrees/s rotation) at a frequency baseline (typically 100–150 Hz in humans) to mimic a spontaneous baseline rate that is otherwise substantially reduced or eliminated in patients with vestibular loss. Rotational velocity is then mapped according to the vestibular axis of rotation and to a pulse rate above or below this baseline rate. In this way, the frequency of the pulses encodes both the direction and strength of the stimulus along each semicircular canal axis of rotation. This stimulation strategy is called either **pulse frequency modulation (PFM)** or **pulse rate modulation (PRM)**. Fig. 16.4 shows an example waveform using this strategy. The velocity of the rotational stimulus can also be co-modulated by varying the amplitude

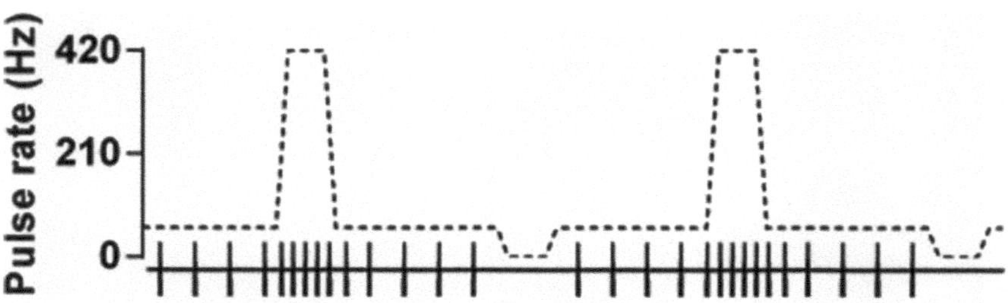

Fig. 16.4 Example of a pulse frequency modulation paradigm. Biphasic pulse rate is maintained at some baseline (in this case, 60 Hz). To deliver an excitatory stimulus this rate is increased, and to deliver an inhibitory stimulus this rate is decreased. This mimics the physiological rate code of the vestibular afferent. *(Figure adapted from Aplin et al. (2019).)*

of the biphasic pulses relative to the stimulus strength; this secondary strategy is called **pulse amplitude modulation (PAM)**. Reported stimulation pulse amplitude perceptual thresholds are in the range of ~100–150 μA with a phase duration of 50–200 μS (determined on a by-patient basis) and no interphase gap.

Clinical outcomes

Vestibular prostheses are currently in the early clinical stage of development and have not yet been approved for commercial use. However, several groups have performed clinical trials demonstrating the viability of vestibular stimulation as a means to restore vestibular function. These studies have also highlighted key steps that are necessary to improve the function of vestibular prostheses moving forward.

The primary method of assessing stimulation outcomes in the clinic is to use compensatory eye movements generated by the vestibulo-ocular reflex (VOR). The main measure of the VOR is how well the compensatory eye vector matches the relative rotation of the head. In normal clinical practice a standard method of quantification is to track eye movements while a subject is rotated in a chair in the dark (to minimize visual/proprioceptive input) or after disturbing the system via hot or cold water irrigation into the ear canal (the **caloric test**). For electrical stimulation it is also possible to achieve this without the need for additional setup by delivering arbitrary stimulation signals not coupled to a motion sensor. The important psychophysical characteristics of this test are the **gain** (the ratio between head velocity, simulated or real, and eye velocity) and the **phase** (how synchronized the eye movement is to the associated stimulus in time). Some studies also consider the **alignment** or **axis** (how closely the direction of eye movement matches the expected direction of a given stimulus) as a measure of the canal specificity of the stimulation. The gain and phase of the VOR are stimulus frequency dependent, meaning that signal-processing standards such as **Bode plots** (amplitude and phase dependence of the signal as a function of frequency) are commonly used to interpret vestibular output. In the dark and for rotation stimulus frequencies at ~1 Hz, normal function should expect a gain of $\sim$0.8 and a phase lead/lag of less than 2 degrees. When visual feedback is available (i.e., in a well-lit environment), normal human VOR gains should be close to one. Vestibular dysfunction lies on a scale of severity, with extreme cases that are considered primary candidates for a vestibular implant having gains of 0.25 or less.

A handful of initial clinical studies and trials published over the past half-decade have reported mostly consistent findings. Implantation surgery was universally uncomplicated and in one chronic study the implants remained post-operatively stable for the trial period (8 weeks). Patients suffered from severe vertigo when the device was initially activated, but rapidly recovered (<5 min upon onset of stimulation). This is an expected consequence of the introduction of the "baseline" pulse rate. Subsequent frequency modulation of one or more semicircular canals produced a VOR response appropriate to the stimulated canal, direction of PFM (increased or decreased stimulation frequency relative to baseline), and frequency/amplitude stimulus intensity. VOR gain showed a significant improvement, with best-case scenario improvements from a preoperative gain of <0.1 to a post-operative gain of $\sim$0.5 during 1 Hz rotations (Fig. 16.5). The critical frequency range for several activities such as walking and gaze stabilization during reading is 0.1–2 Hz. However, there remains limited information about responses at higher frequencies (2–20 Hz), which are still within the range of physiologically relevant head movements. Although the reported post-operative gains are still below normal function, in one study using a chronically activated device, patients qualitatively reported more stable vision and balance as well as the ability to perform many routine tasks that were previously impossible unassisted. These are promising outcomes for initial trials.

There remain some limitations in the reported outcomes. There is an asymmetry in gain, with rotations towards the implanted side (increased stimulation frequency) consistently achieving greater gains and greater dynamic ranges of eye rotational velocity than contralateral rotations (decreased stimulation frequency). This is likely the result of an inherent asymmetry in vestibular physiology: there is a greater dynamic range above baseline ($\sim$300 Hz) than below ($\sim$150 Hz), as it is not possible to modulate frequency below 0 Hz. Increasing the baseline to balance this asymmetry does not result in more balanced gains.

Vestibular and cochlear labyrinths are connected through a structure called ductus reuniens. By that, the endolymph produced in the stria vascularis can also fill the vestibular organ. This, however, also means that any manipulation of the vestibular organ can lead to cochlear damage. Indeed, one clinical study reported complete hearing loss on the implanted side in all patients, although subsequent studies have demonstrated that this is not an inevitable consequence of vestibular implantation surgery. To avoid this, device designs have favored unilateral implantation or co-implantation with a cochlear implant (wherein the patient is already profoundly deaf). Regardless, the risk of hearing loss remains a major regulatory hurdle as well as an ethical and pragmatic consideration for vestibular prostheses.

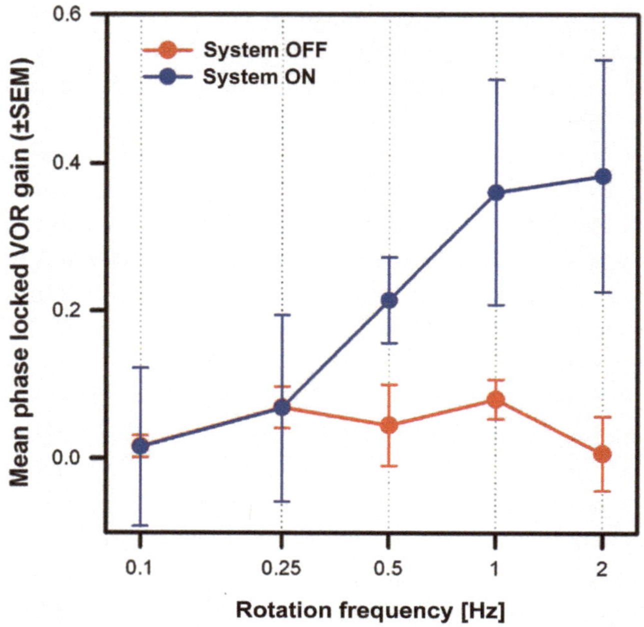

Fig. 16.5 Patient data ($n=3$) from a study using the multichannel vestibular implant shown in Fig. 16.3. The X-axis shows the frequency of VOR rotational stimuli, while the Y-axis shows the resultant VOR gain. There was a clear, albeit highly variable, improvement (*blue vs. red line*) compared to when the device was switched off, demonstrating that the effect is a direct result of the stimulation paradigm and not a training effect or related to the surgical approach. However, the measured improvement still fell below normal functioning mean VOR gain (~0.6). *(Figure from Perez Fornos et al. (2014).)*

The next stage for vestibular implants will be broader clinical trials to prove safety, efficacy, and economic viability on a larger patient population. Further device innovation and optimization is possible if initial designs overcome economic and regulatory hurdles and prove commercially successful. The development and implantation of bilateral implants could improve accuracy and overcome issues with asymmetric gains introduced by unilateral stimulation. The main roadblock for bilateral implantation is the risk of hearing loss. Although it appears that hearing can be preserved directly following implantation, unilateral implant designs will first have to demonstrate that they do not damage hearing over chronic timeframes (years to decades).

Closed-loop stimulation

Another emerging application in neuroprosthetics is closed-loop approaches. Most prosthetic devices discussed in this book have been treated as unidirectional devices: they either stimulate neurons (as in the case of auditory, visual, and vestibular implants or in deep brain stimulation) or record neuronal activity (as discussed in **Chapter 15**). Neither sensory organs nor the motor system is exclusively unidirectional in natural conditions; all receive some kind of feedback. For example, the sensory systems receive extensive efferent (brain to sensory organ) information that can influence the sensitivity and the working mode of the sensory organs. In the example of the auditory system the efferents can set the working point of the organ of Corti and by that affect the sensitivity of the sensing hair cells. This means that under noisy conditions the sensory organ becomes less sensitive and thus less prone to masking effects of the noise without efferent input. Reciprocally, the motor system is tightly interwoven with the somatosensory and proprioceptive feedback from the motor organ. The circuits with the spinal cord can be considered from the perspective of control theory as a servo system setting the length of the muscle and controlling it to secure the length under perturbing influences from the physical world (like passive stretch of the muscle). Under passive stretch the muscle returns to its original length by the action of muscle spindles in the muscle and its feedback through a simple control circuit in the spinal cord. Tight connections between the proprioceptive system, the somatosensory system, and the motor system can be observed at all levels of their architecture. All neural systems are part of some kind of control loop with feedback signals and are thus bidirectionally interconnected. This architecture assures that there is no runaway activity and no instability in function.

It is therefore conceptually misleading to consider a sensory prosthetic device as a unidirectional device, independent from the function of the brain. There are different requirements on prosthetic devices at rest, in sleep, and in activity. We have to consider them as part of a loop with the brain, registering and detecting its current state and adapting the prosthetic function to the recent needs of the subject. Only such a bidirectional connection, with a closed loop between brain and device, allows the optimal replacement of lost functions by a prosthetic device. Closed-loop approaches can be applied to nearly any prosthetic device, many of which have been patented and are currently in clinical trials.

Sensory prostheses in particular can benefit from feedback adaptation. In an auditory prosthesis, a key feedback component is attention (i.e., which auditory stimulus should be heard or ignored). In particular, it is important that auditory attention is directed towards a selected stimulus. For example, in a crowded room it may be more important to focus on speech from a particular individual to the front or side of the listener. It is already possible, using spatially sensitive microphones and beam-forming techniques, to increase the sensitivity of the prosthesis for a particular position in the room. That might partially counterbalance the coarse representation of spectral information in cochlear or brainstem implants that precludes the brain from doing this. Experimentally, there have been attempts to record gaze direction (which often coincides with attentional focus). Recording of EEG activity through the implant (e.g., using the casing of the implant as a recording electrode) is a further technique under exploration in several laboratories.

Present-day cochlear implant devices already include a technique to record the auditory nerve compound action potentials. These are accessible for the clinician and often serve as the first approximation of perceptual threshold currents for implant fitting, particularly important for young deaf children who cannot communicate yet. Many teams around the world currently work on automated implant-fitting procedures using these signals. This is not a simple task, particularly since the compound action potentials are partly covered by large stimulation artifacts. Compound action potential thresholds are greater than perceptual thresholds and thus the procedure further requires an extrapolation technique.

Similarly, feedback is key in prosthetics used for pain relief. Perceived pain fluctuates throughout the day. Thus, stimulation requires adaptation to the moment-to-moment pain intensity. For this, establishing a reliable readout of the perceived pain is required. If such a system could even anticipate an increase in pain before it is perceived it would substantially alleviate the suffering of the subject. Similarly, in deep brain stimulation (Fig. 16.6) the required feedback would be the severity of the tremor, accessible by recording the activity of the neurons in the stimulated region (that are synchronous to the tremor) or alternatively, recording from the affected muscle groups. In cortical implants using electrocorticographic grids, particularly in cases of epilepsy, a closed-loop

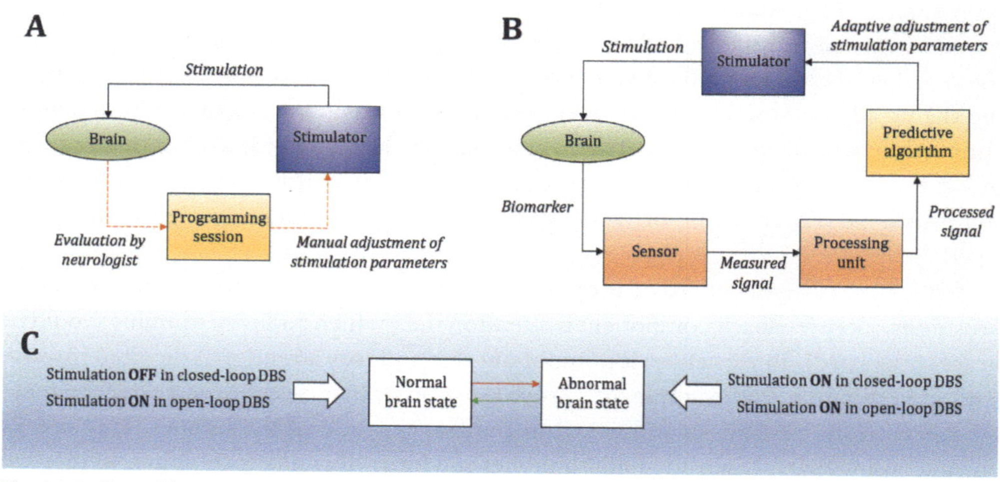

Fig. 16.6 Closed-loop stimulation in DBS. In a standard DBS implant (A), the stimulator is adjusted only during a programming session with a neurologist and cannot adapt to dynamic changes in brain state. In a closed-loop implant (B), sensors can constantly measure relevant biomarkers and can adapt the stimulus. By only stimulating during abnormal brain states (C) closed-loop DBS can be more energy efficient, effective, and less likely to induce unwanted side effects when the patient is healthy. *(Image redrawn from Parastarfeizabadi and Kouzani (2018) under the Creative Commons license. http://creativecommons.org/licenses/by/4.0/.)*

approach might detect epileptic activity and interrupt it before seizures appear and generalize. Such a technique could make surgical removal of the epileptic locus obsolete in the future. It is clear that closed-loop approaches are broadly applicable for virtually all forms of neural prosthetic. Future development will bring more sophisticated implants that use closed-loop techniques to better integrate into the body, and this will further boost functionality and acceptance for users.

Somatosensory and proprioceptive prostheses

One the most integrated and important "closed loops" in the nervous system is the interaction between the motor system and the somatosensory system. In **Chapter 15**, we discussed the use of sensing implants to drive robotics or motor prostheses for patients. These address the acquisition of *motor* commands that can be used to drive prosthetic or robotic limbs or manipulators for amputees or paralyzed patients. As briefly discussed in **Chapter 14**, the somatosensory and proprioceptive ("self" sensing) components are also important facets of motor control as they provide feedback for the position of the body in space. Without these feedback signals, the brain cannot dynamically adjust the force required to grasp or manipulate objects. It also cannot rapidly compensate for errors that occur between the *intended* and *actual* motor outputs due to stochastic error in the neural signal or interference from, for example, an external unexpected resistance or counterforce. A common example of where this dynamic adjustment is a key component of motor control is the manipulation of fragile objects, such as a wine glass or egg; enough force must be applied to maintain friction so that the object does not slip from the grasp, but not so much that the object is destroyed by the grip. Proprioceptive adjustment (the position of the limb in space) can be somewhat compensated for via visual feedback, but the visual system is slow (see **Chapter 12**), unreliable in low-light environments, and mentally taxing (requires conscious effort).

An often-overlooked feature of proprioceptive and somatosensory limb feedback is that it also provides a sense of *embodiment* over a limb. Embodiment is a patient's process of incorporating a prosthesis into their concept of *self-image*, so that they perceive the prosthesis as part of their own body. The human mind instinctively rejects the physical incorporation of objects into itself that it does not recognize as part of its own body (see **Chapter 3**). A common issue during rehabilitation with a prosthetic limb is that the patient refuses to accept their new limb as a part of the body, does not learn to use it effectively, and may continue to feel distressing symptoms such as phantom limbs/pain associated with the lack of the amputated limb. Already used in rehabilitation for amputations or strokes are techniques such as *mirror box therapy*, which crudely "mimic" somatosensory feedback and thus reduce this psychological distress. It should be expected that proper somatosensory integration would thus be even more helpful in eliminating these issues. In combination with the functional limitations of a motor prosthesis without somatosensory feedback control, it is clear that the development of proper somatosensory and proprioceptive feedback for motor prostheses is an important area of innovation for these interventions. This is not a new concept. This field has been active since the beginning of robotic limb prosthesis research. However, due to the complexity of the task, only in the last decade has there been substantial progress towards clinical and commercial translation of integrated motor/sensory prostheses.

Peripheral somatosensory stimulation

The somatosensory, proprioceptive, and nociceptive (pain) systems are a closely interlinked network of mechanoreceptors, thermoreceptors, and chemoreceptors (see **Chapter 14**, Fig. 14.1). These systems overlap in their physical (and sometimes even neural) pathways, further diverging only as the information is classified in the spinal cord and through into the brain. The primary sensory neurons of these systems have their sensory apparatus in the periphery (at the site of sensory detection), but cell bodies located in the dorsal root ganglion at the spinal cord (**Chapter 14**, Fig. 14.3). When a limb is lost the nerve is cut and the peripheral apparatus is lost, but the cell bodies remain along with the surviving length of nerve. Over time and without continued input, these cells will retract their processes and may degenerate, but, fortuitously, there is a timing window after implantation where the still-intact component of the cells can be stimulated to produce sensations perceived as localized within the (now non-existent) limb. By mapping these sensations to artificial receptors on a newly installed prosthetic limb, it is thus possible to "close the loop" between motor and somatosensory systems. The implanted devices used to stimulate the surviving peripheral nerve are called "peripheral nerve interfaces." The biggest limitation of these devices is that, as previously mentioned, neurons in these nerves are in close proximity and are neither topographically nor functionally mapped, except in the crudest sense. This makes the delivery of *precise* sensations (as necessary for feedback) a daunting and complex task. As such, peripheral nerve interface development has focused on optimal electrode position, design, and stimulation parameters that can aid in the discreet stimulation of neurons in the peripheral nerves to produce *localized* percepts with controllable somatosensory properties.

Generally, peripheral nerve interface electrodes are implanted in either *extraneural* or *intraneural* positions, with specific electrode designs optimized for one of these two locations. Extraneural electrodes are implanted so that they are in contact with a peripheral nerve, but do not penetrate the epineurium (Figs. 14.2 and 16.7A). This electrode concept is also often referred to as a *nerve cuff* and has a proven clinical history. The most basic form of cuff electrode is a silicone cuff design with flat, circular electrodes spaced longitudinally along the device. More complex devices increase the available surface area of the electrode by wrapping the contacts around the nerve (Fig 16.7E). Because extraneural electrodes do not penetrate the epineurium, they have the advantage of safety and longevity compared to intraneural electrodes. However, the tradeoff is that they have less

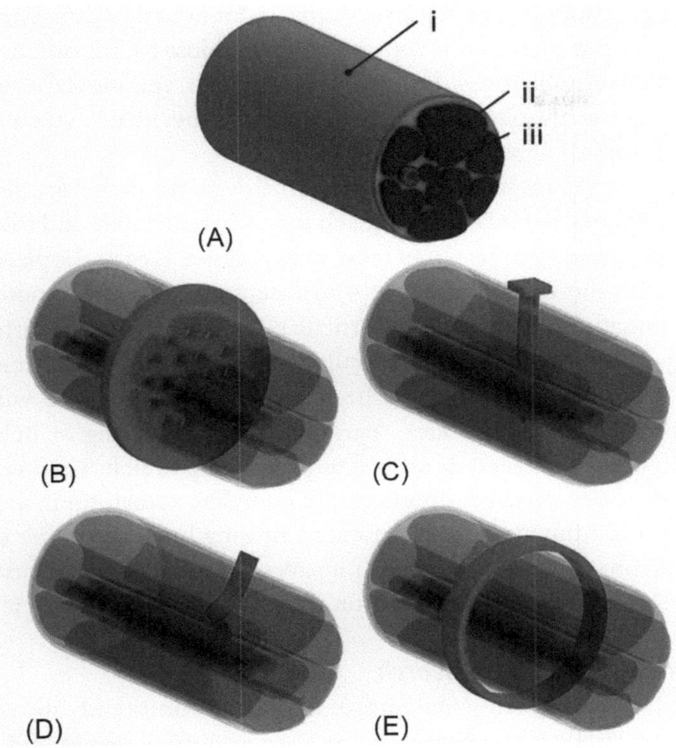

Fig. 16.7 Examples of peripheral recording/sensing electrode designs. (A) Schematic of a peripheral nerve containing an epineurium (i), nerve fascicles (ii), and blood vessels (iii). (B–E) Example simplified designs for peripheral nerve electrodes including the regenerative (B), intrafasicular (C), intraneural (D), and nerve cuff (E). *(Image reproduced from Russell et al. (2019) under the Creative Commons license. http://creativecommons.org/licenses/by/4.0/.)*

specificity as they only have optimal access to nerve fibers on the exterior surface of the nerve and must contend with greater current spread through the non-neural components of the nerve bundles.

Intraneural electrodes are inserted within the nerve itself (i.e., through the epineurium, Fig 16.7D). There is a further subset of these devices that also penetrate the perineurium and are thus in the closest proximity to the neural tissue within the fascicles (Fig 16.7C). These electrodes consist of either rows of penetrating shanks with variable length or "grids" that resemble a sieve. In these grid electrodes the nerve is transected, the electrode implanted, and finally the nerve is sewed together again. The regenerating axons are then allowed to grow back through the electrode for maximal contact area (regenerative arrays; Fig 16.7B). As intraneural electrode approaches penetrate closer to the nerve, they trade greater specificity for greater levels of physiological disruption. The perineurium is not a passive connective tissue but rather a part of the blood–nerve barrier that helps maintain homeostatic mechanisms for neural health. The destruction of perineural integrity can increase the inflammatory response to implantation and degrade neural health, both of which reduce specificity. As such, intraneural electrodes do not always result in better thresholds or perceptual outcomes than extraneural electrodes and the optimal surgical approach remains unclear.

For a patient with damage to the central somatosensory pathways, such as in spinal cord injury, a peripheral stimulation approach is no longer feasible and the task of restoring somatosensory perception becomes more complicated. Electrodes placed in the spinal cord centrally from the injury, or in the somatosensory cortex, can potentially induce somatosensory sensations in this case. In particular, the somatosensory cortex is organized somatotopically so spatially discreet stimulation with intracortical microstimulation (ICMS) arrays can be used to elicit localized perceptions. One issue with these arrays is that they more commonly produce "paresthesia"-type buzzing or itching sensations rather than "physiological" sensations such as pressure or stretch. Furthermore, perceptual mapping appears to produce only partially complete somatotopic maps that would not be able to restore function across an entire missing limb but rather only a random subset of topographic areas. Continued improvements in the specificity and safety of CNS implants should help drive innovation for central somatosensory prostheses.

Clinical outcomes and future research

In the past half-decade, experimental human trials have consistently shown that peripheral somatosensory stimulation approaches are chronically safe, stable, and can elicit consistent and discreet somatosensory percepts that are localized to the "missing" or prosthetic limb. They have demonstrated a reliable reduction in phantom limb pain and mild but significant increases in functional outcomes for prosthetic limb use, encouraging more "naturalistic" reflexive behaviors compared to prosthetic limb use without feedback. The main barrier to more widespread clinical application of current somatosensory prostheses is the limited range of perceptual "space" they can meaningfully generate. Not only does somatosensory stimulation need to evoke responses in space (i.e., across an artificial limb) but it also needs to evoke responses across many different types of sensory perception (i.e., itch, pressure, pinch, etc.) and at a range of perceptual magnitudes. The progress of these devices is slowed down by difficulties in eliciting a large enough perceptual range for commercially relevant use.

Today, research in this area focuses on the development of devices and stimulation strategies that can overcome this limitation. As this field continues to progress, the idea that one electrode equals one percept is rapidly being abandoned for a more nuanced approach to somatosensory control. The most straightforward approach is the creation of devices with greater electrode density and closer physical proximity, so as to increase specificity and dynamic range. While this does not linearly increase the number of available perceptions, due to current spread, more electrodes allow for more manipulation of the summed electrical field, creating opportunities for current steering paradigms as previously discussed in **Chapter 12**. In part, the limited perceptual space occurs because the sensitivity of neurons to pulsed current is primarily a function of the size and myelination of the neurons' axons (see **Chapter 7**). Somatosensory neurons vary in myelination and axon diameter depending on their function, meaning that the larger A-fibers (**Chapter 14**, Fig. 14.1) will always be preferentially stimulated. However, the sensitivity of the axon to current is also a function of membrane channel kinetics, and these properties may be exploitable by modulating the stimulation waveforms. For example, quasi-trapezoidal pulses may reduce the threshold for small axons, or ramped pulses may have lower thresholds for axons further from the electrode location. Furthermore, somatosensory neurons encode information as a function of spike frequency individually, but also via population spike patterns (e.g., relative magnitude or synchrony). The use of more complex "patterned" stimulation frequency and intensity thus holds promise to tease out these population dynamics and thus increase the range of meaningful percepts that can be generated by a single electrode. Taken together these stimulation paradigms hold promise for a dramatic increase in the perceptual space available for somatosensory stimulation. If this promise is realized, it would open the path for widespread viable commercial translation of these technologies.

Vagus nerve stimulation

The vagus nerve (10th cranial nerve) is the largest cranial nerve that extends from the brainstem to the abdomen, enervating many organs including the heart, spleen, liver, gastrointestinal/urogenital tracts, and lungs. It contains both afferent (sensory) and efferent (motor) nerves, but its primary role is the mediation of the parasympathetic nervous system response as part of the autonomic nervous system. The vagus nerve is well known for the regulation of heart rate/blood pressure via innervation of atrial nodes, but it has a wide array of autonomic functions beyond this. Along with direct activation/inhibition of both smooth and striated muscle tissue, the vagus nerve is a major component of the neuro-endocrine-immune axis. It regulates this axis via the hypothalamic pituitary adrenal feedback control and the cholinergic anti-inflammatory pathway, where it releases acetylcholine to downregulate peripheral macrophage activity directly and indirectly via the spleen.

The vagus nerve contains a diverse population of nerve fiber types that vary in axon diameter, myelination, ion channel distributions, function, and location of their synaptic terminals. These are grouped according to their conduction velocity (proportional to axon diameter as discussed in **Chapter 4**) into A-, B-, and C-fibers (see **Chapter 14**). The A-fibers are myelinated fibers that have the largest axonal diameter. Their efferent fibers transmit motor commands and their afferent fibers carry gastrointestinal sensory signals. The B-fibers are small diameter myelinated fibers that are primarily parasympathetic efferents. C-fibers are unmyelinated fibers with small diameter that carry afferent information, most notably visceral pain. The relative distribution of these fibers and their target locations are dependent on the anatomical location of the nerve relative to the brain; various fiber bundles branch off to enervate their target organs as the nerve progresses towards its termination in the lower abdomen. The complex, multi-functional nature of the vagus nerve is both a blessing and curse for neuroprosthetic development. Vagus nerve efferents modulate a wide variety of potential therapeutic targets such as heart rate, the inflammatory immune response, and gastrointestinal motility. Vagus nerve afferents are also implicated in many conditions such as migraine, depression, and epilepsy. However, this wide range of targets also means that achieving therapeutic *specificity* is difficult, and side effects associated with incorrectly calibrated electrical stimulation can be severe, including cardiac arrest. Recently, the shift in focus towards *neuromodulation* in neuroprosthetics, combined with a maturation of peripheral nerve interface technologies and materials, has resulted in a proliferation of more sophisticated approaches to vagus nerve stimulation.

Vagus nerve stimulators

The most basic vagus nerve stimulator design is identical to many other peripheral stimulation devices such as spinal cord stimulators described in **Chapter 14**. It consists of an implanted pulse generator (IPG) usually inserted into the chest cavity, a flexible lead, and a spiral cuff or paddle electrode with one or more contacts that is wrapped directly around the vagus nerve (Fig. 16.8). The most common electrode implantation location is the neck, primarily due to the ease and safety of surgical implantation at this location. More recently there has also been interest in the placement of electrodes closer to the organs that are targeted by the therapy; however, this increases risk of surgical complications, particularly bleedings. Devices deliver monophasic or charge-balanced, biphasic pulses in the range of 0.1–5 mA, a pulse-width of 50–500 μs, and at a rate of 1–300 Hz, depending on the specific device and therapy. Many devices also include a closed-loop feedback component such as heart rate or seizure monitoring, which controls the onset or intensity of the stimulation.

Ultimately, the mechanisms of action behind vagus nerve stimulators are often unclear. While some outcomes and side effects, such as breathing and heart rate changes, have clear causal links, there is no direct explanation (outside of general functional links) for why essentially non-patterned stimulation results in reported outcomes in many applications. Studies have provided evidence for several disparate theories, including generalized inflammatory downregulation, neuromodulation of cortical/subcortical plasticity, and increased blood flow/metabolism, but there is not yet an accepted mechanistic explanation. Given the wide range of proposed applications, and the non-specific positioning of most vagus nerve stimulators in the neck, it is likely that multiple broad mechanisms are at play.

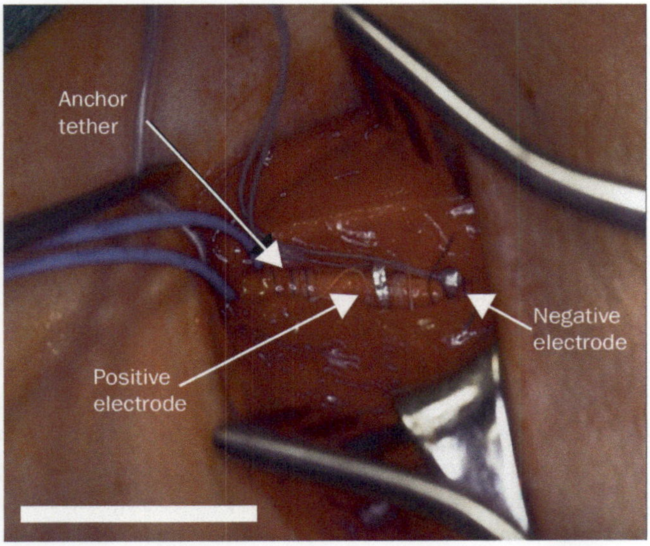

Fig. 16.8 A vagus nerve cuff electrode, consisting of a passive anchor, the stimulating (positive) electrode, and the (negative) return electrode. Scale bar approx. 5 cm. *(Figure adapted from Ben-Menachem (2002).)*

Clinical outcomes and future directions

In the past decade, both preclinical and clinical trials have been performed on vagus nerve stimulators for a wide range of indications, including epilepsy, depression, obesity, insomnia, migraine/cluster headache, addiction, heart failure, and others. The outcomes of these trials have been conflicting and controversial, with epilepsy and heart failure having the most promising results and obesity, depression, and addiction having the most mixed. The general strategy has been to attempt early clinical translation using simplistic approaches in a variety of possible avenues without considering underlying mechanisms, presumably in the hope that the commercial success of one or more of these approaches will then drive increased interest and funding towards a better understanding of the therapeutic mechanism (and from that, further optimization of the stimulation paradigms). It is difficult to tell whether such a scattergun approach has helped this field (by maintaining commercial interest) or hindered it (by casting controversy and thus causative suspicion). The high variability in outcomes are potentially explainable as a function of the complexity of vagus nerve input/output coupled with poorly understood mechanisms that likely involve, motivation, metabolism, and plasticity. That is to say, small variations in study design, patient population, or stimulation parameters may lead to large outcome variations. Vagus nerve stimulation has also been plagued by high rates of serious side effects such as bradycardia (slow heart rate), again with high reported variability between trials. For these reasons, vagus nerve stimulation historically had never managed to penetrate into mainstream accepted use.

It is clear that vagus nerve stimulation *can* produce favorable outcomes in a wide variety of indications, but our limited understanding of the underlying biology and constraints of current clinical technologies hinder precise identification and optimization of these outcomes. As science and technology progresses, the future of vagus nerve neuroprosthesis development thus holds promise. As mentioned, the development of closed-loop approaches that can deliver current only when required may substantially improve the viability of epilepsy and heart failure treatments by increasing their efficacy while reducing associated risks. The success of transcranial direct current stimulation (tDCS) as a non-invasive neuromodulation tool has also generated progress in the development of non-invasive (transcutaneous) vagus nerve stimulation, although the efficacy of this approach is still to be determined. Importantly, the general success of peripheral nerve stimulation (see **Chapter 14** and preceding section on somatosensory implants) has driven innovation in the development of nerve cuff technologies that use soft, flexible materials and miniaturized electrodes. The translation of these technologies to the vagus nerve could allow for the implantation of cuffs in specific vagal nerve branches, which could deliver more functionally focused stimulation. Finally, the development of new stimulation modes beyond standard IPGs are likely to be particularly relevant for vagus nerve neuroprosthetics. These will be outlined more generally in the following section, but in particular, the ability to target neurons by functional category using optogenetics elegantly overcomes the primary confound of vagus nerve stimulation. Direct current stimulation may also be of interest, as the greater range of stimulation waveforms available to that modality may be better fit to the generally neuromodulation-focused vagal nerve therapies. These novel innovations have the potential to drive an even greater expansion of specific vagal modulation targets if they prove to be clinically viable approaches.

Upcoming technological innovations

In the following sections, we discuss technologies currently in early or preclinical development, that in the future may be implemented into clinical neuroprosthetic devices. These innovations have the potential to overcome the present limitations of neural prostheses and thus create opportunities to either improve preexisting approaches or provide entirely new therapeutic directions.

Novel stimulation modes

Neuroprosthetics as a field is historically dominated by the use of pulsed electrical current to stimulate the nervous system (see **Chapter 2**). These types of electrical stimulus have been so successful and prevalent because neurons use electricity to convey information via transmembrane potential changes (action potentials; see **Chapter 7**), and pulsed current can be used to initiate these action potentials to deliver a "rate code" with temporal characteristics that can match physiological conditions. Furthermore, devices that use charge-balanced biphasic current pulses have a long history of chronic safety and stability (due to the associated electrochemistry; see **Chapters 6 and 10**), making them easy to clinically translate.

There are, however, limitations to this standard stimulation modality. Electrical stimulation has high temporal specificity, but often poor spatial specificity. It is difficult to selectively target individual neurons or specific subtypes of neurons in a populated group with the large electrodes that are chronically stable in in vivo preparations, and so functional stimulation relies on some spatially defined functional pattern of the neural population to be available for exploitation (e.g., in the cochlea). In addition to this, while short electrical pulses are efficient for generating increased action potential firing, they cannot normally reduce spontaneous firing or modulate/block incoming neural signals (with exceptions; see high-frequency block in **Chapter 14**). Ultimately, while current pulses have a well-deserved reputation as the "gold standard" by which the majority of neuroprosthetic device development of research is based upon, more sophisticated stimulation models are needed to fully interact with the complexity of many neural systems. In this section we will discuss several such novel stimulation modes that have become increasingly popular as alternative means for nervous system control.

Optogenetic stimulation

Optogenetics uses intrinsically photoreceptive ion channels called "opsins" (ion channels that open in response to light) to transform non-light-sensitive neurons into light-sensitive ones. This is commonly achieved via the use of the adeno-associated virus (AAV), a non-pathogenic virus that can insert genetic material into specific cell populations. This is a widespread technique used in many experimental neuroscience labs that can then use light to activate specific neurons or neural pathways in a controlled fashion in order to interrogate their function (Fig. 16.9). The chemical mechanisms involved in optogenetics are complex and the scientific applications are beyond the scope of this book. However, it is clear that the technique has application in neuroprosthesis research. By virally transfecting photosensitive ion channels into cells in a neural pathway (such as bipolar or ganglion cells in the retina, or inhibitory interneurons/C-fibers in the nociceptive pathway) it is in theory possible to bypass the dysfunctional or destroyed neural tissue without the need for electrical stimulation. The greatest advantage of this approach is that it bypasses a primary limitation of electrical stimulation by allowing for the precise stimulation of otherwise physically collocated neurons with different functional properties. For example, in the nociceptive periphery, Aδ and C-fibers are co-located with lower threshold Aβ fibers, making it hard to electrically modulate one without affecting the other. Similarly, functional areas in the midbrain are often not physically discreet from surrounding structures, and optogenetics may provide an opportunity to stimulate these

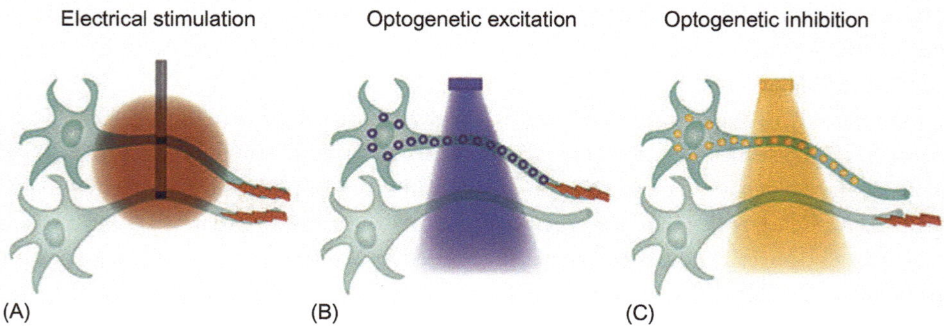

Fig. 16.9 Simple diagram demonstrating the advantages of optogenetic modulation over electrical stimulation. (A) Electrical stimulation excites all neurons as a function of distance from the electrode and (primarily) axonal diameter. (B and C) Optogenetic therapies can target specific cell types and deliver either excitation (B) or inhibition (C) only to these neurons. The combination of wavelengths and associated photosensitive ion channels enables sophisticated neuromodulation paradigms. *(Figure from Tung et al. (2016).)*

areas in a much more precise fashion than the relatively non-specific DBS approaches discussed in **Chapter 13**.

In practice, optogenetic therapies have been difficult to achieve. One key issue is the need to use viral transfection to make the neurons sensitive to light. Not all neurons near the injection site of the virus are transfected with it; rates can be as low as one third. Such transfections have to be repeated every few months, leading to a varied population of light-sensitive neurons. Finally, not every structure is easily accessible for such transfections, as it requires physical penetration and injection. An ideal structure for virus injection is the eye. However, this most obvious use, the restoration of light sensitivity in the dysfunctional retina, has seen little historical success. The luminance levels required to activate currently identified opsins are well beyond physiological levels and are typically narrow band (e.g., requiring high-intensity UV to activate). The timing characteristics of the ion channel kinetics can be too slow for environmentally relevant stimuli. Introducing these opsins into a target cell requires the use of viral vectors (such as the previously mentioned AAV), an as-of-yet unproven technology in the clinic in terms of safety, efficacy, and target specificity. Finally, many of the challenges associated with a remodeled/degenerated retina discussed in **Chapter 12** still exist for optogenetic approaches. Outside of the retina, such approaches also require an implanted device that delivers the necessary light rather than electricity to stimulate the newly photosensitive cells. Miniaturization of the optical light source and power source remains an engineering challenge, however, there are recent advances in LED technology that support this approach. As these technologies progress, optogenetic neuromodulation may have the potential to compete with electrical approaches as another viable form of neuroprosthetic therapy. However, the different strengths of electrical stimulation (fast temporal precision) compared to optogenetics (possibility for high functional/spatial precision) mean that they are likely to be complementary, rather than opposing, methodologies.

Direct current stimulation

Primarily as a consequence of safety limitations (**Chapter 6**) virtually all neuroprostheses use charge-balanced biphasic pulses to excite neurons. While safe and effective, charge-balanced pulses have a relatively constrained set of ways they can influence the transmembrane potential of neurons: typically, they only excite neurons to generate action potentials, although they can in some circumstances be used to interfere with propagation. In theory, the use of non-charge balanced slow-changing analog waveforms ("direct current" [DC] in this context) opens up a much wider array of potential ways to interact with the neural membrane potential, including excitation, inhibition (hyperpolarization), neural block, subthreshold synaptic excitability, and AP conduction velocity. In conjunction, DC waveforms invoke a more stochastic (and thus "naturalistic") change in firing rate and have thresholds that are more dependent on the ion channel distributions of the neurons (rather than just their axonal diameter). The ability to use these effects in vivo would open up the possibility of treating some conditions more efficiently, for example, in the vestibular system (by down-modulating spontaneous firing rate without needing an adapted baseline, Fig. 16.10) or when neural *sensitivity* modulation is the primary goal, such as in neuropathic pain where a total loss (block) of pain signals might be counterproductive if it reduces the functionality of the associate limb.

While there is a wealth of experimental evidence to suggest that DC waveforms would be valuable stimulation modality for neuroprostheses, there are serious technical barriers associated with the delivery of safe, non charge-balanced electrical current. Chemical reactions that occur after the delivery of current for a prolonged duration to a metal electrode implanted in biological tissue effectively prevent standard chronically implanted devices from using DC-based neuromodulation as a stimulation modality. Instead, the use of DC for neural modulation has focused almost entirely around the field of tDCS, which delivers current non-invasively using scalp electrodes. This method has become popular in the past decade, with many potential therapeutic applications. However, like most non-invasive neuromodulation approaches, tDCS suffers from poor specificity and cannot reach deep neural targets. While we will not describe the approach in depth here, an in-depth review is provided in the further reading section. Importantly, the success of transcranial direct-current stimulation (tDCS), coupled with recent technical innovations that have enabled the delivery of current for longer durations, has created a resurgence in interest around the use of DC-based neuromodulation for neuroprostheses.

DC-based in vivo stimulation approaches have focused on either the mitigation or elimination of toxic byproducts generated by chemical reactions at the electrodes.

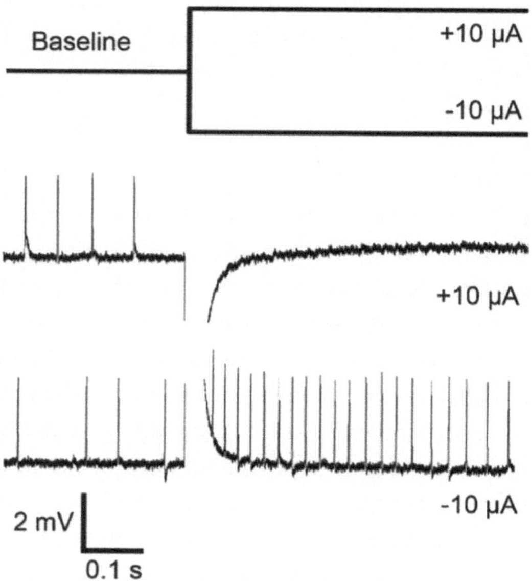

Fig. 16.10 The effect of DC steps on vestibular afferent firing rate in the mouse. Stepped delivery of DC in either the cathodic or anodic direction can excite or inhibit the vestibular afferent, potentially allowing for modulation of firing rate both above and below the spontaneous resting rate. *(Figure adapted from Manca et al. (2019).)*

The most straightforward approach is to generate an electrochemical barrier via the physical separation of the electrode from the tissue via an electrolytic gel. The current is then delivered via a fluidic channel via ions (ionic DC or iDC). An example of this is the Separated Interface Nerve Electrode (SINE), which uses silicone tubing containing filtration barriers that greatly delay the diffusion of byproducts/pH changes and allow for short-term safe delivery of iDC for applications such as opioid-free post-surgical analgesia. For longer-term applications, it is necessary to prevent DC-mediated toxic electrochemical reactions completely. In principle, using ionic conduction through microfluidic channels, it is possible to rectify alternating current at the electrodes into a non-alternating waveform at the load (like a bridge rectifier in an electronic circuit). By rectifying current, charge balance can be maintained at the electrodes while DC is applied to the target neural tissue via a microfluidic channel. This concept is called "Safe Direct Current Stimulation" (SDCS) and has been successfully demonstrated as a proof of concept. These new technologies hold promise for the more widespread application of DC waveforms for neuroprosthetic therapies; however, their novelty means they first must overcome high regulatory barriers. The success of these technologies will depend on whether they can be demonstrated pragmatically as a viable long-term implantable alternative to standard technologies such as IPGs.

Ultrasound stimulation and power delivery

Ultrasound technologies can be used for several applications in neuroprosthetics. As already mentioned in **Chapter 15**, ultrasound can be used for power delivery and bidirectional communication to free-floating sensor elements in the brain. In contrast to high-frequency electromagnetic waves, ultrasound has a higher penetration depth and can be better focused to a specific target. Additionally, since the 1950s it has been known that ultrasound can be used without implanted receivers to stimulate peripheral nerves, increasing spiking/nerve conduction velocity or decreasing spontaneous activity. In humans a tactile sensation can be evoked by 1–100 ms ultrasound pulses to the hand and forearm. One of the advantages of ultrasound is that it enables deep tissue targeting with submillimeter spatial resolution depending on the stimulation frequency. However, the attenuation in biological tissues depends on the ultrasound frequency following a power law $a \sim f^n$ with a factor n varying between 1 and 1.5 depending on the type of tissue. Consequently, high ultrasound frequencies that have a high spatial resolution have a low penetration depth as a drawback.

Precise delivery of ultrasound to a target in the brain would require phased arrays or acoustic lenses inside the cranium, as the skull bone acts as a scattering element and has been considered non-penetrable by ultrasound for a long time. Although the cranium has a large impedance mismatch due to the higher density and sound speed leading to huge reflection losses, it has been demonstrated that frequencies below 1 MHz can be focused to deep-seated targets in the brain. In humans, ultrasound stimulation of the visual system has resulted in the perception of phosphenes and increased responsiveness in coma patients. Motion processing cortical areas have also been shown to be modulated by ultrasound in an experiment identifying the main direction of moving visual dots on a screen. To reach targets through the skull deep in the human brain either phased multi-piezo-arrays or adaptive acoustic lenses can be used to compensate aberrations by the skull bone and to focus onto the intended target. Suppression of pain and epileptic activity, obsessive-compulsive disorder, and depression are suggested as potential applications. Demonstrated effects are mostly transient modulations of activity. Experimentally, modulation could be clearly shown by stimulation of the anterior cingulate cortex in primates while examining the activity in connected areas by functional magnetic resonance imaging (fMRI). Some effects persisted after stimulation, but the exact mechanism of modulation is still unknown. Possible mechanisms of neural stimulation by ultrasound include:

(1) The opening of mechanosensitive channels. In patch clamp experiments with hippocampal pyramidal cells, potassium channels could be modulated by ultrasound, reducing the threshold current. Voltage-gated sodium and calcium channels are also candidates for ultrasound activation.

(2) Capacitive currents by membrane displacement and conformation changes in ultrasound fields altering the transmembrane potential (flexoelectricity).

(3) Thermal effects by absorption of ultrasound energy and local temperature increase as in infrared stimulation (e.g., some ion channels are temperature sensitive).

(4) Sonoporation, which is the formation of pores in cell membranes by ultrasound. Sonoporation may be associated with cavitation when the negative peak phase of the pressure wave exceeds a threshold, forming voids or bubbles that collapse during the positive pressure phase. In one hypothetical model mechanism, neuronal intramembrane cavitation excitation (NICE) ultrasound leads to voids (sonophores) oscillating in the lipid bilayer, inducing transmembrane currents.

The enormous local energy density of cavitation has given rise to other applications of sonoporation. After injection of microbubbles, high intensity low frequency (mechanical index 0.35–0.55 MPa, 400 kHz) ultrasound creates openings in the blood-brain barrier permitting flow and diffusion through the created pores. This results in modulation of sensory evoked potentials that last less than one hour in rats, but this approach has also been suggested as a method for "washing out" proteins that otherwise would not penetrate the blood brain barrier in Alzheimer's and Parkinson's disease. Furthermore, sonoporation can be used similar to electroporation to enable the locally targeted exchange of genes in "sonogenetics." The future development of ultrasound techniques thus clearly has potential for a broad application space not only within neural stimulation but in biological sciences more widely.

Electrophoretic neurotransmitter release

Another alternative approach to neural stimulation is to remove the artificial electrical stimulus entirely, and instead modulate neurons directly via neurotransmitters. This is an attractive potential solution given that inter-neural communication is primarily neurotransmitter based, making this approach more nuanced and "naturalistic." Organic electronic ion pumps (OEIPs) have been developed that use electrophoresis to deliver charged molecules, typically neurotransmitters, directly from a drug reservoir to neural tissue via microfluidic channels (Fig. 16.11). Modulation of neural activity using this approach has been successfully demonstrated in animal models both in vitro and in vivo. OEIPs provide a significantly different mechanism of action compared to electrical stimulation of neurons and open a new creative space for modulation of neural tissues. However, OEIP development also faces significant challenges, including poor temporal resolution and the challenge of refilling empty OEIP neurotransmitter reservoirs in an implanted device. Co-modulation of neurons with excitatory, inhibitory, and/or neuromodulatory transmitters, potentially in conjunction with electrical stimulation, is an exciting future direction for these devices.

Magnetogenetic stimulation

Magnetogenetic neuromodulation as a concept is similar to optogenetics as discussed above, but with the transfection of *magnetically* sensitive ion channels or proteins into

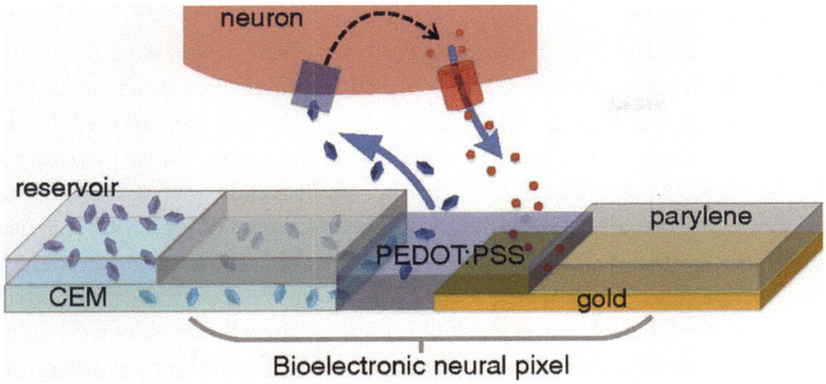

Fig. 16.11 Basic schematic for a dual-purpose stimulation/recording OEIP device (the "bioelectronic neural pixel"). Neurotransmitters or other bioactive molecules are pumped via electrophoresis through a PEDOT:PSS release layer *(left side)* that is co-located with conductive gold contacts that measure the electrochemical potential *(right side)*. The device is encapsulated in an inert parylene layer. *(Figure from Jonsson et al. (2016).)*

target neural populations. This could enable the stimulation (or inhibition) of specific neural networks completely noninvasively using external magnetic fields, in a way that cannot be achieved with electrical stimulation. While the possibilities for this approach are almost boundless, magnetogenetics has generated intense controversy in recent years due to difficulties with the reproducibility of the magnetogenetic transfection methods. Furthermore, due to an exponential reduction in magnetic field strength from the source, it is unclear how useful these approaches might be in vivo for humans given the relatively large physical distance to penetrate through the skull and to non-superficial neural tissue (particularly when compared to preclinical model animals such as mice). Hard limitations imposed by physics thus interfere with the rapid implementation and translation of these technologies into the clinic and will need to be creatively overcome.

Novel electrode and carrier materials

As discussed in **Chapters 5 and 6**, the total charge that can be delivered to neural tissue by a prosthesis is limited by the capacitive and electrochemical properties of the electrode material. Furthermore, the electrode and surrounding carrier materials of an implant, even if not electrically conductive, play an important role in the inflammatory foreign body response to an implanted device (**Chapter 8**). The development of new materials is thus a major component of ongoing and future research in the field of neuroprosthetics, with the overall aim to increase the range of charge capacities available for electrodes and/or to reduce damaging tissue reactions.

Novel electrode materials

Improvements on electrode design have generally focused on increasing the charge injection limits for electrode materials. Charge injection limits are a function of the surface area of an electrode, meaning that larger electrodes of the same material will by definition have greater charge injection capacities. However, increasing electrode size has major drawbacks; specifically, it reduces the current *density* while increasing current *spread*, potentially canceling out any benefit. Thus, the primary goal of electrode material development in neuroprosthesis research is to create materials with increased charge delivery capacity (commonly due to higher capacitance) without increasing the physical size of the electrode. A common way to achieve this is to increase the available electrode surface area via an *electrode surface treatment*. The simplest form of surface treatment is to microscopically roughen the electrode surface using chemical, laser, or plasma etching, which is already commonly performed today. Alternatively, depositing conductive nanoparticles onto the electrode surface can result in a dramatically greater surface area and this is used extensively in non-clinical settings, for example, with platinum black (electroplating fine platinum particulate onto platinum electrodes; see **Chapter 6**). Recent research has shown proof-of-concept creation of extremely complex nanoparticle depositions using nanorods or coated silicon nanowires that can increase charge injection capacities by more than 25 times the base material. Alternatively, non-metallic polymer-based coatings such as PEDOT:PSS can conduct electronic current in a matrix that integrates the surrounding electrolyte, improving the effective surface area of the capacitive interface. While these technologies have existed now for some time, they have historically suffered from a lack of translation into chronic application due to concerns about their stability, fragility, and potential for tissue toxicity. However, recent advances in stability and safety of coating and deposition techniques have been gradually moving these novel materials towards long-term implantation. The next generation of implantable electronics will have an opportunity to make use of these materials to improve the specificity of neural stimulation available to them.

Flexible arrays and electronics

In addition to improving the charge injection capacities of electrodes, another recent material innovation has been the development of *flexible electronics*. The rigidity of metallic electrodes, electrode housing, and electrical components are important factors for the mechanical damage of soft tissues (such as neurons) and the resultant tissue reactions (see **Chapter 8**). While it is still possible to implant rigid electrode arrays chronically, these reactions play a major part in reducing their longevity, particularly in the fragile tissues of the CNS. Historical studies have shown that electrodes integrated into soft polymer or silicone housings, originally as a means to facilitate in vitro cell culture, can reduce the tissue reaction compared to more rigid housings, but this approach is limited in scope. In the past decade there has been further concerted effort to develop neuroprosthetic devices using novel materials and fabrication processes to maximize this mechanical biocompatibility without compromising on the electrochemical stability of the contacts. The ultimate goal of flexible electronics in neuroprosthetics is to design devices that are mechanically and structurally near identical to the tissues they are implanted in, allowing them to integrate seamlessly into the biological tissue and thus retain chronic stability (Fig. 16.12). The development of flexible in vivo electrode arrays has taken three primary forms: microwire arrays, electrode mesh grids, and epidural sheets.

Microwire arrays attempt to overcome the problems associated with traumatic insertion and mechanical micromotion of rigid electrodes by separating out each contact into a

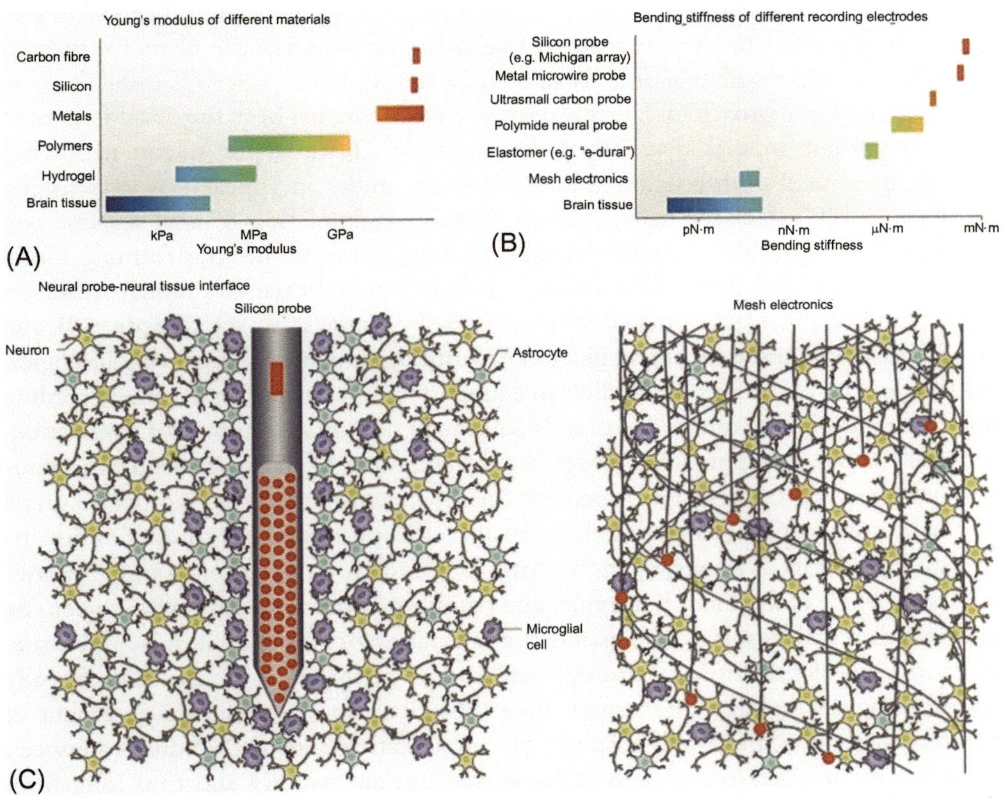

Fig. 16.12 Young's modulus (A) and bending stiffness (B) of various recording electrode materials. Generally, the closer to physiologic tissue a material is, the more physically biocompatible it becomes. However, low modulus values can also make the material sensitive to physical damage or degradation. (C) A schematic comparison of a standard silicon recording probe and a mesh-based probe. Recording contacts are shown as *red dots*. Standard probe designs generate a fibrotic layer that separates them from the neural tissue. In theory, mesh electronics bypass this problem and integrate more seamlessly. *(Figure from Hong and Lieber (2019).)*

flexible fiber microelectrode (i.e., with a form factor more like a bundle of hair than a needle). Fibers can freely bend and shift with the pulsating movements of the brain from circulation and respiration, greatly reducing the chronic inflammatory response. However, the position of the fiber electrode may be more prone to shifting over time as a consequence. The small surface area of fiber electrodes means that the development of materials with high charge injection capacities (as discussed in the previous paragraph) is vital for the continued miniaturization of fiber diameter. For example, 8-μm fibers made from insulating polymer layers and a conductive carbon fiber core, tipped with PEDOT:PSS, have been successfully used to chronically record brain activity in preclinical studies. The biggest limitation of microwire arrays has been the difficulties associated with their implantation. There is a strong tradeoff between the ease and precision of insertion and the free flexibility of the implanted wires. This has been addressed recently by the introduction of coatings that temporarily stiffen the fibers for surgical insertion and then dissolve harmlessly once they are in place.

An alternative approach for laterally dispersed electrodes has been the development of porous electronic meshes that intersperse electrodes (platinum or silicon nanowire) throughout a flexible three-dimensional structure similar in appearance to a fishing net (Fig. 16.12C). Conceptually, a mesh reduces accumulation of glial response on the large planar surface of a conventional planar array, prevents the array forming a solid diffusion "barrier" that limits cell and nutrient dispersion (important for retinal prostheses where blood supply may be isolated from the tissue by a large array; see **Chapter 12**), and encourages neural tissue including glia to grow through the mesh, improving biological integration. Preclinical chronic studies have supported this concept for chronic recording in the brain and retina out to 3–4 months, although not yet as a means for stimulation.

Finally, a popular approach has been the development of planar arrays that can integrate with and/or serve as a replacement for the *dura mater* over the cortex or spinal cord. The cortical surface in particular is an attractive position for recording of distributed neural activity for epilepsy monitoring or feedback control, for example. However, the surface of the brain is irregular and complex, and even small gaps between the array and the cortical surface can enable the infiltration of fluids and non-neural tissue, which quickly degrade the recording performance of the implant. The dura already conforms tightly to the cortex/spine (like "shrink wrap") and the development of implants that can exploit this property via implantation into the epidural (between the layers of the dura mater) allows for better chronic stability and thus long-term recording fidelity over electrodes directly on the cortical surface (see Fig. 16.13). As the epidural space is only a potential space (an area between two adjacent structures that are normally pressed together) these devices must be highly flexible and as thin as possible (1–5 μm) to avoid deformation of the dura. A conceptual step further is the replacement of the dura with "e-dura," an artificial silicone substrate that replaces and mimics the dura mater and that contains both electrodes and microfluidic channels

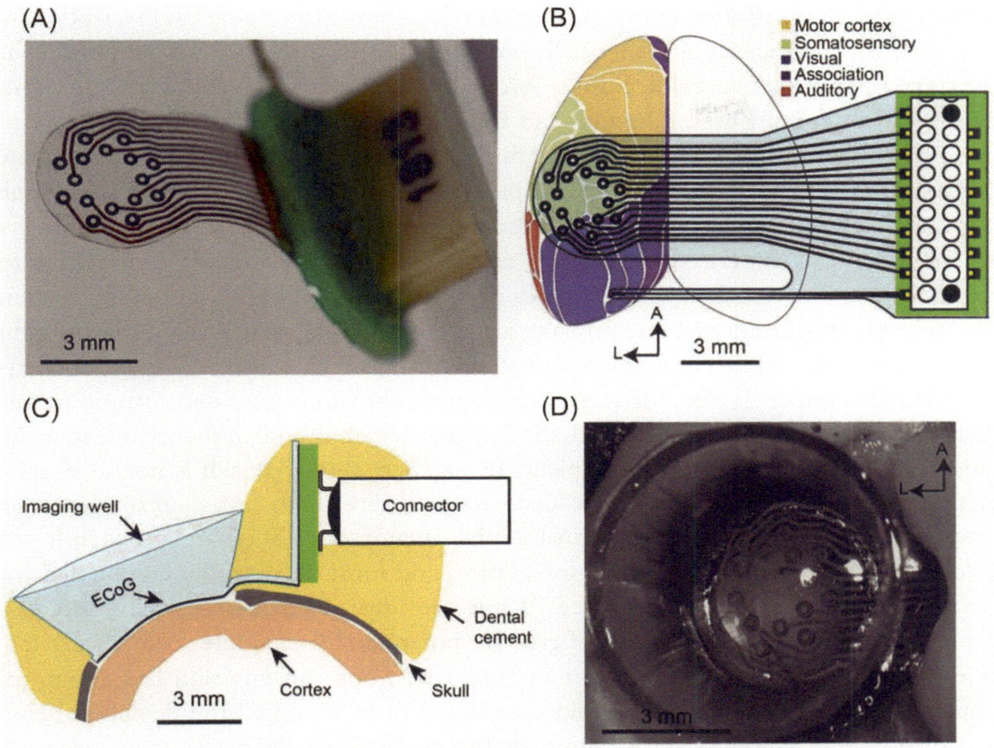

Fig. 16.13 Example of a transparent "e-Dura" ECoG array used for in vivo cortical recording. (A) Image of the recording array. (B) Device schematic relative to the dorsal cortex of the mouse brain. (C) Cross-sectional schematic of the implanted device demonstrating the imaging well and connector for microscope objective. (D) Photograph of the implanted ECoG array in mouse dorsal cortex. *(Figure from Renz et al. (2020).)*

for both electrical recording/stimulation and drug delivery (see also **Chapter 15**). This is potentially highly valuable for spinal cord stimulation approaches where penetrating electrodes have particularly poor stability. Although these technologies are highly promising future directions, the novelty of their approach and materials means that they must be rigorously proven safe in chronic animal models before they can be translated to human patients. If human translation does not produce irreconcilable complications, it is likely that flexible electronic approaches such as these will continue to see further and more widespread adoption in the coming years.

Electrodes as pharmaceutical carriers

In conjunction with advances in device materials and the more widespread adoption of neural implants in the clinic, there has been an increasing interest in the use of neuroprosthetics as **pharmaceutical carriers**. By coating or doping the electrode carrier with a pharmaceutical (potentially encapsulated in a slow-release molecule or matrix), it is possible to deliver drugs locally at the direct site of implantation. This has several important uses. The first and most straightforward is to coat the implant in an anti-inflammatory such as dexamethasone that can release acutely or over time and thus slow the tissue reaction to the implanted electrode array. Local dexamethasone is greatly preferred over systemic administration where possible due to the potentially severe side effects associated with its use, and the low penetrance of systemic drugs to some neural substrates such as the cochlea or retina. This has been successfully used in human patients during cochlear implant surgery, suggesting that this approach might have general applicability; electrodes covered with or capable of releasing other corticoids are also under development. Another approach is to release neurotropic factors that encourage neural growth towards the implant, which should in theory improve the specificity and thresholds of the implant. In practice, this approach is not so simple, as uncontrolled neural growth may decrease *local* thresholds but increase *perceptual* thresholds due to the loss of functional neural organization. Such an approach is not a "catch-all" for improving device integration and must be carefully engineered for the individual use-case of the device. While the idea of pharmaceutically doping a device seems simple, it holds a lot of creative potential: for example, as medical therapies continue to be optimized in individual cases, one can envision the doping of implants with patient-specific protein complexes that "identify" the device as being part of the immunological self to limit the foreign body reaction.

Competing technologies

This book has been focused on the history, theory, and recent developments in neuroprosthetics. As this field continues to grow and sees clinical success, it is important for readers to realize that these interventions do not stand in isolation. Due to the often inherently invasive and high-risk approach of neural implants, clinicians must justify why a neuroprosthetic intervention is the best available option, or else be willing to adopt an alternative intervention when it is not. As a part of a holistic understanding of neural prosthesis research and therapy, it is important that researchers and clinicians are aware of other current and upcoming technologies that may provide alternatives to neuroprosthetics, either as competing technologies or as potential combined/integrated therapies. In the following section, we briefly outline some upcoming fields of medicine that may intersect with the same types of diseases that neuroprosthetics aim to treat, and thus should be considered when developing new technologies.

Genetic therapies and precision medicine

The medical understanding of human genetics has been another rapid area of scientific and technological growth during the twenty-first century. In particular, the underlying genetic mechanisms that cause many inherited or congenital diseases have become well understood and characterized. The identification and development of personalized treatments matched to the genetic or phenotypic specifics of patients is described as **precision medicine** and has become a major topic in medical science and clinical practice. In recent years, the development of gene-editing technologies such as CRISPR-Cas9 has further opened the door for the treatment of individual conditions at their genetic source. It is certainly an exciting (and nervous) time for genetic-based therapeutic approaches, both technically and ethically. How relevant are these approaches for neuroprosthetics research?

It is important to understand that genetic therapies seek to address the *cause* of diseases, while prosthetics seek to replace *loss of function* resulting from an underlying disease process. As such, the two are fundamentally different approaches with many distinct and non-overlapping applications. Where possible, addressing a cause is a better approach than replacing function, and so genetic therapies (if successful) have the potential to replace neuroprostheses as treatments for conditions such as retinitis pigmentosa, or some forms of congenital deafness (**Chapters 11 and 12**). However, this scope is limited: gene therapy can fix an underlying condition only if permanent disability has not already occurred because of that initial genetic error. For example, once a retinitis pigmentosa patient has gone blind, fixing the initial phototransduction pathway errors will not restore sight to the now fundamentally damaged visual system. For congenital diseases, all therapies must consider critical developmental periods (**Chapter 9**) and thus need to be readily applied and quickly effective within early childhood. Injury or disease as a result of environmental factors (e.g., accidents, exposure to neurotoxic drugs such as gentamicin, etc.) cannot be resolved with genetic therapies at all. Neuroprosthetics will thus always have clinical application separate to genetic therapy, meaning that the two approaches will likely coexist. The era of precision medicine may provide great benefit to the field of neuroprosthetics as well: the development of patient-specific stimulation strategies or pharmaceutical implant coatings already holds promise to improve current neural implant function.

Regenerative medicine

As mentioned, neuroprosthetics, by definition, seek to restore or replace lost neural function; the ultimate aim of most neuroprosthetic therapies is for the patient to have the same level of functionality that existed before the disease or injury. Thus, a better solution would be to prevent the functional loss or simply *restore* the original function entirely, rather than replace it with a prosthesis. While genetic therapies may not be able to do this in the case of adult loss of function, regenerative medicine is a field that seeks to do exactly that: to replace organ or tissue loss with artificially regenerated or grown, but otherwise identical, tissues. This field has seen recent success in wound healing and orthopedics, including successful commercial applications. Contemporary research is now focused on artificial growth and transplantation of organs (typically heart, liver, and kidney) and on promoting intrinsic regenerative growth. Given the great potential for this field, are neuroprostheses relevant in a medical environment where diseased organs can be replaced or regenerated biologically? Nervous tissue typically has very low potential for intrinsic regeneration, not least because the *connections* between neurons are as important for function as is the gross *number* of neurons in the tissue. There is an inherent experiential history in many neural tissues that precludes their transplantation or non-selective regeneration (e.g., see information on critical periods in **Chapter 9**). It simply isn't feasible (in fact, it is farcical) to do a "brain transplant" or "spine transplant" in the same manner as a heart or kidney transplant, nor is it possible today to simply "regrow" damaged parts in much of the brain. Neural regeneration of peripheral tissues has seen more success, but even here often the peripheral neural tissue and its development are too complex, and previous attempts at, for example, photoreceptor transplantations in humans have not been successful. Due to these steep challenges, while regenerative medicine may eventually replace neuroprosthesis applications in the future, this is unlikely to occur in any predictable or meaningful timeframe. It is also feasible that prostheses could be used in conjunction with regenerative therapies to help guide (via *neuromodulation*) the functional regrowth of neuronal circuitry. It may also be that as human neuroprosthetics continue to see increased social acceptance, they may shift focus from *replacement* to *enhancement* of human function; however, this currently remains in the realm of science fiction.

Brief summary

- Vestibular prostheses can be used to replace lost vestibular (balance) function. They are on the cusp of commercial translation.
- Closed-loop strategies link neural stimulation to sensing elements for providing feedback. They have seen widespread preclinical adoption and are expected to improve existing device outcomes in the near future.
- Somatosensory prostheses can resolve many outstanding problems for neuroprosthetic limb control by providing closed-loop proprioceptive feedback. Their integration with motor control systems is an essential next step for the success of bionic limb technologies.
- Vagus nerve stimulators have been used to treat a variety of autonomic, metabolic, and mood disorders, albeit with mixed results. Upcoming improvements in cuff electrode design and new stimulation modes may create an opportunity for this field to grow.
- Optogenetics, ionic direct current, electrophoretic neurotransmitter delivery, and magnetogenetics are some of the forthcoming neural stimulation technologies. Rigorous testing of safety and efficacy is necessary before these technologies can see clinical or commercial translation.

- New electrode materials can further enhance existing approaches via the creation of soft, flexible arrays that better integrate into neural tissue.
- Pharmaceutical coatings can be used in conjunction with arrays to further reduce inflammatory responses or encourage neural growth towards the electrode contacts.
- Gene therapy and regenerative medicine are alternative therapeutic strategies. They may provide an opportunity to enhance existing neuroprosthetic approaches, but may also become competing alternative therapies in the future.

Key literature and further reading

Aplin, F.P., et al., 2019. Ionic direct current modulation for combined inhibition/excitation of the vestibular system. IEEE Trans. Biomed. Eng. 66 (3), 775–783.

Aplin, F.P., Fridman, G.Y., 2019. Implantable direct current neural modulation: theory, feasibility and efficacy. Front. Neurosci. 13, 379. https://doi.org/10.3389/fnins.2019.00379.

Ben-Menachem, E., 2002. Vagus-nerve stimulation for the treatment of epilepsy. Lancet Neurol. 1, 477–482.

Boutros, P.J., et al., 2019. Continuous vestibular implant stimulation partially restores eye-stabilizing reflexes. JCI Insight. 4(22), e128397.

Clites, T.R., et al., 2018. Proprioception from a neurally controlled lower-extremity prosthesis. Sci. Transl. Med. 10, 443.

Cywiak, C., et al., 2020. Non-invasive neuromodulation using rTMS and the electromagnetic-perceptive gene (EPG) facilitates plasticity after nerve injury. Brain Stimul. 13 (6), 1773–1783.

Drugger, S.A., et al., 2017. Drug development in the era of precision medicine. Nat. Rev. Drug Discov. 17, 183–196.

Hernandez, V.H., et al., 2014. Optogenetic stimulation of the auditory pathway. J. Clin. Invest. 124, 1114–1129.

Hong, G., Lieber, C.M., 2019. Novel electrode technologies for neural recordings. Nat. Rev. Neurosci. 20 (6), 330–345.

Jakešová, M., et al., 2019. Wireless organic electronic ion pumps driven by photovoltaics. Npj Flex. Electron. 3, 14.

Johnson, R.L., Wilson, C.G., 2018. A review of vagus nerve stimulation as a therapeutic intervention. J. Inflamm. Res. 11, 203–2013.

Jonsson, A., et al., 2016. Bioelectronic neural pixel: chemical stimulation and electrical sensing at the same site. Proc. Natl. Acad. Sci. USA 113 (34), 9440–9445. https://doi.org/10.1073/pnas.1604231113.

Knafo, S., Wyart, C., 2015. Optogenetic neuromodulation: new tools for monitoring and breaking neural circuits. Ann. Phys. Rehabil. Med. 58 (4), 259–264.

Manca, M., et al., 2019. Ionic direct current modulation evokes spike-rate adaptation in the vestibular periphery. Sci. Rep. 9, 18924. https://doi.org/10.1038/s41598-019-55045-6.

Manrique-Huarte, R., et al., 2020. Cochlear implantation with a dexamethasone eluting electrode array: functional and anatomical changes in non-human primates. Otol. Neurotol. 41, e812–e822. https://doi.org/10.1097/MAO.0000000000002686.

Mao, A.S., Mooney, D.J., 2015. Regenerative medicine: current therapies and future directions. Proc. Natl. Acad. Sci. USA 112 (47), 14452–14459.

Marcus, D.C., Wangemann, P., 2009. Cochlear and Vestibular Function and Dysfunction. In: Alvarez-Leefmans, F.J., Delpire, E. Physiology and Pathology of Chloride Transporters and Channels in the Nervous System. Elsevier, Amsterdam, Boston, pp. 425–437.

Nguyen, T.A.K., et al., 2017. Characterization of cochlear, vestibular and cochlear-vestibular electrically evoked compound action potentials in patients with a vestibulo-cochlear implant. Front. Neurosci. 11, 645. https://doi.org/10.3389/fnins.2017.00645.

Parastarfeizabadi, M., Kouzani, A.Z., 2017. Advances in closed-loop deep brain stimulation devices. J. Neuroeng. Rehabil. 14(79). https://doi.org/10.1186/s12984-017-0295-1.

Perez Fornos, A., et al., 2014. Artificial balance: restoration of the vestibulo-ocular reflex in humans with a prototype vestibular neuroprosthesis. Front. Neurol. 5(66). https://doi.org/10.3389/fneur.2014.00066.

Plontke, S.K., et al., 2017. Intracochlear drug delivery in combination with cochlear implants. HNO 65 (Suppl 1), 19–28.

Renz, A.F., et al., 2020. Opto-E-Dura: a soft, stretchable ECoG array for multimodal, multiscale neuroscience. Adv. Healthc. Mater. 9(17), 2000814. https://doi.org/10.1002/adhm.202000814.

Roemer, A., et al., 2016. Biohybrid cochlear implants in human neurosensory restoration. Stem Cell Res. Ther. 7(148). https://doi.org/10.1186/s13287-016-0408-y.

Russell, C., et al., 2019. Peripheral nerve bionic interface: a review of electrodes. Int. J. Intell. Robot. Appl. 3, 11–19.

Shendel, A.A., Eliceiri, K.W., Williams, J.C., 2014. Advanced materials for neural surface electrodes. Curr. Opin. Solid State Mater. Sci. 18 (6), 301–307. https://doi.org/10.1016/j.cossms.2014.09.006.

Tan, D.W., et al., 2015. Stability and selectivity of a chronic, multi-contact cuff electrode from sensory stimulation in human amputees. J. Neural Eng. 12(2), 026002. https://doi.org/10.1088/1741-2560/12/2/026002.

Tung, J.K., Berglund, K., Gross, R.E., 2016. Optogenetic approaches for controlling seizure activity. Brain Stimul. 9 (6), 801–810. https://doi.org/10.1016/j.brs.2016.06.055.

Yang, J., Phi, J.H., 2019. The present and future of vagus nerve stimulation. J. Korean Neurosurg. Soc. 62 (3), 344–352. https://doi.org/10.3340/jkns.2019.0037.

Index

Note: Page numbers followed by *f* indicate figures, *t* indicate tables, and *b* indicate boxes.

A

Access voltage, 141–142
Accommodation, 96, 126
AC/DC stimulation, 102–103
Action potential, 64, 64*f*, 69
Activation function
  anodal surround, 122–123
  cathodic and anodic stimulation, 122–123
  current-distance relations, 124, 125*f*
  distance effect, 124
  strength-duration curve, 125
Active implants, 16–17
  power supply, 43–45, 44*f*
Acute reactions, 135–136
Ag/AgCl electrode, 193–195, 195*f*
Age-related macular degeneration (AMD), 262–263
Aging tests, 46–47
Alternating current, 323–324
Angle-closure glaucoma, 263–264
Anodal surround, 122–123
Anode, 82
Anodic break, 127
Aquaporins, 55–56
Artificial neural networks, 350
Associative learning, 150–151
Auditory neuroprostheses. *See also* Cochlear implants
  auditory brainstem implants (ABIs)
    cochlear nucleus, 242, 243*f*
    complication, 242
    speech outcomes, 244–245, 245*f*
    stimulation strategy, 245–246
    thresholds, 243–244
  central auditory system, 218–219, 218*f*
  cerebral and auditory cortex, 219
  deaf ear, 220–222, 221*f*
  hearing loss, 219–220
  inner ear/cochlea (*see* Inner ear)
  language, 211
  midbrain implants, 246, 247*f*
  peripheral auditory organ, 211–212, 212*f*

B

Bilayer, 55–56, 57*f*. *See also* Electrode bilayer
Biocompatibility, 97–99
Biofilm formation, 145–147, 146*f*
Bipolar configuration, 82–83, 116–117
Boundary effects, 126
Brain-machine interface (BMI)
  arm movement direction, 331–332, 331–332*f*
  artificial neural networks, 350
  body and limb movement, 330–331
  decoders, 346–347
  decoder training, 332–333, 334*f*
  electrocorticography (ECoG), 339–340
  invasive/non-invasive BCIs, 335–338, 337*f*
  Kalman filter (KF), 349–350, 349*f*
  motor coding, 332–333
  neuron dropping curve (NDC), 333–335, 336*f*
  Wiener filter, 348
Brain mapping, 20–21, 21*f*
Buckling, 226, 226*f*
Burst stimulation, 321, 322*f*

C

Capacitive effects, 104
Cardiac pacemaker, 22–23, 23*f*
Cathode, 82
Cell-selective stimulation, 284–286
Central auditory system, 218–219, 218*f*
Central representation of pain, 314
Characteristic frequency, 184–186, 185*f*, 215, 215*f*
Charge-balancing, 103, 127–129, 128*f*
Charge delivery capacity, 104–105, 109
Charge density, 105–110
Chemical surface charges, 182, 183*f*
Chloridization, 91–92
Chronaxies, 230
Chronic neuropathic pain
  heterogeneous, 316–317
  hyperalgesia and allodynia, 315–316, 316*f*
  mechanisms, 317
  nociceptive pain, 315
  plastic adaptation to pain, 314–315
Chronic reactions, 135–136

Clark electrode
  electrode resistance, 193–194
  oxygen concentrations, 204–205, 205*f*
  voltage-current characteristics, 203–204, 204*f*
Clinical trials, 41–42
Closed-loop stimulation
  automated implant-fitting procedures, 362
  bidirectional connection, 361
  deep brain stimulation, 362–363, 362*f*
  feedback adaptation, 361
  pain relief, 362–363, 362*f*
  unidirectional devices, 360–361
Cochlear implants
  circumstances for neuroprosthetic therapy, 222–223
  development, 26–28, 28–29*f*
  electrode
    buckling, 226, 226*f*
    cochlear trauma, 226
    factors to consider, 226–227
    shape, 224–226
  individualization, 239–241, 240*f*
  location, 223, 223*f*
  neurophysiological background
    chronaxies, 230
    dynamic range, 233
    electrical tuning curves, 228, 229*f*
    electric and acoustic stimulation (EAS), 228–230, 230*f*
    implanted electrode impedance, 231–233, 232*f*
    loudness, growth function, 233
    one-channel stimulation, 227
    pitch perception, 233
    power delivery/implant positioning, 234–235, 234*f*
    processor and transmitter coil, 235
    scala tympani, 235
    spectral information, 228
    speech signals, 227
    stimulus phase, 231, 231*f*
  processor
    multichannel coding strategies, 236, 237*f*
    speech coding, 235
  as recording devices, 239
  scala tympani conductivity, 224
  speech perception
    localization precision, 238
    multichannel, 238
    signal-to-noise ratio, 238
    single syllable recognition, 239
    speech-coding strategies, 238–239
    speech understanding, 236
  tripolar stimulation, 224, 225*f*
  type I ganglion cells, 224
Cochlear trauma, 226
Conductive hearing loss, 220
Conductometric titration, 176–178, 178*f*
Cone-rod dystrophies, 262
Congenital deafness, 158–159, 160*f*
Contemporary neuroprostheses, 28–30
Continuous interleaved sampling, 236, 237*f*
Corrosion, 45, 102
Cortical and LGN visual implants, 278
Cortical stimulation, 20
Counter electrode, 82
Cranial neuromodulation implants, 324–325
Critical periods, 160, 162
Current and voltage source, 79*b*
Current focusing, 82–83, 117–118, 228, 238, 248
Current source, 79–80, 79*b*, 142–143, 142*f*
Current steering, 284, 285*f*
Cyclic voltammetry, 145

D

Deafness, 220–222, 221*f*
Debye length, 180, 181*f*, 181*t*
Decoders, 346–347
Decoder training, 332–333, 334*f*
Deep brain stimulation (DBS), 21–22, 24
  basal ganglia, 292–294, 293*f*
  circuit of Papez, 301
  clinical approaches, 300–301
  closed-loop stimulation, 302, 362–363, 362*f*
  configuration, 299–300
  direct and indirect pathway, 294
  dystonia, 301
  electrode, 299, 299*f*
  functional inactivation, 302
  implantable pulse generator (IPG), 298
  innate action patterns, 292–293
  lesion and functional suppression, 301–302
  mechanism, 296–297, 298*f*
  motor cortex, 291–292, 292*f*
  motor system, 291
  muscle regulation, 291
  Parkinson's disease, 294–296, 295*f*, 300

stimulator design, 298
Deficiency ions, 86
Delamination, 45, 101
Delayed rectifiers, 64–65
Depolarization block, 127
Diabetic retinopathy (DR), 264
Dielectric breakdown, 104
Diffuse layer, 179–180
Diffusion potential, 197–199, 198*f*, 199*t*
Dignity, 34
Direct current, 373–374, 374*f*
Displacement current, 87–88
Dissolution, 102
Distance effect, 124
Donnan potential, 200–203, 200–201*f*
Double-layer, 86, 87*f*, 179
Durability of device, 45–46, 46*f*
Dynamic range, 233
Dystonia, 301

E

Early brain prostheses, 25–26
Elderly subjects, 163
Electrical instability, 88–89
Electrical stimulation
electricity *vs.* human perception, 19
melancholy, 19–20
Electrical tuning curves, 228, 229*f*
Electrochemical cell, 188–189
Electrocorticographic (ECoG) and endovascular recording, 338–340
Electrode bilayer
capacitive/displacement currents, 87–88
current crossing, 92
electrical instability, 88–89
electric models
equivalent circuit, 89–90, 90*f*
ideal non-polarized electrode, 91–92
ideal polarized electrode, 91
leakage resistance (R_e) and series resistance (R_s), 89–90
RC circuit, 90
tissue-electrode interface, 90–91, 91*f*
Faradaic reactions, 92
Helmholtz-Debye double-layer, 86, 87*f*
non-Faradaic reactions, 92
overpotential, 88
polarized and non-polarized electrodes, 89
recessed electrodes, 88–89
Electrode dissolution, 102
Electrode potential, 85–86
Electrodes and electrolytes
Ag/AgCl electrode, 193–195, 195*f*
chemical reactions at electrodes, 167, 169*f*
chemical surface charges, 182, 183*f*
Clark electrode, 203–205, 203–205*f*
conductometric titration, 176–178, 178*f*
diffusion potential, 197–199, 198*f*, 199*t*
Donnan potential, 200–203, 200–201*f*
electric conduction, 168
electric models, 182–184, 184*f*
electrochemical processes (*see* tissue-electrode interface)
electron transfer, 191*b*
Faraday constant, 168–169
Hittorf transport numbers, 176, 177*f*
interface impedance
Faraday currents, 188
frequency dependence, 187–188
surface area *vs.* capacitance and conductance, 186–187
ion conductivity and mobility, 175
Nernst equation, 189–191, 194*f*
non-polarizing electrodes, 188–189, 189*f*
pH electrode, 205–207, 206*f*
redox reaction, 192
reference electrode, 195–197, 196*f*
solvation of ions, 174–175, 174*t*
specific conductivity, 169–170
standard electrode potentials, 192–193, 193*t*
strong and weak electrolytes, 171–173
strong electrolytes conductivity, 170–171, 172*f*
tissue-electrode interface
Debye length, 180, 181*f*, 181*t*
diffuse layer, 179–180
double-layer, 179
Gouy-Chapman layer, 179–180
Helmholtz layer, 179
potential difference, 182
Electrode surface and electrode impedance, 110–111
Electrode-tissue interface. *See also* Electrodes and electrolytes; Tissue-electrode interface
constant current source, 79–80, 79*b*
constant voltage source, 77–79, 79*b*
current and voltage source, 79*b*

Electrode-tissue interface *(Continued)*
current conduction in electrolytes, 83–84, 84*f*
electrical fields, 77
electrode bilayer
capacitive/displacement currents, 87–88
current crossing, 92
electrical instability, 88–89
electric models, 89–92, 90–91*f*
Helmholtz-Debye double-layer, 86, 87*f*
overpotential, 88
polarized and non-polarized electrodes, 89
recessed electrodes, 88–89
electrode configurations
current flow, 82
monopolar and bipolar, 82–83
return/counter electrode, 82
stimulation configuration, 82–83
stimulation/working electrode, 82
tripolar/multipolar, 82–83
electrode-electrolyte reactions
chemical batteries, 86
electrode potential, 85–86
ionic and electrolyte concentrations, 84–85
standard hydrogen electrode (SHE), 85–86
impedance, 77
resistance, 77
water hose analogy, 80–81, 81*f*
Electrolyte, 83–84, 143. *See also* Electrodes and electrolytes; Electrode-tissue interface
Electrolytic cell, 188–189
Electron transfer, 191*b*
Electrophoretic neurotransmitter release, 376, 377*f*
Electrophysiology
action potentials, 15
bioelectricity, 12–13, 13–14*f*
electro-encephalogram, 14–15
language function, 15
Electrotaxis, 144
Electrotonic propagation, 65
Epiretinal prostheses, 274, 275*f*
Equilibrium potentials, 58–61, 58*t*, 60*b*
Ethics
brain implants as human extension
androids, 48
integrity, 49
interventions, 49–50
transhumanism, 48–49
durability, device, 45–46, 46*f*
free will/decision, 34–35
general design considerations, 43
human dignity, 34
informed consent, 35
medical practice, 34
medical technology
balancing costs against risks and benefits, 37–38
clinical trials, 41–42
post-market clinical follow-up (PMCF), 42–43
preclinical testing, 38–39, 39*f*, 40*t*
risk management, 42–43
moral agency, 35
power supply in active implants, 43–45, 44*f*
technology development
complications, 36
explantation criteria/termination criteria, 36
lifetime medical and technical care, 36
technological safety, 35–36
technology readiness level (TRL), 36–37
Excess ions, 86
Excitatory postsynaptic potentials, 65–66, 66*f*
Excitotoxicity, 154
Explantation criteria/termination criteria, 36

F

Failed back surgery syndrome (FBSS), 318
Faradaic charge transfer
corrosion of platinum electrodes, 102
dissolution of the electrode, 102
H-atom-plating, 100–101
irreversible reactions, 101–102
oxidation of chloride ions, 102
oxidation of water, 102
oxide formation, 100–101
reversible reactions, 100–101
Faradaic reactions, 92
Faraday constant, 168–169
Feedthrough, 44–45, 243*f*
Flexible electronics
chronic stability, 378–379, 379*f*
microwire arrays, 379–380
planar arrays/epidural sheets, 380–381, 381*f*
porous electronic meshes, 380
Foreign body reaction
immune reaction, 135–136, 136*f*
implant mechanical instability, 136
injury/infection, 136–137

Functional Low-Vision Observer Rated Assessment (FLORA), 287–288
Functional mapping, 20–21

G

Galvanic cell (element), 188–189
Galvani potential, 190
Gate control theory of pain, 312–313, 312*f*, 320–321
Gated/adult plasticity, 153
General design considerations, 43
Genetic therapies, 382–383
Geometric surface area, 107–108, 108*f*
Glaucoma, 263–264
Glia cells, 55
Gliosis, 265–266
Gouy-Chapman layer, 179–180

H

Hair cells (inner and outer), 217–218
Half-reactions, 192
H-atom-plating, 100–101
Hearing loss, sensory, conductive, mixed, 219–220
Helmholtz-Debye double-layer, 86, 87*f*
Helmholtz layer, 179–180
Hermeticity failure, 45
High-frequency spinal cord stimulation (HFS), 321–323
History
  biomedical technology, 4–5, 4*f*
  computer technology
    binary calculus, 11–12
    clay tablets, 5
    information flow, 9–12
    Jacquard loom, 6–7, 6*f*
    machine code, 7, 8*f*
    neuronal activity, 12
    real computing machines, 7, 9*f*
    software/programming language, 7–8, 10*f*
    virtual machine/universal Turing machine, 8–9
  electrophysiology, 12–15, 13–14*f*
  neural prosthesis, 15–17
Hittorf transport numbers, 176, 177*f*
Homeostatic plasticity, 153
Homosynaptic and heterosynaptic plasticity, 151

I

Impedance, 77, 110–111, 126, 186–188, 231–233, 232*f*
Implantable pacemaker, 22–25, 23*f*
Implantable pulse generator (IPG), 298
Inactivation, 63, 126, 302, 323–324
Inactivation gate, 127
Infection
  bacteria adherence, 146–147
  biofilm, 145, 146*f*
  clinical symptoms, 147
  colloidal adhesion, 146
  complications, 147
  prevention, 147
Informed consent, 35
Inhibitory neuron, 153, 155, 157, 244–245, 312, 371–372
Injury-related plasticity, 153–154
Inner ear. *See also* Cochlear implants
  anatomy, 212–214, 213*f*
  auditory nerve, 217–218
  basilar membrane vibration, 214–215
  hair cells, 217–218
  organ of Corti, 214
  place code, 215, 215*f*
  sensory organ, 212–214
  sound pressure level, 217
  temporal code, 216, 216*f*
  transduction, 214
Interface impedance. *See also* Electrode-tissue interface
  circuit impedance, 184–186, 185–186*f*
  Faraday currents, 188
  frequency dependence, 187–188
  surface area *vs.* capacitance and conductance, 186–187
Intracortical microstimulation (ICMS) arrays, 366
Intraneural electrodes, 365–366
Invasive brain-computer interfaces (BCIs), 338
Ion conductivity and mobility, 175
Ionic channels, 56–57
Ion mobility, 173–174, 174*t*

J

Juvenile plasticity, 151–153

K

Kalman filter (KF), 349–350, 349*f*
Kennard principle, 159
Kilohertz frequency alternating current (KHFAC), 323–324
Kohlrausch's law, 170–171, 172*f*
Koniocellular system, 258

L

Leakage potassium channels, 56
Leakage resistance, 89–90
Length constant, 70, 72*f*
Lifetime medical and technical care, 36
Ligand-gated channels, 62–63
Lobotomy, 21–22
Local current, 67–69
Long-term potentiation (LTP), 151, 152*f*, 313–314
Loudness, growth function, 233
Low-frequency spinal cord stimulation, 320–321, 320*f*

M

Macular dystrophies, 262–263
Magnetic stimulation, 28–29
Magnetogenetic stimulation, 376–377
Magnocellular system, 258
Materials
  biocompatibility, 97–99
  electrochemical reactions, 99
  electrode impedance measurement, 99–100
  insulating materials, 100
  metal properties, 97–98, 97*t*
  silver chloride, 99
  stainless steel, 98
Mechanotransduction, 305, 306*f*
Michigan probe/NeuroNexus probe, 342
Microelectrodes, 109–110
Microwire recordings, 342–344, 343*f*
Monopolar configuration, 82–83, 115–116, 116*f*
Moral agency, 35
Motor commands
  nervous system signals, 330
  spared muscle signals, 329
Multichannel coding strategies, 236, 237*f*
Multipolar configurations, 82–83
Myelin, 55, 68, 68*f*
Myelination, 68, 68*f*

N

Nernst equation, 189–191, 194*f*
Neural dust electrodes, 345
Neuromodulation, 317–318
Neuronal excitation
  action potential, 64, 64*f*
  ionic concentrations, 65
  ligand-gated channels, 62–63
  membrane dynamic properties
    length constant, 70, 72*f*
    step-like depolarizing current effects, 70, 71*f*
    strength-duration curve, 70, 71*f*
  nervous system macroanatomy, 73–74
  postinhibitory rebound, 63
  potassium channels, 64
  propagation
    action potentials, 69
    active propagation, 67
    excitatory postsynaptic potentials, 65–66, 66*f*
    membrane parameters, 67–68, 67*t*
    myelination, 68, 68*f*
    passive (electrotonic) propagation, 65
    saltatory conduction, 68–69
  refractory period, 65
  synapse, 62, 62*f*
  thresholds, 73
  voltage-sensitive sodium channels, 63
Neuronal plasticity
  adaptive process, 150
  in adult age, 162–163
  aging/elderly subjects, 163
  associative learning, 150–151
  cerebral cortex, 155–157, 156*f*
  definition, 149
  forms
    adaptation and sensitization, 151
    excitotoxicity, 154
    gated/adult plasticity, 153
    homeostatic plasticity, 153
    homosynaptic and heterosynaptic plasticity, 151
    injury-related plasticity, 153–154
    juvenile plasticity, 151–153
    long-term depression, 151
    long-term potentiation, 151, 152*f*
    short-term plasticity, 151
    synaptic effects, 150–151
  loss of function, 149

neuroprosthetic devices
adaptations and maladaptations, 163–164
adverse effects/maladaptive plasticity, 150
beneficial effects, 150
non-plastic synapses, 154–155
physiology, 149
plastic synapses, 155
prosthetic therapy outcomes
abnormal brain activity, 158
brain injury, 159
cochlear implants, 158–159
congenital deafness, 158–159, 160*f*
critical period for therapy, 160, 162
developmental brain changes, 162
inducing pathology, 157
maturational changes, 159–160, 161*f*
single-sided deafness, 160–162
Neuron dropping curve (NDC), 333–335, 336*f*
Neurons
glia cells, 55
morphology, 55, 56*f*
neuronal membrane
depolarization and hyperpolarization, 61
equilibrium potentials, 58–61, 58*t*, 60*b*
equivalent circuitry, 61, 61*f*
ionic channels, 56–57
ionic concentrations, 57–58, 58*t*
osmotic pressure, 57
phospholipid bilayer, 55–56, 57*f*
resting potential, 58
Neuropathic pain, 314–317, 316*f*
Neuropil, 55
Neuroprostheses
concept, 15–17
history
brain mapping, 20–21, 21*f*
cochlear implant, 26–28, 28–29*f*
contemporary neuroprostheses, 28–30
deep brain stimulation (DBS), 21–22
early brain prostheses, 25–26
electrical stimulation, 19–20
implantable pacemaker, 22–25, 23*f*
Neurotrophic factors, 345–346
Non-invasive brain-computer interfaces (BCIs), 335–338, 337*f*
Non-polarizing electrodes, 188–189, 189*f*
Non-proliferative diabetic retinopathy (NPDR), 264

O

Open-angle glaucoma, 263–264
Optic nerve implants, 277–278
Optogenetics, 371–373, 372*f*
Organic electronic ion pumps (OEIPs), 376, 377*f*
Osmotic pressure, 57
Ostwald's dilution law, 173
Overpotential, 88

P

Parkinson's disease
cog wheel phenomenon, 294–295
deep brain stimulation, 298*f*
dopamine, 296
inhibiting effect, 296
spiking activity, 294–295, 295*f*
targets, 300
Parvocellular system, 258
Passivation, 99–100
Perceptual thresholds vs. frequency, 95, 96*f*
Period histogram, 216, 216*f*, 230*f*
Peripheral auditory organ, 211–212, 212*f*
Peripheral nerve and spinal stimulation
burst stimulation, 321, 322*f*
central control, 314
chronic neuropathic pain, 314–317, 316*f*
clinical outcomes
behavioral responses, 326
multidimensional questionnaires, 326
pain reduction measures, 327
self-reporting, 325–326
unidimensional questionnaires, 326
cranial neuromodulation implants, 324–325
dorsal horn, 309–311, 310*f*
failed back surgery syndrome (FBSS), 318
gate control theory, 312–313, 312*f*
high-frequency spinal cord stimulation, 321–323
information processing, 311
low-frequency spinal cord stimulation, 320–321, 320*f*
nociceptive and somatosensory periphery
epineurium, 305–307, 307*f*
information transmission, 307–308
mechanoreceptors, 305, 306*f*
pH-sensitive chemoreceptors, 305
polymodal receptors, 305
thermoreceptors, 305

Peripheral nerve and spinal stimulation *(Continued)*
  pain neuromodulation, 317–318
  peripheral nerve block, 323–324
  principles of operation, 318–319, 319*f*
  short-term and long-term plasticity, 313–314
  spinal neuroanatomy, 308–309, 309*f*
  targets for peripheral neuromodulation, 324–325
  vagal nerve neuromodulation, 325
Peripheral nerve block, 323–324
Pharmaceutical carriers, 381–382
Phase locking, 130
pH electrode, 205–207, 206*f*
Phosphene, 271–272
Photodiode arrays, 276–277
Photoreceptor degenerations, 261
pH-sensitive chemoreceptors, 305
Pitch perception, 233
Platinum black, 98, 111
Polarized electrode, 89, 91
Polymer microelectrodes, 344–345, 344*f*
Population vector, 347–348
Postinhibitory rebound, 63, 127
Post-market clinical follow-up (PMCF), 42–43
Post-retinal visual pathway, 258
Postsynaptic potential, 65–66, 66*f*
Precision medicine, 382–383
Preclinical testing, 38–39, 39*f*, 40*t*
Pre-implant data processing, 283–284
Proliferative diabetic retinopathy (PDR), 264
Proprioceptors, 329
Pulsatile stimulation, 96–97

R

RC circuit, 90
Reactive effects, 97–98
Recessed electrodes, 88–89
Redox couple, 190–191
Redox reaction, 192
Reference electrode, 195–197, 196*f*
Refractory period (phase), 65, 126
Regenerative medicine, 383–384
Resistance, 77, 89–90, 143, 193–194
Resting potential, 58
Retina
  anatomy, 251, 252*f*
  area centralis, 254, 255*f*
  function, 253–254
  optic disc, 254, 255*f*
  photoreceptor, 251–253, 253*f*
  retinal pigment epithelium (RPE), 254
  rods and cones, 251
  tapetum lucidum, 254
Retinal remodelling
  histological example, 265, 266*f*
  phases, 265
  progression, 266
  visual rescue strategies, 265–266
Retinitis pigmentosa (RP), 261–262, 262*f*
Retinotopy, 20–21
Return electrode, 115–118, 116*f*
Risk management, 42–43
Robotic placement of probes, 345
Rod-cone dystrophies, 261–262, 262*f*

S

Safety limits
  capacitive effects, 104
  charge delivery capacity, 104–105, 109
  charge density safety limit, 107
  dielectric breakdown, 104
  faradaic vs. non-faradaic charge transfer, 105, 106*f*
  faradaic reaction limit, 109, 109*f*
  geometric surface area, 107–108, 108*f*
  safety threshold vs. excitation threshold, 107
  Shannon formula, 108–109
Saltatory conduction, 68–69
Scala tympani, 224, 235
Sensing implants
  artificial neural networks, 350
  brain-machine interface (BMI)
    arm movement direction, 331–332, 331–332*f*
    body and limb movement, 330–331
    decoder training, 332–333, 334*f*
    motor coding, 332–333
    neuron dropping curve (NDC), 333–335, 336*f*
    prerequisites, 333
  decoders, 346–347
  electrocorticographic and endovascular recording, 338–340
  motor commands
    nervous system signals, 330
    spared muscle signals, 329
  neural dust electrodes, 345
  neurotrophic factors, 345–346
  polymer microelectrodes, 344–345, 344*f*
  population vector, 347–348

proprioceptors, 329
robotic placement of probes, 345
Sensory hearing loss, 220
Series resistance, 89–90
Shannon formula, 108–109
Short-term potentiation (STP), 151, 313–314
Signal-to-noise ratio, 238
Silicon microarrays, 340–342, 340*f*
Single-sided deafness, 160–162
Single-unit recording arrays, 340
Solvation of ions, 174–175, 174*t*
Somatosensory and proprioceptive prostheses
clinical outcomes, 366–367
embodiment, 363–364
feedback signals, 363
peripheral somatosensory stimulation
intracortical microstimulation (ICMS) arrays, 366
intraneural electrodes, 365–366
peripheral nerve interface electrodes, 364–365, 365*f*
Spatial summation, 65–66
Specific conductivity, 169–170
Speech perception
localization precision, 238
multichannel, 238
signal-to-noise ratio, 238
single syllable recognition, 239
speech-coding strategies, 238–239
speech understanding, 236
Spike-rate adaptation, 126
Spinal cord stimulators (SCS), 320–321. *See also* Peripheral nerve and spinal stimulation
Standard electrode potentials, 192–193, 193*t*. *See also* Standard hydrogen electrode
Standard hydrogen electrode (SHE), 85–86
Stereotactic frames, 22
Stimulation rules
electric field geometry and neurons
activation function, 121–125, 122–123*f*, 125*f*
bipolar configuration, 116–117
boundary effects, 126
electrode/tissue orientation, 118, 119*f*, 121, 121*b*
monopolar configuration, 115–116, 116*f*
tissue impedance, 126
tripolar configuration, 117–118
working position and return electrode, 115–118, 116*f*
energy requirements, 132–133
signal forms
biphasic stimulation, 127–128
interphase gap, 129
monophasic pulses, 128
pseudomonophasic pulses, 128*f*, 129
pulsatile stimulation, 127–129
sinusoidal stimulation, 129–130
symmetrical biphasic pulses, 128, 128*f*
suprathreshold responses
dynamic range, 130–132, 131*f*
intracortical stimulation, 132
phase locking, 130
rate-level functions, 130–131, 131*f*
temporal adaptation phenomena
anodic break, 127
depolarization block, 127
electrical accommodation, 126
hyperpolarization, 127
postinhibitory rebound, 127
refractory period, 126
spike-rate adaptation, 126
Strength-duration curve, 70, 71*f*, 125
Strong and weak electrolytes, 170–173, 172*f*
Subretinal prostheses, 274–276
Suprachoroidal prostheses, 276
Surface materials, 111
Synapse, 62, 62*f*

T

Technological innovations
electrode materials, 378
flexible arrays and electronics
chronic stability, 378–379, 379*f*
microwire arrays, 379–380
planar arrays/epidural sheets, 380–381, 381*f*
porous electronic meshes, 380
pharmaceutical carriers, 381–382
stimulation modes
direct current stimulation, 373–374, 374*f*
electrophoretic neurotransmitter release, 376, 377*f*
magnetogenetic stimulation, 376–377
optogenetic stimulation, 371–373, 372*f*

Technological innovations *(Continued)*
ultrasound stimulation and power delivery, 375–376
Technological safety, 35–36
Technology readiness level (TRL), 36–37
Temporal adaptation phenomena
anodic break, 127
depolarization block, 127
electrical accommodation, 126
hyperpolarization, 127
postinhibitory rebound, 127
refractory period, 126
spike-rate adaptation, 126
Temporal summation, 65–66
Thermoreceptors, 305
Time constant, 70, 72
Tissue-electrode interface, 178–180, 181*f*, 181*t*, 182. *See also* Electrode-tissue interface
Tissue impedance, 126
Tissue reaction
acute and chronic reactions, 135–136
electrode impedance
access voltage, 141–142
cell adhesion, 143
compliance limits of current source, 142–143, 142*f*
current and voltage curve, 140–142, 141*f*
cyclic voltammetry, 145
electrolyte composition, 143
electrotaxis, 144
extracellular matrix, 144
frequency-dependent resistance function, 137–139, 138*f*
integrity checking, 137
resistance information, 143
simplified circuit, 138*f*
transimpedance measurement, 144–145
voltage measurement, 139–140, 140*f*
infection, 145–147, 146*f*
passive reactions, 135
surrounding tissue adaptations, 135–137, 136*f*
Tonotopy, 223
Toxic effects, 97–98, 102–103
Toxicity, 38–39, 154, 267–268, 273, 315, 373–374, 378
Transhumanism, 48–49
Transimpedance measurement, 144–145
Traveling wave, 214, 217
Tripolar configuration, 82–83, 117–118

U

Ultrasound stimulation, 375–376
Universal Turing machine, 8–9
Utah array, 340–342, 340*f*
Utilitarian ethics, 34

V

Vagus nerve stimulation, 325
anatomy and function, 367–368
clinical outcomes, 369–370
mechanisms of action, 368
stimulator design, 368, 369*f*
Vestibular protheses
clinical outcomes
bilateral implantation, 360
limitations, 359
vestibulo-ocular reflex (VOR) response, 358–359, 360*f*
designs, 357, 357*f*
pulse amplitude modulation (PAM), 357–358
pulse frequency modulation (PFM)/pulse rate modulation (PRM), 357–358, 358*f*
spontaneous baseline of activity, 357–358
stimulation strategy, 357–358
vestibular system physiology
anatomy, 353, 354*f*
sensory mechanism, 354–355, 355*f*
vestibulo-ocular reflex (VOR), 356
Vision loss, 260–261
Visual neuroprostheses
age-related macular degeneration (AMD), 262–263
animal models, 267, 268*t*
cell-selective stimulation, 284–286
clinical outcomes
Functional Low-Vision Observer Rated Assessment (FLORA), 287–288
functional outcomes, 286
functional vision tests, 287–288
motion detection, 287
perimetry, 287
qualitative tests, 286–287
regulatory threshold for safety and efficacy, 288
visual acuity, 287
common materials and stimulation parameters, 272–273, 272*f*, 274*f*
cone-rod dystrophies, 262
cortical and LGN visual implants, 278

current steering, 284, 285*f*
data processing and stimulation strategies, 282–283
diabetic retinopathy (DR), 264
epiretinal prostheses, 274, 275*f*
glaucoma, 263–264
information processing
center-surround processing, 256, 257*f*
contrast sensitivity, 256
edge detection, 256
receptive fields, 255–256
spatial and temporal resolution, 256–258
koniocellular system, 258
lateral geniculate nucleus (LGN)
anatomy, 258–260, 259*f*
prostheses, 279, 280*f*
macular dystrophies, 262–263
magnocellular system, 258
non-proliferative diabetic retinopathy (NPDR), 264
operational flow, 269, 270*f*
optic chiasm, 258
optic nerve prostheses/implants, 277–278
parvocellular system, 258
pharmacological models, 267–268
phosphene, 271–272
photodiode arrays, 276–277
photoreceptor degenerations, 261
post-retinal visual pathway, 258
pre-implant data processing, 283–284
primary visual cortex (V1)
anatomy, 260
orientation selectivity, 260
prostheses, 279–282, 281*f*
proliferative diabetic retinopathy (PDR), 264
retina (*see* Retina)
retinal remodeling
histological example, 265, 266*f*
phases, 265
progression, 266
visual rescue strategies, 265–266
retinitis pigmentosa (RP), 261–262, 262*f*
retinotopic organization, 258
rod-cone dystrophies, 261–262, 262*f*
subretinal prostheses, 274–276
suprachoroidal prostheses, 276
vision loss, 260–261
Voltage gated channel, 64, 67, 70, 73
Voltage-sensitive channels, 63–64
Voltage source, 77–79, 79*b*

W

Warburg region, 138*f*, 139–140
Water window, 102
Wiener filter, 348

Kolibri 360 GmbH
Ferdinand-Jühlke-Straße 7
99095 Erfurt, Deutschland
produktsicherheit@kolibri360.de